Diagnostic Ultrasonics
Principles and Use of Instruments

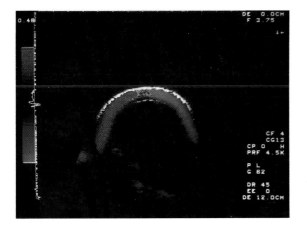

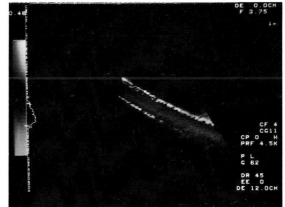

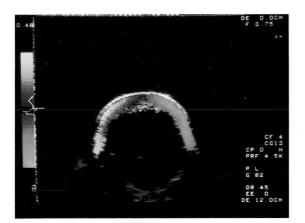

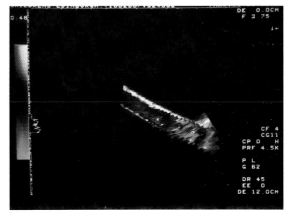

Plate 1 Colour flow images from a curved tube. Top: colour saturation related to power of echo signal, colour related to direction. Bottom: hue of colour is related to size of velocity component along beam. *Note*: at top of arch, beam-to-vessel angle is 90° and Doppler signal is poor.

Plate 2 Top: parabolic flow in tube; bottom: stenosis in tube causes turbulence.

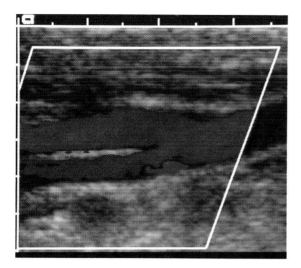

Plate 3 Carotid artery flow; localised reverse flow in blue region. Beam-to-vessel angle is similar at all points (courtesy of Acuson).

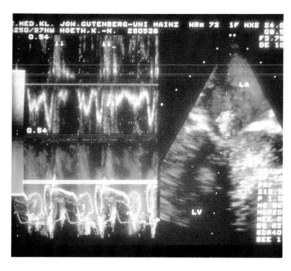

Plate 4 Simultaneous presentation of anatomical grey tone image, colour flow image, sonogram (top left) and colour-coded Doppler M-scan (bottom left) (courtesy of Toshiba).

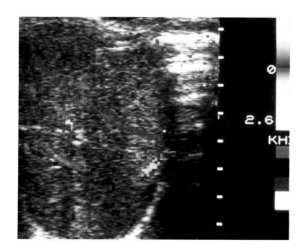

Plate 5 Grey tone image of liver plus flow in hepatic vessels (courtesy of Acuson).

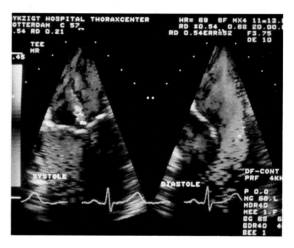

Plate 9 Transoesophageal colour flow image of mild mitral regurgitation in systole and diastole (courtesy of Toshiba).

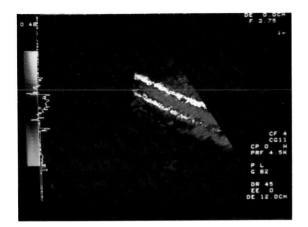

Plate 6 'Leakage' of blood flow colour-coding to weak signals outside tube.

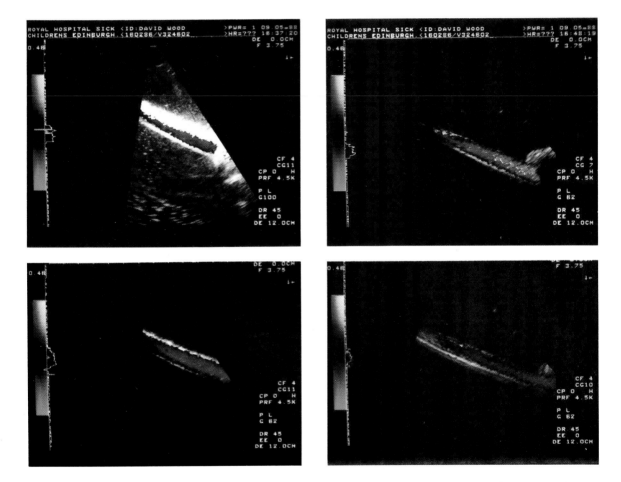

Plate 7 Bottom: parabolic flow in tube; top: high gain producing wall echo saturation and artefactual reduction of tube internal diameter.

Plate 8 Bottom: parabolic flow in tube; top: increased velocity of flow causing aliaising with resultant error in colour-coding.

Diagnostic Ultrasonics
Principles and Use of Instruments

W. N. McDicken BSc PhD FIPSM
Professor of Medical Physics and Medical Engineering
Department of Medical Physics and Medical Engineering
The Royal Infirmary
Edinburgh

THIRD EDITION

CHURCHILL LIVINGSTONE
EDINBURGH LONDON MELBOURNE AND NEW YORK 1991

CHURCHILL LIVINGSTONE
Medical Division of Longman Group UK Limited

Distributed in the United States of America by Churchill
Livingstone Inc., 1560 Broadway, New York, N.Y. 10036,
and by associated companies, branches and representatives
throughout the world.

First edition 1976
Second edition 1981
Third edition 1991

ISBN 0 443 041326

British Library Cataloguing in Publication Data
McDicken, W. N.
    Diagnostic ultrasonics. — 3rd. ed.
    1. Medicine. Diagnosis. Ultrasonography
    I. Title
    616.07543

Library of Congress Cataloging in Publication Data
McDicken, W. N.
    Diagnostic ultrasonics: principles and use of instruments / W. N.
McDicken. — 3rd ed.
        p.   cm.
    Includes bibliographical references.
    ISBN 0-443-04132-6
    1. Diagnosis, Ultrasonic. 2. Diagnosis, Ultrasonic — Instruments.
    I. Title.
    [DNLM: 1. Ultrasonic Diagnosis — instrumentation. 2. Ultrasonics.
WB 289 M134d]
RC78.7.U4M3   1990
616.07′543 — dc20
DNLM/DLC
for Library of Congress   89-70802

Produced by Longman Group (F.E.) Ltd
Printed in Hong Kong

Preface to the Third Edition

Since the second edition was published there have been advances in the technology and quality of real-time B-scan imaging; invasive techniques have become widespread and the use of Doppler instrumentation has increased dramatically. Over the last decade there has also been increased discussion and investigation of the safety of diagnostic ultrasound. Our knowledge of the propagation of ultrasound in tissue has improved as has our ability to specify and measure the output parameters of machines. The range and complexity of clinical applications make it desirable for the users of ultrasonic instrumentation to base their expertise on a good understanding of the scientific and technical principles. It is hoped that by presenting these principles in conjunction with practical information that they will be helpful to the medical user and remove any mystique which need not exist in the subject. Just as for pulsed-echo imaging all of the new Doppler techniques can be understood by a gradual accumulation of knowledge rather than by a blinding flash of enlightenment.

I am indebted to my physics and medical colleagues in Edinburgh for their contributions to this edition and for creating an atmosphere in which I could learn from their knowledge and practice. Tom Anderson, Peter Hoskins, Thanasis Loupas and Steve Pye have contributed to, and criticised initial drafts of, large portions of the text. I am also indebted to others in the UK and abroad who have supplied me with material and permitted me to reproduce results from their publications. The skill and efficiency of the staff of the Medical Illustration Department of the Western General Hospital, Edinburgh have greatly eased the task of producing the manuscript. Finally, I would like to acknowledge the work of the staff of Churchill Livingstone in turning the manuscript into a book.

Edinburgh 1991   W. N. McDicken

Contents

1. Introduction to diagnostic ultrasonics

Ultrasonic diagnostic techniques have been shown to be powerful, versatile, and well suited to medical practice. Growth of application continues both in established techniques and in new fields. These techniques employ ultrasound as a means of obtaining information about the structure of organs and the cardiovascular function of the body. Ultrasound is the transmission of mechanical vibrations through matter. The phenomenon of ultrasound is similar to that of normal audible sound. 'Ultrasound' is the term used to describe sound when the pitch is too high for us to hear it.

One of the most important applications of ultrasound is to produce images of soft-tissue structures. Images are created by transmitting ultrasound into the body and detecting echoes which are produced by reflection at tissue boundaries. From these images, it is possible to determine both the size and the nature of the structures. The abdomen is a particularly fruitful area of application, as are the heart, eye, neck, limbs, and infant brain. We will see that blood flow is also studied extensively by non-invasive ultrasonic methods.

The interaction of ultrasound with tissue structures gives rise to information that is directly related to the acoustic (i.e. ultrasonic) properties of the tissues and is essentially different from that supplied by other diagnostic techniques such as roentgenography, computed axial tomography, magnetic resonance imaging, or isotope imaging. In the competition among these methodologies, diagnostic ultrasound has several strings to its bow and, hence, an increasingly important role in the difficult business of examining the body by non-invasive and invasive methods.

Over the past three decades, diagnostic ultrasonic instruments have developed from basic units designed for industrial flaw-detection to the present generation of sophisticated medical instruments. Simultaneously with this development has come the establishment of diagnostic ultrasound in medical disciplines such as obstetrics and gynaecology, radiology, paediatrics, ophthalmology, neurology, and the cardiovascular field. The use of ultrasound in other fields of medicine is being explored.

AIM OF THIS TEXT

To get the best from diagnostic ultrasonic techniques, it is essential for an investigator to have a reasonable knowledge of how the instruments work. In ultrasonic scanning, the highest quality results are achieved only by the logical and scientific manipulation of the scanning head and the machine controls. Ultrasonic scanning involves subtle man–machine interactions in which preliminary scans and adjustments lead to the final images being recorded. This aspect of the procedure is not fully emphasized in the research literature. Anyone intending to use ultrasonic scanning should, at an early stage, be sure to see the techniques being applied. The aim of this text is to assist medically orientated personnel to become familiar with the various technical points that arise during use of the instruments. In addition, I hope that it will provide a firm foundation for an understanding of future developments.

This text originated in a series of courses conducted for medical personnel on the scientific and technical principles of diagnostic ultrasound. I hope that the experience I have gained in these courses and in practical situations has enabled me to present the material in a form acceptable to the reader. I have tried to avoid the pitfalls of using unexplained terms and jargon, or of assuming prior knowledge. During the courses mentioned, participants found it useful to scan simple objects. This allowed the effects of individual factors to be studied separately. A few of these objects are described in Appendices 1 and 2.

In these days of the 'information explosion', time is at a premium. By studying, from the outset, the technical aspects of the subject, however, the reader should save a great deal of time and effort in subsequent years of clinical application.

Lastly, although ultrasound has applications in surgery and therapy, it is only the diagnostic use that will be considered here.

ULTRASOUND

The transmission of mechanical vibrations through matter

Ultrasound is the transmission of mechanical vibrations through matter. These vibrations are not random, as in thermal vibrations, but are orderly, oscillatory motions generated by an external source. A typical source (called a 'transducer') is one or more crystals driven electrically to vibrate and placed in contact with the outside surface of the body. As soon as the surface particles move, the net force on their neighbouring particles alters so that they also begin to move. In this way, the mechanical vibrations pass very quickly through the material (Fig. 1.1a).

The word 'particle' is used to describe a very small volume of matter in which all the atoms can be considered to be experiencing the same physical forces. The terms 'molecule' or 'atom' could be used as well. If the motion of a particle in matter transmitting ultrasound is examined in detail, the particle is seen to be moving backward and forward by small amounts. A common form of vibration is simple harmonic motion or sinusoidal motion. Then the motion of each particle is similar to that of the weight on the end of a long pendulum, although the distances actually moved are microscopic (e.g. one-millionth of a centimetre).

Frequency

Frequency is an important quantity in relation to the motion just described. The frequency of ultrasound is the number of oscillations per second performed by particles of the matter in which the ultrasound is propagating. The frequency has a great influence on the final result of a clinical examination and is one of the quantities that is selected by the operator.

The following nomenclature is used for the unit of frequency:

1 oscillation/second(s) = 1 cycle/s = 1 hertz (1 Hz)
1000 oscillations/s = 1 kilocycle/s = 1 kilohertz (1 kHz)

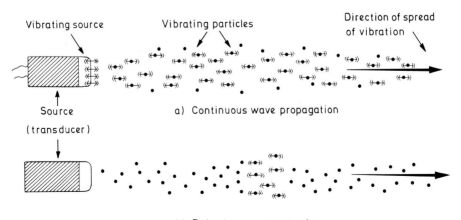

a) Continuous wave propagation

b) Pulsed wave propagation

Fig. 1.1   The propagation of continuous- and pulsed-wave sonic vibrations.

1 000 000 oscillations/s = 1 megacycle/s = 1 megahertz (1 MHz)

The unit 'hertz' is the agreed international standard; however, 'cycle/sec' (c/s) is found in the older literature.

It is possible at present to generate sound over a range of frequencies from less than 1 Hz to 10 000 MHz. Audible sounds are in the range 20 Hz to about 18 kHz. Above 18 kHz, the term 'ultrasound' is used to describe the wave phenomena. In other words, the term refers merely to sound of a frequency above that audible to the human ear. In diagnostic ultrasonics, frequencies in the range 0.5–25 MHz are used. More commonly, the range used is 1–10 MHz; for example, 3 MHz for abdominal scanning, or 10 MHz for eye work.

The frequency of ultrasound is measured by converting the mechanical oscillations into voltage oscillations using an ultrasound transducer which acts as a pressure detector. The voltage oscillations are then displayed on an oscilloscope and the number of oscillations per second counted. Alternatively, the voltage oscillations are fed into a frequency meter that electronically detects and counts the number of complete oscillations per second. At present, there are few techniques in diagnostic ultrasonics that require an ultrasonic frequency to be measured, though frequency in the audible range is often measured when Doppler blood-flow techniques are employed. Special instruments called 'spectrum analysers' are made for this purpose (Ch. 21).

It is interesting to note that ultrasound, unlike ionizing radiation, does not occur extensively in nature except at low frequencies. Bats and porpoises can transmit and receive ultrasound at frequencies up to 120 kHz. Grasshoppers can generate 100 kHz ultrasound. Fracturing rocks emit low-intensity ultrasound in the MHz region. The lack of a natural background level creates difficulties when hazards are being investigated, since we have little experience of the long-term effect of ultrasound on humans.

THE CASE FOR DIAGNOSTIC ULTRASOUND

Before proceeding further, let us consider what diagnostic ultrasonic techniques actually have to offer. We will also examine some of the present difficulties.

The case for employing ultrasound is usually a combination of some of the following considerations:

1. Tissue structures can be imaged in detail. This is particularly true of soft tissues, which are difficult to depict by conventional X-ray techniques.
2. Movement of tissues within the body can be presented on display screens and chart recorders.
3. Rapid examinations are possible with relatively inexpensive equipment.
4. Portable instruments are available.
5. Blood flow can be recorded using the Doppler effect and, in some instances, measured quantitatively (see Ch. 2).
6. Regions of blood flow can be visualized and related to the vascular structure.
7. No harmful effects have been shown to be associated with diagnostic ultrasound. In addition, there is no risk to the operator.
8. Many examinations are non-invasive and do not distress the patient. Repeated examinations can therefore be made.
9. Treatment can be monitored.
10. Transducers can be made small and suitable for invasive applications.
11. Needles and catheters can be directed under ultrasonic guidance.
12. Information can be obtained about the nature of a tissue from its effect on the ultrasonic beam. This type of information is being gained more often as techniques are refined.
13. Quantitative measurements can be made of structures within the body. For example, the biparietal diameter of a fetal head, the volume of a liver, or the movement of cardiac structures can be quantified.

Of the difficulties that may arise, the following are most likely to trouble a new participant in the field:

1. Some instruments have a large number of controls. This may make the instrument of value in a wide range of applications. Systematic study overcomes this problem.

2. Interpretation of ultrasonic images can be difficult. Initially, this is due to lack of familiarity with the images, but even after considerable experience has been gained, problems of interpretation arise. Herein lies a challenge for the operator.

3. Difficulty can be experienced in locating some structures of interest, for example, the pancreas or pulmonary heart valve.

4. Although image detail is surprisingly good, it is still coarse compared to many anatomic features.

5. Gas, bone, and fat can present major problems for ultrasonic imaging.

6. Blood flow is affected by several physiologic parameters; therefore, Doppler signals have to be interpreted with care.

7. Tissue movements may make the detection of Doppler signals difficult.

Some of these problems will, no doubt, be solved by future developments. Even with these limitations, ultrasound is a powerful tool for the investigation of soft tissues.

ULTRASONIC BEAM, FIELD, AND ZONE

Virtually all established diagnostic techniques depend on an ultrasound beam being directed into tissues. The term 'beam' is used in two ways in medical ultrasonics. This can be confusing. One definition of ultrasonic beam is 'the pattern in front of a transducer of the intensity of the transmitted vibrations'. However, it is better to talk of the ultrasonic 'field', rather than 'beam', when referring to transmitted vibrations.

A transducer also has a region in front of it from which it can detect ultrasonic vibrations, i.e. the reception zone. This zone often has a shape similar to that of the transmission field, but not always, particularly with modern, multi-element transducers. When a transducer is used to transmit ultrasound into an object and to receive echoes from internal structures, the region from which echoes are detected depends on the shapes of both the transmission field and the reception zone (Fig. 1.2).

A second definition of ultrasonic beam is 'the pattern in front of a transducer related to the mag-

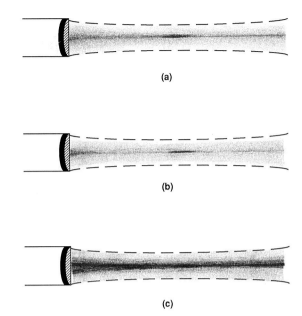

Fig. 1.2 (a) Transmission field, (b) reception zone, (c) ultrasonic beam — the combination of the field and zone.

nitude of the echo detected from a standard target at each point when the transducer is operating in the transmit–receive mode'.

The first definition is appropriate to the study of bio-effects and in other situations where the output of transducers is being considered in detail. The second is, by far, the most relevant when imaging or Doppler techniques are being discussed.

In this text, 'field' will refer to transmission, 'zone' to reception, and 'beam' to transmission–reception.

An essential feature of most ultrasonic instruments is the ability to produce a narrow, ultrasonic transmission field. This field can be considered the acoustic equivalent of a miniature searchlight or hand lamp. In some instruments ultrasound is transmitted continuously (Fig. 1.1a), while in others it is in the form of short, regular pulses. In this context, 'pulse' denotes a short burst of vibration that passes through the medium, influencing only a limited region at each instant. Typically, in an abdominal examination, an ultrasonic pulse travelling through tissue will influence, at each instant, a layer 1 or 2 mm thick (Fig. 1.1b).

Everyday experience of audible sounds spreading out in all directions may make one wonder if reasonably directional ultrasonic fields can be produced. Fortunately, at the high frequencies used in diagnostic ultrasound, well-directed fields can be generated by small transducers. For the moment, we shall consider one or two standard types of transducer (also called 'probe') that will be sufficient for our initial studies. Chapters 5, 11, and 27 give more detailed discussion of transducers and ultrasonic fields.

Single-element transducer

A basic ultrasonic transducer for diagnostic applications takes the form of a small cylindrical tube with a disc-shaped active element covering one end. The active element is either ceramic crystal or plastic material. Thin, metallic electrodes are evaporated on the front and back faces of the element. If the transducer is to be used to generate short pulses of vibrations, material is bonded to the back face of the element to dampen the vibrations quickly after excitation (Fig. 1.3).

Materials suitable for transducer elements exhibit the piezoelectric effect — the appearance of electric voltage on the faces of the material when pressure is applied. The converse of the piezoelectric effect is the change in thickness of the material when an electric voltage is applied across it. In the detection of ultrasound, the mechanical vibrations strike the element and cause small fluctuating voltages to appear on its surfaces.

To generate ultrasound, one applies a fluctuating voltage to the element, causing it to vibrate.

Most ultrasonic transducers can be conveniently held in the hand and applied to the patient's skin. The same element is used for the generation and detection of pulsed ultrasound. Figure 1.4 shows a 3.5 MHz transducer that has a crystal diameter of 13 mm.

The frequency of ultrasound generated by a transducer is determined by three factors: the frequency of the excitation voltage, the thickness of the element, and the structure of the transducer. An example of the thickness of an element is 0.54 mm for a 3.5 MHz ceramic crystal. A few 'broad band' transducers can be made to function at a number of different frequencies. In Figure 1.4, the transmitted field shape can be considered to be a cylinder gradually tapered to a distance of about 9 cm from the crystal face, after which it slowly diverges. The magnitude of the transmitted vibrations is greatest at the central axis and falls off toward the edge. The reception zone has a similar shape.

Focusing

The ability to see small structures in an ultrasonic image depends, to a large extent, on the width of the transmission–reception beam that interrogates the tissues. One way of reducing the beam width

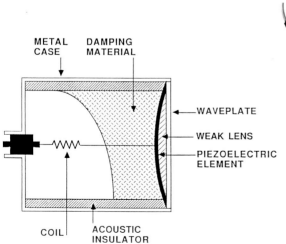

Fig. 1.3 The structure of a basic, single-element ultrasonic transducer.

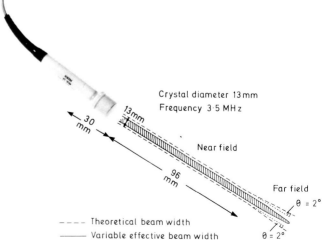

Fig. 1.4 A diagnostic ultrasound transducer and its beam. The concept of effective beam width is discussed in Ch. 12.

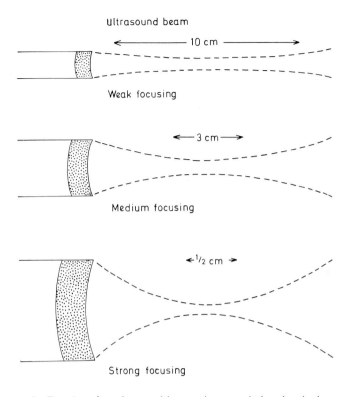

Fig. 1.5 Focusing of an ultrasound beam using curved piezoelectric elements.

is to focus it. It is possible to focus an ultrasound beam by using concave elements or by placing the acoustic equivalent of an optical lens in front of a flat element. Note that this focuses both the transmission field and reception zone. Focusing is usually described as weak, medium, or strong (Fig. 1.5). Weak focusing helps to produce a narrow beam over a useful range and is employed in diagnostic units. Medium focusing gives a narrower beam over a limited range (e.g. 3 cm) and a reasonable width outside the focal zone; it also finds application in medical instrumentation. Strong focusing results in a very narrow beam in a small region (e.g. 0.5 cm) and is rarely used in diagnostic ultrasonics.

Multi-element transducers

In many ultrasonic instruments, it is necessary and advantageous to construct the transducer from a number of small elements that act together to produce a beam. Consider a transducer composed of five strip elements. When these elements are ac-

tivated in unison, they produce a beam that has a shape similar to that from a single element of the same dimensions as the five elements placed side by side (Fig. 1.6a). An attraction of this approach is that, if a large array is constructed of elements placed side by side, a beam can be produced from any point in the array by electronically arranging to activate the appropriate group of neighbouring elements. It is possible, therefore, to alter very rapidly the source of the ultrasound beam and, hence, its path into the body. Later we will see that multi-element transducers are also employed to focus the beam. The focusing potential of multi-element transducers is further exploited by using concentric annular elements (Fig. 1.6b).

DETECTION, LOCALIZATION, AND IDENTIFICATION OF TISSUE INTERFACES

The examination of tissues with ultrasound can be considered in three parts.

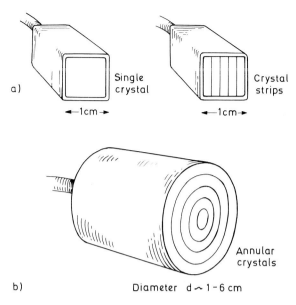

Fig. 1.6 Multi-element transducers constructed from several piezoelectric elements.

1. A tissue interface is detected if it reflects part of an incident ultrasound beam back to the transducer.

2. An interface is located by noting the direction of the beam and, in the case of pulsed ultrasound, the time taken for the echo to return to the transducer.

3. Identification of tissue may be achieved by studying the magnitude of the returned echo and the depth of the reflecting interface. A more reliable way of identifying structures is to use the echo magnitude and depth information from several directions to produce images. Moving blood may be identified by noting the change in frequency of the reflected ultrasound due to the Doppler effect (Ch. 2 and 18).

Detection

Reflection of ultrasound from a large smooth-tissue boundary is the same phenomenon as that observed when audible sound is reflected from a large flat surface such as a wall. The main difference is that 99.9% of the incident vibrational energy is reflected from a wall, whereas less than 1% is reflected from a typical soft-tissue interface. The fraction of the incident beam energy reflected from a flat, soft-tissue interface depends on the difference between the acoustic impedances of the two media forming the boundary. Acoustic impedance is a property of a medium related to its density and elasticity.

Modern ultrasonic instruments are highly sensitive and can also detect ultrasound scattered from small internal discontinuities in organ tissue. The received echo signals from within organs are of the order of 1/50 of that from flat, soft-tissue boundaries. Scattering is a complex process; it is further considered in Chapter 4. Many of the major surfaces within the body appear to reflect ultrasound as from a flat surface, but still have sufficient irregularities on them to produce a scattered component.

When pulsed ultrasound is used, tissue interfaces are detected as follows. A transducer is placed in contact with the outside skin surface so that ultrasound can pass from the element into the body. Let the body contain the structures A, B, C, D, and E as shown in Figure 1.7. A short pulse of ultrasound is transmitted and travels at high speed toward surface A. On reaching A, a small echo is produced and the rest of the incident pulse carries on toward B. At B, a second echo is generated. Since the transmitted pulse strikes the surfaces A and B almost perpendicularly, the

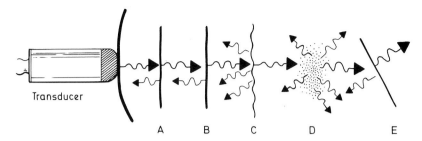

Fig. 1.7 The generation of echoes at reflecting and scattering interfaces.

echoes travel back to the transducer and are detected.

Surfaces A and B are flat and smooth; therefore, reflection occurs in a manner analogous to reflection of light on a smooth glass plate. Most of the interfaces within the body are not so simple. For example, surface C illustrates a rough surface that scatters some of the reflected energy. At D, a region of small, closely packed discontinuities scatters sound in many directions. An interface can be detected if it returns an ultrasonic echo of sufficient magnitude to the transducer. With an instrument of correctly adjusted sensitivity, all of the above structures can be detected. Surface E illustrates the case of a large surface at an angle to the beam. Because the major fraction of the reflected signal does not travel back to the transducer, the returned signal may be too weak for detection. The reflecting properties of tissues play an important part in the design of ultrasonic instrumentation.

Localization

When an echo returns to the transducer, two quantities are recorded that allow the reflecting interface to be located. One is the direction of the beam; the other is the time from the instant of pulse transmission until the returning echo strikes the element, the go–return time. Only a very short time is required for echoes to be received, since, on average, the velocity of sound in soft tissue is 1540 m/s. Having measured the go–return time, one can easily calculate the depth of the interface. For example, consider an echo received after 80-millionths of a second, that is, a go–return time of 80×10^{-6} s. The depth of the surface is given by:

$$\text{Depth} = \frac{\text{velocity of}}{\text{ultrasound}} \times \frac{(\text{go–return time})}{2}$$

$$= 1540 \times \frac{(80 \times 10^{-6})}{2}$$

$$= 0.062 \text{ m} = 6.2 \text{ cm}$$

Medical instruments are all calibrated to read depth automatically. Note that instruments actually measure the time from which depth is calculated, using an assumed value for the velocity of sound. This point will be relevant when we discuss a few situations where it is inadequate to assume an average value for the velocity of sound in tissue, e.g. measurement of dimensions in the eye.

Identification

When a narrow ultrasound beam is directed along a fixed line through tissue structures, examination of the echo magnitudes and the ranges of the echo-producing interfaces may allow structures to be identified if the anatomy is relatively simple. In the vast majority of cases, however, the anatomic structures are very complex, so identification is accomplished by using the echo information to produce images.

The most common way to generate images with echo information is to gather echo data from a large number of ultrasound beam paths through the body. The beam paths are usually restricted so as to lie in a selected plane section through the tissues of interest. For each ultrasound beam direction, the echo signals are depicted as spots on a related line on a display screen. The position of each spot on the line corresponds to the depth of

Sample beam directions   Sample lines of echo

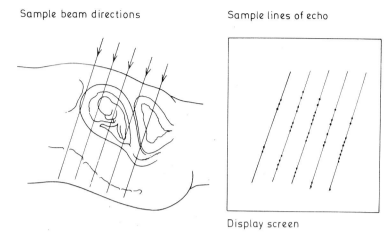

Display screen

Fig. 1.8 The basic method of image production using echoes from tissues.

the tissue interface that produced the echo, and the brightness of the spot corresponds to the magnitude of the echo (Fig. 1.8).

This approach to imaging is used in techniques known as 'static B-scanning' and 'real-time B-scanning'. The former is now rarely used, having been replaced by the latter as a means to depict both static and moving structures.

Ultrasonic data can be used in other ways to make images. We shall study these more specialized approaches later in the text.

Identification of structures is also assisted by movement. Repeated interrogation of a heart valve with a fixed ultrasound beam path produces echoes at rapidly changing depths. These echoes can be employed to draw a trace of the position of the valve versus time. Such a trace is known as an M-scan.

The echoes received from a moving structure have experienced a slight alteration in their ultrasonic frequency. This change in frequency is an example of the Doppler effect, which enables flowing blood to be identified and, in fact, provides a great deal of information about the velocities of the cells. The site of the flowing blood can be localized and, hence, images of regions of flow produced. Doppler devices are considered briefly in Chapter 2 and more fully in Chapters 18–24.

SENSITIVITY OF ECHO-DETECTING INSTRUMENTS

The magnitude of a received echo from an interface within the body is obviously related to the magnitude of the ultrasonic pulse transmitted into the body. It is also greatly dependent on the attenuation processes (e.g. absorption, scattering, and beam divergence) to which the transmitted pulse and the returning echoes are subjected in tissue. To produce echo signals of an acceptable size in an imaging system and to compensate for the attenuation processes, the operator manipulates two or three sensitivity controls on the instrument.

For the moment we will identify the basic sensitivity controls and indicate how they are used. More detailed discussion of them is deferred until Chapter 7.

Manual control of sensitivity

The sensitivity controls include:

1. *Frequency.* The lower the frequency selected, the greater is the penetration achieved into tissue. Each transducer operates at a particular frequency. When a transducer is selected, the receiving amplifier is tuned either automatically or manually to that frequency.

2. *Transmitted output power or intensity.* This determines the size of the transmitted pulse.

3. *Overall gain.* This controls the amplification applied to all the received echoes.

4. *Time-gain compensation* (TGC; this is also called swept gain). The total attenuation affecting the magnitude of a received echo increases with the depth of the reflecting surface. Since the echo-return time is related to the depth of the reflector, it is possible to compensate for increased attenuation with depth by steadily increasing the gain of the receiving amplifier as echoes from deeper and deeper regions return. In some basic instruments there are two controls in the TGC group. The 'near gain' reduces the sensitivity at the instant of pulse transmission; the 'slope' fixes the rate of increase of gain with time, that is, with depth (Fig. 7.2a). In other instruments, there is a batch of around 10 controls in which each one influences the amplification over a different depth range (Fig. 7.2b).

5. *Suppression* (reject). This sets a variable threshold for the rejection of weak signals.

You will note that the amplifier is controlled by the overall gain and TGC group acting simultaneously. For instance, if the TGC has been set to provide a particular compensation, the gain can be manipulated to increase the overall echo signal level without altering the TGC.

The output power and gain controls are sometimes labelled in decibels (dB), and the TGC slope in decibels per centimetre. For introductory purposes, we will regard the decibel labels as a measure of output power or amplifier gain. Indeed, for many applications the operator regards decibels in this way when operating equipment in the practical situation. The decibel notation is discussed in Appendix 3.

These sensitivity controls collectively influence the final echo pattern obtained when a pulsed beam of ultrasound is directed into the body. They have to be used in a logical and related fashion. A simple operating procedure allows baseline settings to be established for those controls available on each instrument (Ch. 7).

Automatic control of sensitivity (adaptive gain control, automatic TGC)

The manner in which sensitivity controls are set manually by the operator has been referred to. It is possible, however, to build into the machine circuitry to sense the general decrease in echo size with depth and to apply the appropriate compensation (Fig. 1.9). This approach is known as automatic or adaptive gain control (AGC). Simple forms of AGC are found in a range of equipment at present. Their performance is close to that of an experienced operator. Some care has to be exercised in assessing each automatic control system; for example, the lack of echoes from fluid may cause the gain to be raised in that region with a generation of noise signals in the image. Since diagnostic information is often based on the recognition of clear-fluid structures, this noise is obviously not desirable. For well-established tasks, such as fetal head measurements, basic AGC works well. It is also of value for rapid searching through tissues, since the sensitivity quickly receives some optimization for each plane of scan. The full potential of automatic sensitivity control is very great, since compensation can be applied during the scanning process as the ultrasonic beam sweeps through the body. Systems of this type are now being introduced into commercial scanners. Accurate automatic compensation is desirable because it allows the operator to concentrate on the business of diagnosis. We shall return to the topic of automatic sensitivity control in Chapter 7.

STORAGE AND DISPLAY OF ULTRASONIC INFORMATION

Scan-converter memory

After the echo signals have been amplified to a few volts they are stored in a computer memory, commonly called the scan converter. Scan converters are discussed in more detail in Chapter 10. Some numeric manipulation may be performed on the echo signals while they are in the scan converter, but the main value of this store is that the signals can be read out rapidly on a TV display giving a flicker-free image.

Cathode-ray tube (TV tube)

The echo voltage signals produced by the transducer are electronically stored and presented on a display in such a way that the operator can

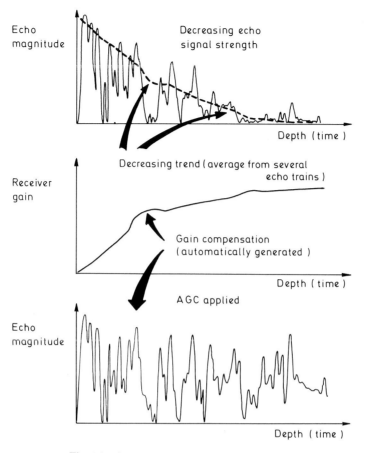

Fig. 1.9 Automatic TGC (adaptive gain control).

relate them to tissue structures. In almost all cases, a cathode-ray tube (CRT) is used as the means of displaying echoes. CRTs are commonly encountered in oscilloscopes, television sets, and patient-monitoring equipment. Tubes vary in their design, but this need not concern the operator, who requires only knowledge sufficient to understand the way in which the echo data is being presented and to optimize the displayed image. We will consider here the basic form of a CRT (Fig. 1.10).

The glass vessel shown in the figure has a high voltage (e.g. 10 000 volts) applied over its length. The electron gun, located at one end of the tube, is heated electrically, producing free electrons from the cathode filament. These electrons are then accelerated along the vessel under the influence of the high voltage and strike the phosphor

material on the screen, causing it to emit light. To make possible the writing of patterns and images, we bring the paths of the electrons down the tube to a point focus on the screen phosphor, generating a bright spot. Focusing is achieved by passing the electrons through an electrostatic or electromagnetic lens in which an electric or magnetic field forces the electrons along the desired path. Rapid manipulation of the position and the brilliance of the spot is necessary. Its position can be altered by applying voltages to the X- and Y-plates in order to deflect the beam with an electric field. Alternatively, it is common practice to deflect the beam by a magnetic field generated by an electric current in coils placed outside the tube. Spot brilliance is controlled by applying a voltage to the cathode or control grid to influence the number of electrons passing down the tube, or, in

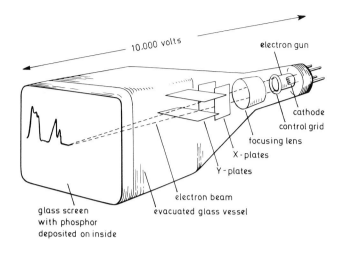

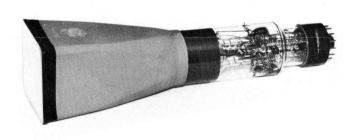

Fig. 1.10 The basic structure of a cathode-ray tube.

other words, to control the electron-beam current.

Echo signals are presented on a CRT screen by two mechanisms. In one mode, the bright spot is made to travel at a uniformly high speed across the screen in the X-direction. During this traverse, echo-voltage signals, as they are detected, are applied directly to the Y-plates and cause the spot to be deflected vertically for the duration of each echo. The size of the deflection is a measure of the echo magnitude (Fig. 1.11); this is known as the 'A-scope presentation'. In 'B-scope presentation', the echo signals are read from the scan-converter memory and applied to the cathode to increase the brilliance of the moving spot. The brightness of each spot is governed by the echo size (Fig. 1.11). By applying the requisite voltage

signals to the X- and Y-plates, one can place this straight line of bright echo spots in any direction across the screen.

Television raster presentation

A television picture is presented on a CRT display tube as a number of closely spaced horizontal lines (e.g. 625 or 525 lines). The first line of the image is produced by sweeping a spot across the top of the screen from left to right. The spot is then moved a small distance down the screen and swept again to give another line, and so on down the screen. The electron beam in the tube is said to be scanning the screen in a raster. The brilliance of the spot is varied to produce an image. A signal

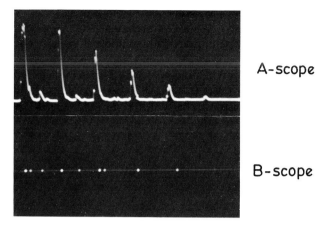

A-scope

B-scope

Fig. 1.11 Presentation of echo signals, A-scope and B-scope.

that controls the spot brilliance is called the 'video signal' and is usually supplied from either a television camera, a video-tape recorder, or an electronic scan-converter memory.

Since the electron beam can move very rapidly, line sweeps are completed in about 60 μs. A complete picture, one image frame, is generated in around 40 ms. A combination of 25 such images per second and the persistence of human vision gives the illusion of a constantly presented picture. In fact, the television raster does not scan lines in the order 1, 2, 3, and so forth, but rather does 1, 3, 5 . . . to the bottom of the screen and then jumps back to the top and does 2, 4, 6 . . . This interlacing of lines reduces image flicker.

Colour-television displays are described in Chapter 26.

UNITS AND SYMBOLS

SI units are used throughout this text. The reader is likely to be well acquainted with most units; for example, metre (m), centimetre (cm), gram (g), kilogram (kg), second (s), and watt (W). The units of force, energy, and pressure may be unfamiliar; namely, newton (N), joule (J), and pascal (Pa), respectively.

1 N = 1 newton = 0.225 lb weight = 0.102 kg weight
1 J = 1 joule = 0.24 calorie
1 Pa = 1 pascal = 1 N/m² = 0.00001 atmospheric pressure

A number of prefixes and symbols are used, as found in the scientific literature:

One million $\equiv 10^6 \equiv$ mega $\equiv$ M
  e.g. one million hertz $\equiv 10^6$ Hz $\equiv 1$ MHz
One thousand $\equiv 10^3 \equiv$ kilo $\equiv$ k
  e.g. one thousand grams $\equiv 10^3$ g $\equiv 1$ kg
One-thousandth $\equiv 10^{-3} \equiv$ milli $\equiv$ m
  e.g. one-thousandth of a metre $\equiv 10^{-3}$ m $\equiv$ 1 mm
One-millionth $\equiv 10^{-6} \equiv$ micro $\equiv \mu$
  e.g. one-millionth of a second $\equiv 10^{-6}$ s $\equiv 1$ μs

Finally, the following method of writing units often occurs in the printed literature:

Velocity: m/s $\equiv$ ms^{-1}
Density: g/cm³ $\equiv$ gcm^{-3}
Pressure: N/m² $\equiv$ Nm^{-2}

SUMMARY

1. Ultrasound is now a widely applied tool for the examination of soft tissue and blood flow.

2. A systematic study of the subject distinguishes the amateur from the professional.

3. Ultrasound is the transmission of high-frequency vibrations through a medium; through tissue in the case of medical applications.

4. There are at least 13 reasons for the application of ultrasound in medical diagnosis. This number is growing. Little progress has been made

in tackling the basic problems of bone, gas, and fat.

5. It is worthwhile to distinguish the definitions of ultrasonic field and beam.

6. Transducers can be made small for holding in the hand.

7. Ultrasound beams can be made narrow. This is probably the most crucial fact in the technology of ultrasound.

8. Echoes are generated in tissue by reflection and scattering at boundaries and points where there is a change in acoustic impedance. Note that it is the size of the change that determines the size of the echo and not the individual values.

9. Since our brains are so powerful in the interpretation of images, ultrasonic-echo and blood-flow information is probably best presented in this form.

10. The sensitivity controls on each machine should be carefully identified.

11. Scan-converter computer memories play a central role in the functioning of most machines.

12. It is easy to take the fast performance of CRTs for granted, but they are remarkable instruments.

13. Take care to attribute the correct units to each physical quantity and you will impress your friends.

REFERENCES

Clinics in Diagnostic Ultrasound. Churchill Livingstone, New York (Large series of clinical texts)
Cosgrove D O, McCready V R 1982 Ultrasound imaging. Wiley, Chichester, England
Evans D H, McDicken W N, Skidmore R, Woodcock J P 1989 Doppler ultrasound: Physics, instrumentation and clinical applications. Wiley, Chichester, England
Meire H B, Farrant P 1982 Basic clinical ultrasound. British Institute of Radiology, London
Feigenbaum H 1986 Echocardiography, 5th edn. Lea and Febiger, Philadelphia
Hatle L, Angelson B 1985 Doppler ultrasound in cardiology, 2nd edn. Lea and Febiger, Philadelphia
Hill C R (ed) 1986 Physical principles of medical ultrasonics. Ellis Horwood, Chichester, England
Hansmann M, Hackeloer B J, Staudach A 1985 Ultrasound diagnosis in obstetrics and gynecology. Springer, Berlin
Holm H H, Kristensen P 1981 Ultrasonically guided puncture technique. Saunders, Philadelphia
Hussey M 1985 Basic physics and technology of medical diagnosis. Macmillan, London
Hykes D, Hedrick W R, Starchman D E 1985 Ultrasound physics and instrumentation. Churchill Livingstone, New York
Journal of Clinical Ultrasound. John Wiley, New York (largely medical articles)
Kisslo J, Adams D B, Belkin R N 1988 Doppler color flow imaging. Churchill Livingstone, New York

Kremkau F W 1989 Diagnostic ultrasound: principles, instruments and exercises, 3rd edn. Saunders, Philadelphia
Lerski R A (ed) 1988 Practical ultrasound. IRL Press, Oxford
Meltzer R S, Roelandt J (eds) 1982 Contrast echocardiography. Martinus Nijhoff, The Hague
Omoto R (ed) 1987 Color atlas of real-time two-dimensional Doppler echocardiography, 2nd edn. Shindan-To-Chiryo, Tokyo
Powis R L, Powis W J 1984 A thinker's guide to ultrasonic imaging. Urban and Schwarzenberg, Baltimore
Repacholi M H, Benwell D A 1982 Essentials of medical ultrasound. Humana, Clifton, USA
Silk M G 1984 Ultrasonic transducers for nondestructive testing. Adam Hilger, Bristol
Taylor K J W, Strandness D E (eds) 1990 Duplex Doppler ultrasound. Churchill Livingstone, New York
Taylor K J W 1985 Atlas of gray scale ultrasonography, 2nd edn. Churchill Livingstone, Edinburgh
Taylor K J W, Burns P N, Wells P N T 1988 Clinical applications of Doppler ultrasound. Raven Press, New York
Timor-Tritsch I E, Rottem S 1987 Transvaginal sonography. Elsevier, New York
Ultrasound in Medicine and Biology. Pergamon, Oxford (medical, technical, and biological articles; also very extensive bibliography)
Wells P N T 1977 Biomedical ultrasonics. Academic Press, New York
Woodcock J P 1979 Ultrasonics. Adam Hilger, Bristol

2. Basic ultrasonic instruments

This account of the principles and use of ultrasonic instruments in their simplest form will provide an introduction to the basic ideas of such machines. A second aim of this chapter is to assist readers in the scientific use of equipment that may be deceptively simple in appearance, but which can provide results that are difficult to interpret. This is particularly true of some real-time scanning machines, which, being relatively inexpensive, are finding application in many diverse situations. It is hoped that this introduction will help operators in the initial application of these machines and encourage them to read further on the subject of diagnostic ultrasound.

Many ultrasonic techniques employ the same means of collecting ultrasonic information in the form of echoes. Variations are often found only in the way the ultrasound beam is directed into the body or in the presentation of the echo signals on a display. Familiarity with one technique gives insight into another.

A-SCAN (A-MODE)

The simplest technique is called 'A-scanning'. A transducer, acting as both transmitter and receiver, is pointed in the direction of interest through the body, and echoes are detected from interfaces that intersect the beam. Since only those surfaces lying within the beam are recorded, this is a one-dimensional scan (Fig. 2.1).

An A-scan trace can be produced in the following manner. Simultaneously with the ultrasound pulse being transmitted into the body, the bright spot on the CRT screen starts to sweep horizontally at a fast uniform speed across the screen from the left-hand side. This is done by applying a

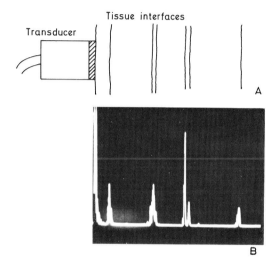

Fig. 2.1 An A-scan trace and related reflecting surfaces.

steadily increasing voltage across the X-plates. During this sweep, echoes are received, amplified, and applied as voltage pulses to the Y-plates. The spot is therefore deflected from the horizontal baseline for the duration of each echo signal. The size of a vertical deflection is a measure of the size of the echo signal, provided the echo is not too large, in which case the receiver is saturated, and the deflection is limited. The position of a deflection along the horizontal trace is a measure of the time taken for the echo to return, that is, a measure of the depth of the reflecting surface.

The A-scan mode on its own is not widely used, although basic instruments are relatively inexpensive. A-scanning can be usefully employed only where the anatomic structures are not complex, allowing one to identify the interfaces that give rise to the echoes. Examples are examination of the

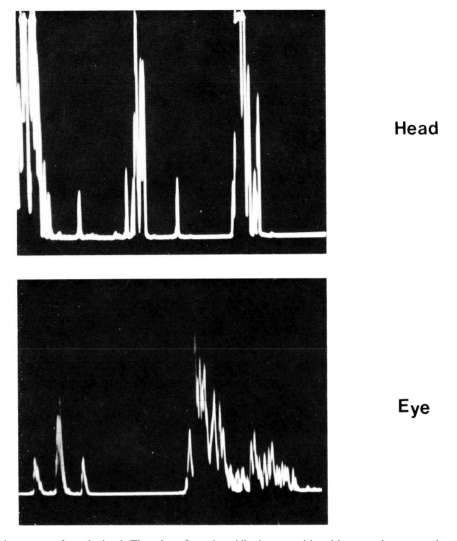

Head

Eye

Fig. 2.2 An A-scan trace from the head. The echoes from the midbrain are positioned between the strong echoes from the skull. An A-scan trace from the eye shows cornea and lens echoes on the left and orbital echoes on the right.

midline of the brain or the bulb of the eye (Fig. 2.2).

When an A-scan instrument is in use, the transducer is held fixed pointing into the region of interest. The A-scan pattern on the screen is then interpreted in terms of echo magnitudes and positions of reflecting interfaces. Skill in the technique involves recognizing patterns that correlate with anatomic structures and lesions. Basic instruments have few controls, and sensitivity is likely to be adjusted by an overall gain and a simple TGC arrangement. Oil or gel is used to ensure good acoustic coupling between the transducer and the patient. Oil or gel is required since it is difficult

to transmit high-frequency ultrasound through even a thin layer of air.

The A-scan mode of echo presentation is sometimes found as an additional feature of a real-time B-scanner.

REAL-TIME B-SCAN

Grey-shade image production

Owing to the ambiguity that often arises in A-scanning, imaging techniques have been developed to provide a pictorial representation of anatomic sections. As we noted earlier, to create such images, one makes the ultrasonic beam sweep in a plane section through the body. For each beam position, tissue structures are located by determining the times of return of the echoes and the beam direction.

Consider, initially, that the beam is directed into the right-hand side of the region to be scanned (Fig. 2.3a). The beam is then made to move while pointing into the tissue structures. Echoes detected at each beam position are displayed on a CRT screen as bright spots along a line, the scan line. The direction and position of each scan line on the display screen are accurately related to the direction and position of the ultrasound beam in the patient. By sweeping the ultrasonic beam across the scan plane, we obtain many lines of echoes, and they combine to delineate the internal structures of the body (Fig. 2.3b, 2.3c). During the above process, the echo signals are actually stored in an electronic scan-converter memory before passing on to the display screen.

On the display screen, the brightness of each spot is a measure of the magnitude of its echo signal. This is known as grey-shade imaging. To obtain high-quality grey-tone images, the electronic system and display module make great effort to present echo information in the most suitable manner. For instance, more of the available shades of grey are allocated to the weak echoes from within organs than to stronger signals from major tissue boundaries. This is usually described as logarithmic processing of the data. Great care is taken to construct transducers and amplifiers that detect weak echoes. Appreciation of the importance of grey shades and weak echoes led to a major advance in diagnostic ultrasound in the 1970s.

Principles of real-time B-scanners

Since the speed of sound in tissue is very high, namely 1540 m/s, each line of echoes is collected in less than a millisecond. The beam can therefore be moved quickly to collect the next line of echoes. When the beam has swept across the scan plane, i.e. across the field of view, the procedure is immediately repeated. Complete images can be produced in a fraction of a second; typically 25 images are generated per second. This is one of the main attractions of real-time B-scanners. It means

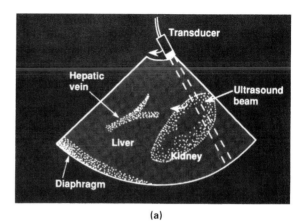

(a)

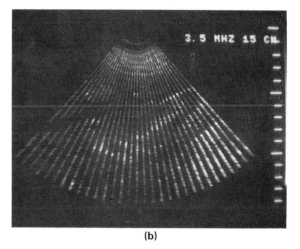

(b)

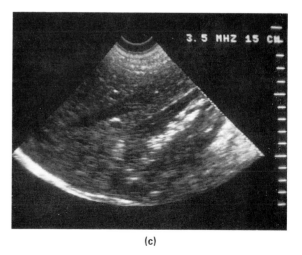

(c)

Fig. 2.3 (a) The sweep of an ultrasound beam through tissues, (b) sample lines of echo information, (c) many lines of echo information merged to form a complete image.

that the motion of organs such as the heart can be observed, since echoes are being continually gathered from tissues in their new positions and the whole image is continually being refreshed. Equally important, it means that the scan plane can be quickly altered, allowing the operator to search through the anatomy. A third attraction of real-time B-scanners is that the transducers can be made small for holding in the hand, resulting in great flexibility in their use.

Simple linear or radial (sector) sweeps are commonly performed by the ultrasonic beams of real-time instruments. The number of images generated per second varies from 5 to about 40 per second, depending on the scanner and its intended field of application. The number of lines of echoes in an image varies from about 50 to 200.

Real-time B-scanners consist of a transducer assembly, which sends the beam along rapidly changing directions, and an electronics-plus-display system. Several transducers may be available for different applications. The scanners are often small and portable (Fig. 2.4). More complex instruments with added peripherals are less mobile. They will be discussed in later chapters.

10 groups. No generally accepted classification or nomenclature exists for instruments. In this text, the following will be used:

1. Mechanical sector oscillator
2. Mechanical linear oscillator
3. Mechanical rotator
4. Electronic linear array
5. Electronic curved array
6. Electronic sector scanner (phased array)
7. Water-bath scanner
8. Small-parts scanner
9. Invasive scanner
10. Compound scanner

In one common form of simple mechanical scanner, a single-element transducer is pivoted at its front face and made to rock rapidly (Fig. 2.5a). In another type of oscillating mechanism, the transducer reciprocates on a line with its beam always pointing in the same direction (Fig. 2.5b).

(a) **Oscillating transducer**

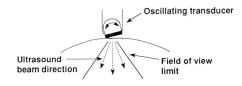

(b) **Reciprocating transducer**

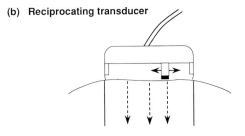

(c) **Rotating transducer**

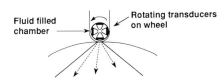

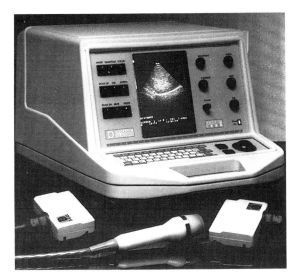

Fig. 2.4 A portable, ultrasonic, real-time B-scanner with three transducer assemblies (courtesy of Dynamic Imaging).

Types of real-time scanner

Real-time scanners may be roughly classified into

Fig. 2.5 Three mechanical systems for sweeping the beam in real-time B-scanners.

(a) **Linear array**

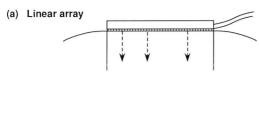

(b) **Curved array**

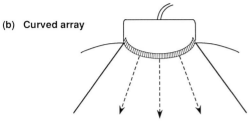

(c) **Phased array**

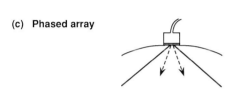

Fig. 2.6 Three electronic systems for sweeping the beam in real-time B-scanners.

Alternatively, several transducers are mounted on a wheel that rotates (Fig. 2.5c).

One basic form of electronic real-time scanner has a transducer assembly consisting of a linear array of small elements (Fig. 2.6a). Groups of neighbouring elements are activated in turn to give a narrow ultrasonic beam. In this way, parallel beams interrogate the tissues, and images are produced without moving any part of the transducer. A modification of this approach is to use an array of elements which is curved outwards (Fig. 2.6b). Contact on the skin is easier with this sort of array in some situations, and the field of view is increased since the beam paths diverge in the body.

Another approach to real-time scanning, which depends wholly on electronic means for moving the beam, is the electronic phased array. In this device, the transducer head is constructed from a number of very thin element strips placed side by side (Fig. 2.6c). The element strips are excited almost simultaneously to generate the transmitted ultrasonic field. By introducing slight time delays,

i.e. phase differences, between their excitation signals, we can control the direction of the resultant field. Each direction corresponds to a particular set of delays. To sweep the field through a sector, we systematically alter the delays between each transmission. The direction of the reception zone is altered by introducing similar delays to the echo signals at each element strip before they are combined to form the total signal. Both transmission and reception directions are therefore made to coincide and form a scanning beam in the normal manner. The physics of the process by which contributions from each strip combine at transmission or reception to form a narrow field or zone is discussed in Chapter 5. A small, stationary transducer head, 1.5 cm wide, constructed from 64 strips, can generate a pulsed beam of ultrasound that scans through a 90° sector.

In a number of real-time B-scanning units, a water-bath is placed between the transducer assembly and the patient. The combination of water-bath and transducer assembly may result in a fairly large scanning head being in contact with the patient. On the other hand, removing the patient from the immediate vicinity of the transducer allows greater variety in transducer assembly design, e.g. more than one transducer incorporated in the head or motorized control of the scan-plane position. The stand-off water-bath aids imaging of superficial regions just under the skin, since they are no longer very close to the transducer where the beam properties are not optimum. High-frequency linear arrays can often image superficial structures without the help of a water-bath. Another approach is to use a piece of jelly material, which is commercially available, as a stand-off layer.

High-frequency transducers, operating at 5 to 10 MHz, with or without a water-bath and based on any of the above scanning principles, are often called 'small-parts scanners'.

Basic mechanical and electronic scanners are relatively inexpensive and are finding many applications. We shall now study them in more detail, emphasizing the salient points and indicating topics that are worth further study.

Mechanical scanner

A mechanical scanner of the rotating-wheel variety

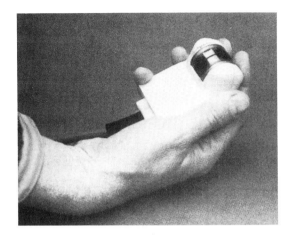

Fig. 2.7 A mechanical transducer assembly in which four transducers rotate in a thin-walled oil-bath (courtesy of BCF).

is shown in Figure 2.7. Four standard transducers are mounted with their beam axes directed outward radially from the centre of the wheel. Each ultrasonic beam is directed at an angle of 90° to the axes of adjacent beams. This assembly of transducers is supported inside an oil-filled cylinder. The curved wall of the cylinder is thin and normally made of plastic or rubber. Rotation is achieved by linking the transducer wheel to a small motor.

With all four transducers in operation, each is activated as it passes through a 90° sector at the plastic window, providing a 90° field of view. With two transducers in use, each is activated over 180° with a corresponding field of view. Electric contact is made with the transducers via small devices (e.g. slip-rings or rotating transformers), which maintain contact while the wheel rotates continuously. Similarly, the position of the wheel is measured by types of angle resolvers that can cope with high-speed continuous rotation.

The transducers are of fixed frequency and fixed focal length. For example, 3 MHz transducers may be focused at a depth of 8 cm. Changing the frequency of ultrasound normally involves changing the entire transducer assembly. At least one device has a wheel of sufficiently large diameter to accommodate a range of transducers of different frequency. It is a feature of real-time scanners that altering the frequency is somewhat limited, in practice, by the cost of transducer heads.

A liberal amount of fluid and a slight pressure of application on the skin surface ensure good acoustic coupling and, in turn, a large field of view. It should be noted that static recordings of real-time images do not have the same information content as the actual screen image. Several factors contribute to this degradation in image quality. In the real-time image, movement of tissues, small and large, helps to identify genuine tissue structures and reduces the significance of spurious, artefact echoes. Slight changes in the scan plane aid in the identification of reflecting interfaces.

Oscillating transducer scanners have a construction similar to that of rotating devices. Their field of view is often less than 90°; on the other hand, since they require only one transducer, it is easier to incorporate an annular array transducer (Fig. 2.8).

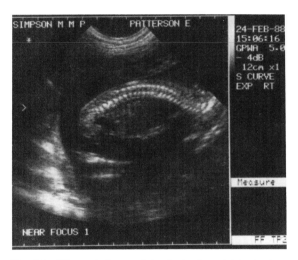

Fig. 2.8 Ultrasonic image of the fetal spine, obtained using an annular array (courtesy of Chambers S).

Electronic linear array

Present-day basic linear arrays are typically constructed from 150 piezoelectric-element strips of dimensions 10 mm × 1 mm, rather than 15 strips of dimensions 10 mm × 10 mm, as was the case in very early units. The strip elements are fired in small groups (e.g. 10) so that the effective source of ultrasound is similar to that of a standard single-element transducer. Later we will see that if a source is made too small, the ultrasonic beam spreads out rapidly and lacks good directional characteristics. The advantage of making the array from small strip elements is that the groups can be excited in the following sequence. First, elements 1, 2, 3, . . . 9, 10 are activated to transmit and receive echoes. This is immediately followed by 2, 3, 4 . . . 10, 11, then 3, 4, 5 . . . 11, 12, and so on. The ultrasonic beam is therefore displaced in 1 mm steps, and it sweeps through the plane of scan. With 15 independent elements, there would be 15 lines of echo information in the image; with 150 strip elements in an array of the same length, there are 141 lines in the image.

Beam focusing to reduce the thickness of the tissue slice examined, that is, perpendicularly to the plane of scan, can be achieved by making the strip elements concave or by placing a cylindrical lens along the array. To obtain focusing in the plane of scan, one should include electronic focusing techniques in the processing of the signals of each element. These techniques are now commonly used in the construction of basic array scanners; they are discussed in Chapter 5.

Selection of an ultrasonic frequency involves selection of a particular transducer array. Manufacturers generally offer a few arrays of different frequencies, for example, 3, 5, and 7 MHz. Figure 2.9 shows an image from a linear array. Note that the width of the field of view is determined by the length of the array. Curved arrays which also work on the above described principles increase the field of view and are, in fact, more popular than exactly straight arrays for obstetric imaging (Fig. 2.10).

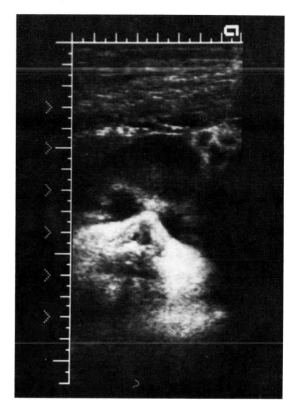

Fig. 2.9 Ultrasonic image of a fetal face, obtained with a linear array (courtesy of Acuson).

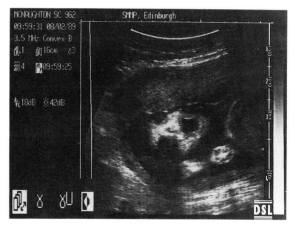

Fig. 2.10 Image of the fetal face, limbs, and part of the thorax lying below the placenta (courtesy of Diagnostic Sonar).

Resolution in real-time B-scanning

With any imaging technique it is important to have a reasonable idea of the smallest detail that the instrument can depict. Resolution may be defined as a measure of the ability of a scanner to display structural detail in its images. Three fundamental components of overall resolution are axial, lateral, and contrast resolution.

1. Axial resolution is a measure of the ability of the instrument to produce separate echoes from structures lying closely, one behind another along the beam. It depends on the length of the transmitted ultrasonic pulse — the shorter the pulse, the better the axial resolution.

2. Lateral resolution is a measure of the ability of the instrument to display separate echoes from

structures lying closely, side by side, across the ultrasonic beam. As might be expected, it depends on the effective width of the ultrasound beam at the structures.

3. Contrast resolution is a measure of the ability of the instrument to display tissues of neighbouring reflectivity as different shades of grey. It depends on the noise in the image, since this makes the distinction of small changes in grey shade difficult to identify.

As the frequency of ultrasound is increased, it is possible to make the transmitted pulse shorter and the beam width narrower. A fundamental fact in diagnostic ultrasound is that the higher the frequency, the better the resolution. A 3 MHz scanner might have an axial resolution of 1.0 mm and a lateral resolution of 3 mm; a 5 MHz device may have corresponding values of 0.5 mm and 2 mm. It is unfortunate that attenuation of ultrasound in tissue increases with frequency. The dependence of contrast resolution on frequency is not marked, but this topic has not been fully studied. Typically, the minimum change in reflectivity which can be observed in an image is around 10%.

The temporal resolution of a real-time B-scanner, that is, its ability to separate events in time, depends on the frame rate of the scanner. A frame rate of 30 images per second is adequate for most motions within the body except the more rapid cardiac actions, such as the flutter of a mitral valve.

Display of real-time images

Display screens on instruments are found with a wide range in dimensions, for example, from 3 × 4 cm to 30 × 40 cm. Large screens are convenient for viewing and for detecting small motions; small screens have some advantages since they are portable. A display monitor with a white phosphor screen and a small spot size is generally recommended for presenting high-quality grey-tone images. The assessment of grey-tone presentation is rather subjective. It can be made more rigorous, however, by carefully setting up the brilliance and contrast controls while observing a test pattern. Grey-shade patterns are often available as a feature of the scanner.

Measurement with a real-time B-scanner

Dimensions of structures can be measured from ultrasonic images. Most commonly measured are linear dimensions, for example, the biparietal diameter of a fetal head or the diameter of a blood vessel. Measurement is accomplished by introducing electronic calliper markers onto the display screen and superimposing them on the dimension of interest in the image. There is a variety of types of calliper. Simplest to use are the omnidirectional ones with which the markers can be placed anywhere on the screen (Fig. 2.11). The distance between the markers is presented on a numeric display in millimetres of tissue.

The accuracy of an electronic calliper is high and may be a small fraction of a millimetre. The overall accuracy of any measurement, however, is much more dependent on other sources of error, for example, uncertainty in the selection of the dimension to be measured. The error in a careful measurement of length is likely to be 1 or 2%, e.g. 1 or 2 mm in 10 cm.

It should be noted that a value for the velocity of sound is assumed in the calibration of a calliper in millimetres of tissue. We saw earlier that distance is obtained from echo information by using echo-return time and the velocity of ultrasound. Two-dimensional images are also constructed by incorporating into the machine design a scale factor depending on the average velocity of ultrasound in tissue. If the calliper and the imag-

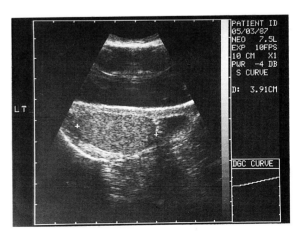

Fig. 2.11 Image of a testicle, obtained with a small-parts, water-bath scanner operating at 7.5 MHz (courtesy of Wild SR).

ing system are used for general soft-tissue work, the velocity of sound for both is usually set to 1540 m/s. Adjustment of the calliper velocity may be possible by an external or internal instrument control. Should measured dimensions be compared to data, such as growth curves from the scientific literature, care should be taken to ensure that the calliper velocity is the same as that employed to produce the reference data in the literature.

From ultrasonic images, cross-sectional areas can be measured with an error of around ±5%. Facilities are incorporated in most instruments to allow this to be done routinely. From a number of cross-sectional areas through an organ, its volume may be derived with reasonable accuracy by using an appropriate formula, e.g. ±15%.

Quantification of the motion of tissue structures is made relatively simple by real-time B-scanning. The most obvious technique is to record a series of image frames and to make measurements of lengths and areas from them. This is particularly applicable in cardiology, where heart walls and valves can be studied. A potent combination of ultrasonic methods is real-time B-scanning plus M-scanning. The latter produces traces of the position of structures versus time. From these traces one may calculate range of movement, velocity, and acceleration. The M-scan mode is described in the next section of this chapter.

The ease of searching through anatomy with real-time instruments helps the selection of the relevant tissue sections. A feature known as the image frame-freeze mode is of considerable value in the measurement procedure as it allows any image to be instantly stored.

Limitations and artefacts

The greatest limitation is the virtually total reflection that occurs at tissue/gas boundaries. Access to the heart is limited by the lungs. A frustrating problem can arise as a result of bowel gas acting as a barrier to parts of the abdomen. Bone is also very different acoustically from soft tissue and causes penetration problems.

A common artefact is the shadowing that occurs when soft tissues lie behind a strong reflector or attenuator that reduces the interrogating field and the echo signals. On the other hand, this artefact may provide diagnostic information. The shadow cast by gallstones often aids diagnosis.

Another familiar artefact results from multiple reflection of an ultrasonic pulse. Because echoes return to the transducer by an indirect route involving more than one reflection, non-existent tissue interfaces may be depicted in the image. 'Ghost' surfaces at the top of the bladder are a very clear example of the artefact. They result from the sound pulse bouncing around in the tissue layer between the transducer and the top of the bladder.

Difficulty is usually experienced in setting the sensitivity controls of a scanner to exact correctness. In fact, this is more or less impossible. If they are set poorly, part of the image may be overemphasized or, conversely, presented as a weak echo pattern. This is especially true of badly adjusted TGC. In other words, electronic processing can introduce artefacts to the image.

Knowledge of artefacts is of paramount importance to the user of ultrasonic equipment. Chapter 15 is devoted to this subject.

Use of basic real-time B-scanners

The type of scanner best suited to each application depends primarily on the ease of access of ultrasound to the underlying tissues. Generally, if access to the region of interest is unrestricted, then all scanners will function; when access is restricted by gas or bone, sector scanners that act from a single point on the skin surface are most successful. The shape of the field of view and the ease of manipulation of the transducer also influence the choice of scanner.

Let us consider some points of importance for the routine use of a scanner. Unless there is some overriding reason, the transducer assembly should be of the highest frequency which can give the necessary penetration, since the higher the frequency the smaller the detail seen in an image. It is important to ensure that the skin surface is never dry where ultrasound is to pass between the transducer and the patient. Having located the scan plane through the region of interest, one arranges the sensitivity control to provide a well-balanced image (see Ch. 7). Any doubts about the settings of the display controls should be resolved by adjusting brilliance and contrast while observing a grey-tone test pattern or a set of echoes from a test-object or familiar section (App. 1).

Recording techniques come in many forms: simple Polaroid cameras, thermal printers, multi-format film cameras, video-tape recorders, etc. A simple photographic technique may be sufficient for record-keeping purposes, but it is not a good record of a real-time scan examination.

A word of warning concerning possible damage to the transducer assembly: a violent mechanical shock could destroy some of the many components in these devices. Advice should be sought if transducers are to be used with water-baths, because of the possibility of electric hazard or corrosion.

With the continuing advances in integrated circuit electronics, more and more features will be available at low cost. Chapters 10, 11, 12, and 13 contain details of scanner features.

M-SCAN (TIME–MOTION SCAN, T–M SCAN, TIME–POSITION SCAN)

M-scanning employs pulsed ultrasound to detect and record the motion of tissues. Just as in A-scanning, a single ultrasound beam is directed through the structures of interest. When an echo from a heart structure is detected, it can be observed on an A-scan display moving toward and away from the transducer. A more meaningful record is obtained if the echo signals are displayed as a line of bright B-scope spots that is made to sweep across a display screen. This produces traces of the positions of echoes versus time (Fig. 2.12). To record more cycles of motion than can be conveniently stored on a display screen or film, we add a fibre-optic chart recorder to the system (Fig. 16.4). The display screen showing repetitive M-scan sweeps is then used to monitor echo information that is fed into the fibre-optic recorder.

An example of a trace from a chart recorder is shown in Figure 2.13. It should be noted from this figure that the ultrasonic beam can be moved slowly during a recording to provide information on the movement of adjacent structures, for example, the aortic root, mitral valve, and left ventricular wall. This technique introduces an element of two-dimensional imaging to the M-mode.

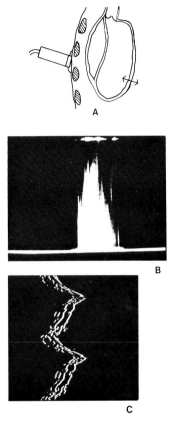

Fig. 2.12 Principle of M-scanning. (**a**) Transducer directed at moving structure of interest and held fixed, (**b**) echoes may be observed on an A-scan display but this does not give a record of motion, (**c**) echo dots sweep up the screen to provide a trace of position versus time.

Recording paper can preserve about five grey tones of echo-magnitude information. More expensive papers can approach photographic quality. The chart-recorder paper also has sufficient width to permit the recording of the ECG and other physiologic signals along with the echoes.

M-scanning is mostly used as an additional facility of real-time scan instruments. The images are used to identify a suitable beam direction for making a trace, for example, through the fetal heart in early pregnancy or the mitral valve in cardiac studies (Fig. 2.14).

M-scanning has been highly developed for use in cardiology. Experience and considerable thought need to be applied to the interpretation of the traces produced. Chapter 16 deals further with the detail of this modality.

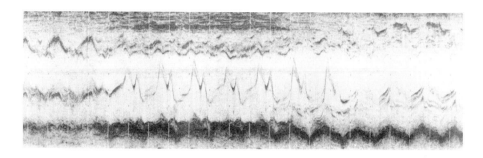

a

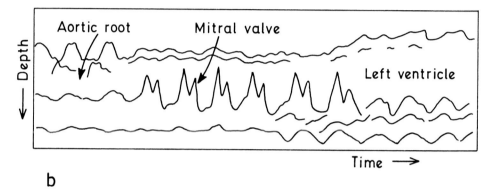

b

Fig. 2.13 Adult heart action recorded by M-scanning: write-out on a fibre-optic chart recorder. The direction of the beam was slowly altered during the recording.

DOPPLER SCAN

Principles of basic Doppler instruments

The Doppler effect in sound is the dependence of the observed pitch (i.e. frequency) of sound on the motion of the source or the observer. The observed frequency of the sound from a motor car travelling at speed is higher when it is approaching the observer than when receding. Reflection of sound at a moving interface also causes a Doppler effect. Consider the idealized arrangement in which blood is flowing along a tube at a uniform speed, u, and where a continuous beam of ultrasound of a well-defined frequency, f_1, intersects the flow at an angle θ (Fig. 2.15). The moving blood cells scatter some of the ultrasound in all directions. Consider the ultrasound sent back toward the transmitter and detected by an adjacent receiving element. This signal will have a Doppler shifted frequency, f_2.

The actual Doppler shift, $f_1 - f_2$, is given by the formula:

$$\text{Doppler shift } (f_D) = f_1 - f_2 = f_1 \frac{2u \cos \theta}{c}$$

where c = velocity of sound.

This arrangement is similar to that used in basic ultrasonic blood-flow detectors. Two transducer elements are necessary. One is driven continuously to generate ultrasound and the other is used continuously for reception, unlike the pulsed scanning modes we have been considering up until now.

The above formula indicates some basic points relevant to the use of blood-flow detectors.

1. The Doppler shift depends on the component of the velocity along the ultrasonic beam, i.e. on $u \cos \theta$ (Fig. 18.9 and Fig. 24.9). Note, therefore, that, in their basic form, ultrasonic Doppler instruments essentially measure velocity.

2. When numeric values are put into the for-

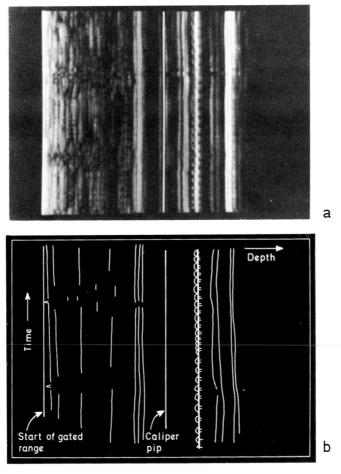

Fig. 2.14   Fetal heart motion recorded by M-scanning and photographed from a display screen (courtesy of Young G B).

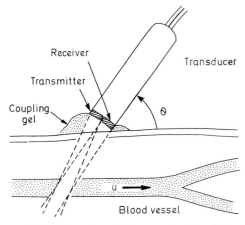

Fig. 2.15   Basic Doppler-technique examination of blood flow in a vessel.

mula, we find that the Doppler frequency shift, f_D, is small and in the audible range, for example, in the range 0 to 10 kHz for typical arterial blood-flow studies. After electronic extraction of the shift by comparing f_1 and f_2, it can be fed into a loudspeaker or earphones. The greater the velocity of the moving reflector, the higher is the pitch heard.

3. In the above model, all of the blood cells were considered to move with one velocity, u, which resulted in one Doppler shift, f_D. In practice, however the cells move with many velocities, each of which gives rise to a Doppler shift. The output from the instrument is therefore not a single note, f_D, but a spectrum of notes, each of which corresponds to a particular velocity of cells

in the blood vessel. The complex output signal can, in fact, be further analysed to yield information on the number of cells moving with each velocity i.e. to produce a 'sonogram' (see Ch. 21).

4. The direction of blood flow with respect to the transducer can be determined. Flow toward the transducer makes f_2 greater than f_1, and for flow away from the transducer, f_2 is less than f_1. Instruments sensitive to direction are very useful in blood-flow studies where reversal of flow can be detected.

Further sophistication of Doppler units involves detecting the frequency shift in reflected pulses of ultrasound. With pulsed techniques, both the range and velocity of the moving reflectors can be determined. Imaging Doppler systems are also available that depict regions of blood flow. This is known as 'colour-flow imaging' or 'colour-flow mapping' (Ch. 20).

The combination of a real-time B-scanner and a Doppler unit is known as a 'duplex Doppler system' (Fig. 2.16). Such a combination allows a blood vessel to be located and the Doppler beam to be directed toward it. The source of the Doppler signal is then known. The vessel diameter can be measured from the image and used along with the velocity information to calculate blood flow quantitatively in units of ml/min. However, it is much more common and fruitful, at present, to study the pattern of blood velocity through the cardiac cycle.

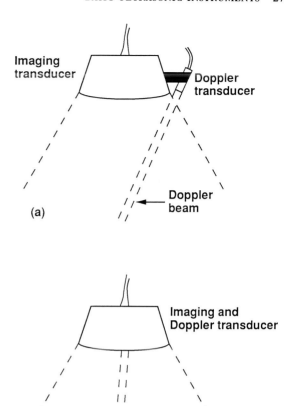

Fig. 2.16 Examples of the combination of real-time B-scanning and Doppler scanning to form duplex systems.

Use of basic Doppler instruments

Basic Doppler instruments find two main applications – the detection of fetal heartbeats and the study of flow patterns in readily identified vessels.

Fetal heart detectors normally utilize 2 MHz ultrasound to provide adequate penetration into the abdomen. The narrow ultrasonic beam is swept systematically through the pregnant uterus until the distinct, crisp beat of the fetal heart is heard. The sensitivity controls of this type of instrument are usually reduced to one gain control. Since a continuous beam of ultrasound is used, compensation for attenuation with depth (TGC) is not feasible. Good acoustic coupling with gel or oil between the transducer and skin is important.

When one searches for weak pulsations, the gain of the device should be high and the rate of sweeping of the ultrasonic beam slow. As the beam is moved through the tissues, static tissues move with respect to the transducer and produce strong, low-frequency Doppler shifts (e.g. of 100 Hz). The instrument filters out frequencies below about 200 Hz so that they do not mask the signals from genuine tissue movements. Blood flow in the umbilical arteries can also be readily detected with basic 2 and 4 MHz Doppler units.

Studies of blood flow in superficial vessels use ultrasound in the frequency range 4 to 10 MHz. The narrow beam of ultrasound is directed to intersect the vessel at a suitable angle. With gel coupling fluid, 45° is a convenient angle. In theory, the largest Doppler shift is obtained at 0°, and zero shift occurs at 90°. The former angle is not practical, and, in the 90° case, a weak signal is obtained since the ultrasonic beam is, in fact, slightly divergent.

For reproducible results, the site of the examination and the angle of the beam are noted carefully. The Doppler signal level is maximized by moving the beam across the vessel. It may be possible to exclude contributions from other arteries or veins by redirecting the beam. It is important to remember that the audible volume of the Doppler signal is related to the number of moving reflectors detected, whereas the pitch is related to their velocity. Even when these steps are taken, quantification of Doppler signals is not simple. For example, uncertainty exists as to the characteristics of the ultrasonic beam at the vessel. The angle of the vessel to the beam has not been determined precisely. More complex systems are required to quantify Doppler signals, particularly if volume flow is to be ascertained. The combination of real-time, B-scan imaging and Doppler techniques is proving fruitful in this field. Basic Doppler instruments are inexpensive devices that can quickly provide diagnostic information, although it is unwise to try to read too much into the information they supply.

SUMMARY

In this chapter, the way in which ultrasound is used was briefly introduced to set the stage for more detailed study. The A-scan was described as a basic way of collecting echo data. Ten types of real-time B-scanner were listed. Mechanical scanners and also electronic-linear and phased-array scanners were considered. The components of resolution – axial, lateral, and contrast – were seen to determine the detail in images. Since ultrasonic images depict interfaces, callipers can be readily employed to measure length, circumference, area, and volume. The topic of image artefacts was introduced. Methods were explained for the measurement of tissue motion and blood flow, namely the M-scan and the Doppler scan. The four Doppler techniques (CW, PW, duplex, and colour-flow imaging) are extremely powerful ways of examining blood flow. The basic Doppler equation provided guidance as to the interpretation of flow signals.

3. The nature of ultrasound

In this chapter, we will discuss ultrasound in more detail. The capabilities and limitations of ultrasonic techniques can be appreciated only by understanding the properties of ultrasound. Physics is not everyone's favourite subject, but when related to an application much of it becomes common sense, and it will probably give you unlimited pleasure.

THE WAVE CONCEPT

Ultrasound is often referred to as a wave. There are many phenomena that can be described in terms of waves, such as radio waves, light waves, X-rays, and even heat waves. This concept greatly improves our understanding of the properties of transmitted ultrasonic vibrations. To clarify the idea, we will first consider waves that are readily visualized, such as waves on the surface of water.

Waves on the surface of water

Imagine a plunger placed on the surface of water and forced to move up and down in a regular fashion. By mechanical interaction, the particles of water on the surface next to the plunger also start an upward and downward motion. These particles immediately cause their neighbours to start moving in a vertical direction from their rest position. A mechanical vibration, or ripple, therefore passes out from the plunger across the surface of the liquid (Fig. 3.1).

Let us now look in more detail at the oscillatory motion of the particles by examining those lying on a line, PX, across the surface (Fig. 3.1). These particles are only displaced in a vertical direction. It is also apparent that, although each has the same

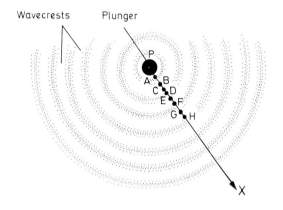

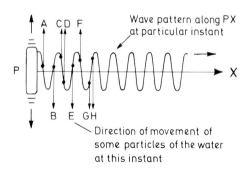

Fig. 3.1 The related movement of particles on the surface of water. The line *PX* is selected for more detailed examination.

motion as that of its neighbours, it is always at a different stage in the oscillatory cycle. It appears that each particle continually passes on to its immediate neighbour, on the side away from the source, its degree of displacement from the rest position. The plunger is said to generate a 'waveform' or 'wave' that passes out from it and dictates, at each instant, the vertical displacement of each particle. By thinking of mechanical vibrations as waves, we can more readily study the phenomena that arise as they pass through tissue.

We have chosen the displacement of particles from the rest position as the means of describing their motion. Another description in terms of the forces acting on the particles or the velocity of the particles about their rest positions would have been just as adequate. The descriptions would have involved the concept of a force wave or a particle-velocity wave moving out from the source and dictating the forces acting on the particles or the velocities of the particles at each instant.

Before leaving waves on water, let us consider what happens when the plunger is made to perform a short burst or pulse of two or three oscillations before coming to rest. In this case, a short ripple passes from the source across the surface of the liquid. In other words, the source has generated a pulsed wave that moves through the medium, influencing a limited number of particles at any particular time.

The movement of the particles is at right angles to the direction of wave propagation, so waves on water are called 'transverse waves'. As we will see below, sound waves are longitudinal waves; that is, the motion of the particles of the transmitting medium is parallel to the direction of wave travel. Waves on water differ from those of ultrasound in two other ways: for waves on the surface of water, velocity of propagation is much slower and the distance between crests is usually much larger.

Sound waves

Consider a pulsating object coupled to a medium so that it pushes and pulls on its neighbouring particles. These particles are made to oscillate and cause their neighbours to oscillate. In this way, a mechanical vibration travels from the object through the medium. Owing to the push-and-pull action of the source, the particles of the medium are made to perform orderly oscillations about their rest position. Again, the process can be described in terms of a wave travelling from its source and dictating to each particle where it should be at each instant. In contrast with waves

on water, the push-and-pull action of the source means that the motion of the oscillating particles is parallel to the direction of wave propagation. For ease of representation, however, a sound wave is drawn as an oscillatory trace in which positive parts represent displacements in one direction, and negative parts represent displacements in the opposite direction (Fig. 3.2a). This type of wave is called a 'longitudinal' or 'compressional' wave. The ear is sensitive to such waves, which are thus known as sound waves, or ultrasound waves if their rate of oscillation is too high to be heard.

The oscillation of particles subjected to a sound wave produces regions of high and low pressure (compression and decompression) along the wave at each instant (Fig. 3.2b). These regions of high and low pressure move outwards from the source. We say, therefore, that a pressure wave is generated by the source. Pressure is commonly used to describe sound waves since the transducers used to detect sound or ultrasound are most often sensitive to pressure.

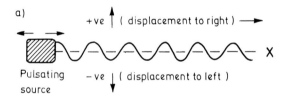

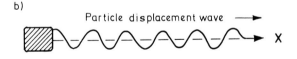

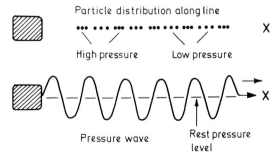

Fig. 3.2 (**a**) The generation of a continuous wave by a push-pull source, (**b**) the resulting particle distribution and pressure variation at a particular instant.

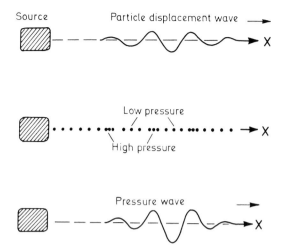

Fig. 3.3 Particle distribution and related pressure variation at a particular instant for a pulsed sound wave.

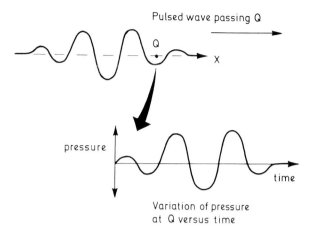

Fig. 3.4 Variation of pressure at point Q as an ultrasonic wave passes it.

If the piston in Figure 3.3 is made to perform a short burst of vibration, a pulsed sound wave is generated. At each instant, only a limited range of particles is influenced by the pulsed wave. For example, a pulse of 3 MHz ultrasound from an echo-imaging instrument might be 2 mm in length and contain 4 cycles of oscillation. On the other hand, instruments using the Doppler effect generate continuous- or pulsed-wave ultrasound, depending on the mode of operation.

The velocity, c, of the sound wave passing through the medium should not be confused with the velocity of the particles moving about their rest position, that is, the particle velocity, u.

When a wave passes a point, the particle at that point experiences cyclic pressure fluctuations, as illustrated in Figure 3.4, in which the pressure at a point is plotted against time. In order to detect a wave, the operator places a transducer at some suitable point and records the variation in pressure with time. The output signal from the transducer is an electric voltage that varies with time in a manner directly related to the pressure fluctuations.

When a waveform is drawn in a diagram, it is always worth noting whether the horizontal axis is labelled 'time' or 'distance'. If it is labelled 'time', the waveform represents the variations in pressure at a point in the medium. If it is labelled 'distance', the waveform represents the variations in pressure along a line through the medium.

The unit of pressure is the 'pascal' (Pa).

1 million pascals (MPa) = 10 × atmospheric pressure

Typically, in medical ultrasonics, a pulse may cause a maximum pressure fluctuation of 2 MPa, a very considerable fluctuation.

WAVE FRONTS

So far, the action of a wave has been examined along one line through the medium. A more complete picture is obtained by taking into account the three-dimensional volume of the transmitting medium. Instead of points of high and low pressure moving away from the source, there are, in fact, surfaces of high and low pressure. Figure 3.5 illustrates this for a continuous wave generated by a basic type of source used in diagnostic ultrasound, that is, a flat, circular disc oscillating like a piston. Here, the source has produced planes of high and low pressure moving away from it. This type of wave is said to have a 'plane wave front'. When pulsed waves are generated in diagnostic ultrasound, only three or four planes of high and low pressure exist as the pulsed wave passes from the transducer. Perfect plane waves are never encountered in practice, since a transmitted wave

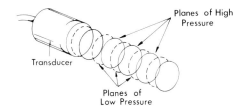

Fig. 3.5 Generation of a plane wave by a flat, oscillating source.

front is concave when it is moving toward a focus and convex as it diverges beyond it.

Spherical wave fronts are generated either by spherical sources or point sources. They are of interest because they result from a wave that is reflected or scattered from small tissue structures or blood cells, which act as small point sources.

Cylindrical wave fronts are created by cylindrical sources oscillating radially about their long axis. Many shapes of wave front can be generated using the appropriate shape of source or reflecting interface.

WAVE PARAMETERS (AMPLITUDE AND WAVELENGTH)

Consider now two parameters that allow a continuous waveform to be accurately specified (Fig. 3.6a).

Wave amplitude

The amplitude of a wave, p_0, is the maximum change is pressure caused by the wave and is related to the intensity of the ultrasonic radiation. As the intensity increases, the amplitude also increases. The term 'amplitude' is also used to describe the magnitude of an echo signal (Fig. 3.6b). Sometimes, in hazard studies, the maximum positive pressure amplitude, p_0^+, is considered separately from the maximum-negative pressure amplitude, p_0^- since they are often not equal and have different effects on tissue.

Wavelength

The wavelength, λ, is the distance between two

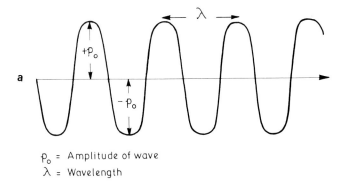

p_0 = Amplitude of wave
λ = Wavelength

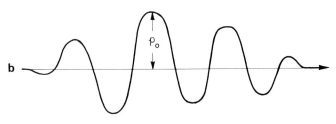

p_0 = Pulse amplitude

Fig. 3.6 (a) The amplitude and wavelength of a sinusoidal continuous wave, (b) the amplitude of an echo signal.

consecutive, identical points on the waveform (Fig. 3.6a). We will see that wavelength plays an important part in determining ultrasonic beam widths and pulse lengths, and, thus, greatly influences the detail that can be obtained in an image.

Wavelength (λ), frequency (f), and speed (c) of ultrasound are related as follows:

$$c = f\lambda$$

This can be deduced easily by considering a point in the medium and noting that the speed of sound equals the number of wavelengths which pass the point in 1 second multiplied by the wavelength (Fig. 3.7). From this formula, we can see that, since the speed of sound is a constant for each medium, there is a single wavelength for each frequency.

We can thus calculate the wavelengths corresponding to the frequencies used in diagnostic ultrasound. Assume the average velocity of sound in tissue to be 1540 m/s. Thus, at 1 MHz,

$$1540 = 1 \times 10^6 \times \lambda.$$

Therefore, $\lambda = 0.00154$ m $= 1.54$ mm.

Similarly, at

2 MHz, $\lambda = 0.77$ mm;
5 MHz, $\lambda = 0.31$ mm;
10 MHz, $\lambda = 0.15$ mm;

15 MHz, $\lambda = 0.10$ mm;
20 MHz, $\lambda = 0.08$ mm.

The distance between identical points on an ultrasonic wave in tissue is, therefore, typically about 1 mm or less. Note also that the higher the frequency, the smaller the wavelength. This results in better image detail at higher frequencies, a fact which will become increasingly obvious as we study the application of ultrasound.

To specify a pulsed wave, we require a few additional parameters. Their meanings are fairly obvious. For example, the pulse-repetition frequency is the rate of generation of ultrasonic pulses. Other parameters are defined in Figure 3.8. The frequency parameter as applied to a pulse is discussed further in Chapter 6.

PHASE OF A WAVE

The concept of phase is encountered in one or two techniques of diagnostic ultrasound. It arises in electronic focusing and steering of ultrasonic beams and also in the detection of direction of flow by Doppler methods. Consider a point, P, in a medium in which an ultrasonic wave is being propagated. The phase of the wave at point P, at any instant, is the stage reached in the cycle of oscillation. Thus, although the term 'phase' may seem imprecise when applied to waves, it is, in

|← Distance travelled by wave in 1 second →|
= Velocity of wave = c

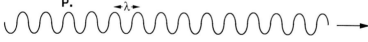

P. ←λ→

Wavelength   = λ

Number of wavelengths past P per second
    = Number of wave cycles experienced by P per second
    = Frequency
    = f

Distance travelled by wave per second (c) = Number of wavelengths past P per second (f) x λ

Hence   c = f λ

Fig. 3.7 Derivation of the relationship among speed of ultrasound, frequency, and wavelength.

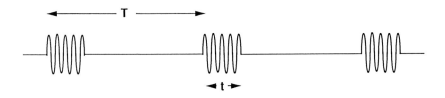

Pulse repetition period = T
Pulse repetition rate = Pulse repetition frequency (PRF) = $\frac{1}{T}$
Pulse duration = Pulse length = t
Duty cycle = $\frac{t}{T}$ x 100%

Fig. 3.8 Temporal parameters which define a pulse sequence.

fact, a familiar usage of the word. In any series of consecutive events, for example, construction of a building, the stage reached can be called the phase of the project. This is obviously similar to looking at a point in a medium and observing the phase reached in the wave cycle.

Phase is often quoted as an angle, since one complete cycle can be considered to be a revolution of 360°. For example, at a phase of 60°, one-sixth of the wave cycle has been performed. Phase also appears as an angle in the formulae used to describe waves mathematically.

Phase difference

When a wave is considered at two different times, the change in phase at a point is called the 'phase difference' between the two times.

It is possible for two waves to be transmitted into the same medium. The resultant pressure fluctuation due to the two waves, at any point, is obtained by adding the pressure fluctuation of one wave to that of the other. This phenomenon is known as the 'interference of waves'; it will be studied in Chapter 5. The term 'phase difference' is also applied when two waves are present in the same medium. At any point in the medium, the phase difference is the difference between the phases of the two waves at that point.

DIFFRACTION

Consider a small piston source transmitting ultrasonic vibrations into a medium. Let the diameter of the piston be equal in size to about 1

wavelength of the ultrasound in the medium (Fig. 3.9a). The mechanical vibrations diverge rapidly from the central axis as they pass through the medium. This spreading out of an ultrasonic field

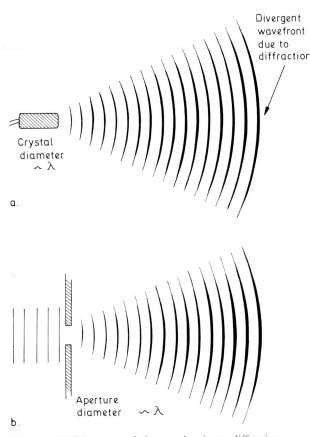

Fig. 3.9 (a) Divergence of ultrasound owing to diffraction is more easily observed when a small source is employed. (b) divergence of ultrasound owing to diffraction is also more easily observed when a small aperture is employed.

is called 'diffraction'. Diffraction can be readily observed when the dimensions of the source are of the order of a wavelength. Standard transducers are designed to be many wavelengths in diameter, for example, 20. In Chapter 5, we will see that they can be regarded as being composed of many small sources whose divergent fields largely cancel out one another except along the main field axis. In some directions where cancellation is not complete, weak side-lobes can be detected in the transmitted field.

Diffraction is also observed when a wave front passes through a small aperture that partially blocks it. The small aperture is then effectively a small source and the field diverges as in Figure 3.9b. A large aperture is analogous to a large source, so the diffraction effect is less obvious. Diffraction at a regularly shaped object or aperture may be considered to be a special case of the scattering process which describes interaction of waves with irregular structures (Ch. 4).

Diffraction is commonly encountered with audible sounds. In air, a 300 Hz sound has a wavelength of 100 cm. This is similar to the dimensions of doors and windows; therefore, sound is observed to diffract around corners.

ULTRASONIC INTENSITY, POWER, AND PRESSURE AMPLITUDE

Users of ultrasound should have accurate scientific information on the output intensity, power, and pressure amplitude of their equipment.

Intensity

When an ultrasonic transducer in contact with tissue is activated, the vibrating crystal quickly produces oscillations of the particles of the tissue medium. The particles of tissue then possess energy due to their oscillation. It can thus be seen that when an ultrasonic wave is generated, energy passes from the source to the tissue. The rate of flow of energy is called the 'intensity' of the field. To be more precise, the intensity of an ultrasonic field at a point is the rate of flow of energy through unit area (e.g. 1 cm^2) orientated perpendicularly to the field at that point (Fig. 3.10). During ultrasonic scanning, the output intensity of many instru-

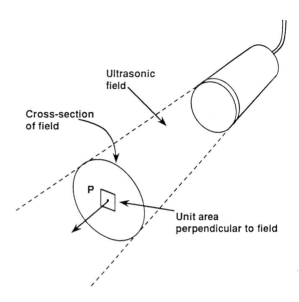

Fig. 3.10   The quantities 'cross section' and 'unit area' used to define power and intensity, respectively.

ments plays a prime role in determining the sensitivity of the instrument, that is, in determining the number and sizes of echoes recorded. Studies of the safety of ultrasonic techniques also require accurate knowledge of the intensities involved. When the intensity of a wave is increased, the physical quantities that we use to describe the wave fluctuate through greater ranges. There is an increase in the pressure amplitude, the particle displacement amplitude, and the particle velocity amplitude. Thus, increased intensity is associated with increased vigour in the mechanical vibrations of the tissue particles.

Three formulae are of interest for relating intensity, I, to the pressure amplitude, p_0, the particle displacement amplitude, x_0, and the particle velocity amplitude, u_0:

$$I = \tfrac{1}{2}\left(\frac{p_0{}^2}{\rho c}\right)$$

$$I = \tfrac{1}{2}\rho c\,(2\pi f)^2 x_0^2$$

$$I = \tfrac{1}{2}\rho c\,u_0^2$$

Here ρ is the density of the medium, and f is the frequency of ultrasound. Later in this chapter, we will use these formulae to acquire an understanding of the magnitudes of the physical quantities associated with ultrasonic waves in tissue.

In discussions of the biological effects of ultrasound and safety, it is necessary to specify intensity more exactly. For example, we may be interested in the peak value of intensity in the field, averaged over a time which includes several pulses. In this case, we would label the calculated intensity 'Ispta' (*I* *spatial* *peak*, *temporal* *average*). The peak-intensity value often occurs at the focus, but not always, particularly in an attenuating medium. Other similar intensity values are specified in Chapter 8.

In Chapter 7, manipulation of the instrument control governing output intensity and power will be discussed. The decibel notation applied to intensity will also be studied in Appendix 3. Appendix 4 contains a brief description of methods for measuring intensity.

Power

The intensity and power of an ultrasonic field are not identical quantities, although the two terms are loosely interchanged at times. The ultrasonic intensity is the rate of flow of energy through unit area, for example, 1 cm^2; the ultrasonic power is the rate of flow of energy through the whole cross section of the field (Fig. 3.10). Thus, for uniform plane wave fields, the following holds true:

ultrasonic power (W) = ultrasonic intensity (W/cm^2) × cross-sectional area of the field (cm^2)

For non-uniform fields, variations in the intensity within the field must be taken into account when power is calculated. Ultrasonic fields used in pulsed scanning have fairly well-known patterns of intensity; power can be calculated if average intensity is measured at points across the field.

The output powers and intensities of commercial echo imaging and Doppler equipment are quoted in Chapter 8.

No discussion of acoustic intensity is complete without reference to the remarkable performance of the human ear. The ear can detect sound waves down to intensities of 10^{-16} W/cm^2 and cope with a range of intensities up to 10^{14} times this value.

Pressure amplitude

It is now felt that potential hazards are more likely

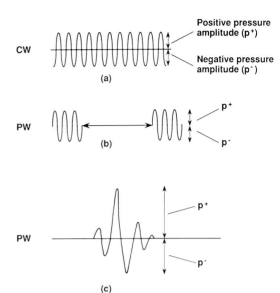

Fig. 3.11 The positive and negative amplitudes of continuous and pulsed ultrasound.

to be related to pressure fluctuations than to heating. It is therefore desirable to specify wave-pressure amplitudes. With continuous-wave ultrasound as used in diagnosis, the waveform is usually symmetrical about the average pressure level. With pulsed-wave devices, this symmetry cannot be assumed, and the peak positive and negative pressure amplitudes are often quoted (Fig. 3.11).

NON-LINEAR PROPAGATION OF WAVES

In our treatment of the subject so far, we have assumed that the shape of the continuous or pulsed wave does not alter as it passes through the propagating medium. This is an oversimplification. One process which alters the shape of a wave is called non-linear propagation.

A medium is said to respond linearly to a wave if the particle-velocity amplitude, i.e. the maximum particle velocity, changes in proportion to the particle-pressure amplitude. This relation between velocity amplitude and pressure amplitude is illustrated in Figure 3.12. The relationship is, in fact, linear for only very low amplitude waves. In reality, velocity amplitude does not change in proportion to pressure amplitude, i.e. the relation-

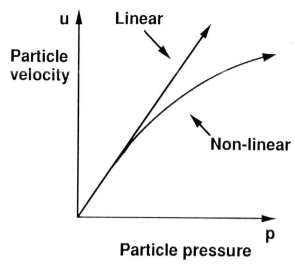

Fig. 3.12 Linear and non-linear relationships between particle velocity and particle pressure shown as graphical plots.

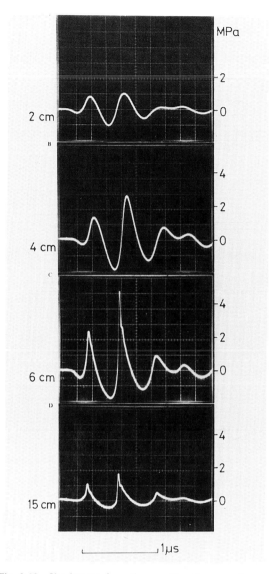

Fig. 3.13 Shock-wave formation resulting from non-linear propagation in water. The 2 MHz pulse clearly shows sharp discontinuities by the time it reaches a depth of 6 cm (courtesy of Duck F A & Starrit H 1984 British Journal of Radiology 57: 231–240).

ship is non-linear (Fig. 3.12). For example, doubling a low value of the pressure amplitude results in a doubling of the velocity amplitude, but this is not the case at higher amplitudes, where doubling of the pressure results in a smaller change in velocity.

The theory of sound waves which takes this non-linear behaviour into account indicates that the velocity of sound in the positive pressure part of the waves (the compressional half-cycle) is higher than that in the negative pressure part (the decompressional half-cycle). As the wave passes through the medium, the positive parts of the waveform move slightly faster than the negative parts, and the waveform becomes distorted (Fig. 3.13). When the waveform exhibits a spiked discontinuity, a shock wave is said to be formed. With the size of pulses used in imaging, this shock-wave formation occurs within a few centimetres of the transducer face, e.g. at 4 cm for a 5 MHz pulse of intensity 20 W/cm^2 (Isptp) in water (see Ch. 8 for the definition of Isptp). As the pulse passes further into the medium, the sharpness of the spike increases.

The theory also indicates several points about non-linear propagation:

1. The larger the amplitude of the initial pulse, the sooner shock waves are formed.

2. The higher the frequency, the sooner shock waves are formed.

3. The distance required to form a shock wave depends on the propagating medium.

The presence of shock waves raises questions concerning the safety of ultrasound (Ch. 8). Experimental investigations have demonstrated the presence of non-linear effects in tissues such as liver and muscle. However, in many situations shock waves may not be a problem since absorption of the ultrasonic energy by the tissues smooths the discontinuities (Ch. 4).

NUMERIC VALUES OF WAVE PARAMETERS IN TISSUE

So far, we have studied the phenomenon of waves and the physical parameters associated with them. To understand what happens when a wave of ultrasound passes through tissue, we must look at the numeric values of the wave parameters. In diagnostic ultrasound, the frequency range is 1 to 20 MHz, and the range of peak intensity is typically 10 mW/cm^2 to 100 W/cm^2 (Isptp). Table 3.1 gives the wave parameters calculated for these limits in the intensity range and for commonly used frequencies.

From these values, it is evident that during a cycle of vibration, the maximum distance moved by a particle is very small, as little as 10^{-8} cm, about the diameter of an atom. The maximum particle velocity is also only a few centimetres per second.

The pressure amplitude, on the other hand, is large. As shown previously, in the distance of half a wavelength along a waveform, the pressure varies from $+p_0$ to $-p_0$, about the average level. We note, therefore, that large pressure changes occur in distances less than 1 mm. Associated with these large pressure changes are very large accelerations.

THE SAFETY OF DIAGNOSTIC ULTRASOUND

The possibility of risk in applying ultrasound for diagnosis is under continual scrutiny. Difficulties arise from a lack of information on the interaction of ultrasound with complex biological systems and are likely to be fully resolved only after many years of investigation. Users of diagnostic ultrasound must therefore keep up to date with current publications to ensure that acceptable exposures are employed. Chapter 8 is devoted to the question of safety.

At present, although several million fetuses have been examined with ultrasound, no confirmed harmful effect has been attributed to ultrasound. In addition, no significant biological effects have been detected for ultrasonic intensities (Ispta) of less than 100 mW/cm^2.

SUMMARY

It is important for users of ultrasound to have an accurate understanding of the nature of ultrasound if they are to apply the techniques well, read the scientific literature, and communicate with their colleagues. From this chapter, the reader should have gleaned information on:

1. The physical phenomenon of sound and ultrasound.
2. The shorthand way of describing mechanical vibrations passing through a medium as waves, in particular, pressure waves of a continuous and pulsed form.

Table 3.1 Numeric values of ultrasonic wave parameters in tissue ($c = 1540$ m/s, density of soft tissue $= 1$ g/ml)

	Particle-displacement amplitude, x_0 cm	Particle-velocity amplitude, u_0 cm/s	Particle-pressure amplitude, p_0 Pa^2 (atm)
2.5 MHz			
10 mW/cm^2	7.3×10^{-8}	1.14	17 600 (0.176)
1 W/cm^2	7.3×10^{-7}	11.40	176 000 (1.760)
100 W/cm^2	7.3×10^{-6}	114.00	1 760 000 (17.600)
10 MHz			
10 mW/cm^2	1.8×10^{-8}	1.14	17 600 (0.176)
1 W/cm^2	1.8×10^{-7}	11.40	176 000 (1.760)
100 W/cm^2	1.8×10^{-6}	114.00	1 760 000 (17.600)

3. Amplitude, wavelength, and phase.

4. Diffraction and non-linear propagation. These are perhaps slightly esoteric phenomena, but they do remind us that a very simple picture of a narrow beam directed through tissue is not the whole story.

5. Intensity and power.

6. Numeric values of the various parameters such as intensity and wavelength. Just as you would carefully distinguish between 1° and 1000° on a temperature scale, you should recognise the difference between milliwatts and watts.

4. Ultrasound in tissue

We will now go beyond the basic properties of ultrasound as a wave, and examine various phenomena associated with such waves as they propagate through tissue. An understanding of these phenomena will be most helpful in our study of techniques in the rest of the text.

SPEED OF ULTRASOUND

The speed, c, at which ultrasonic vibrations are transmitted through a medium depends on the density, ρ and compressibility, κ, of the material:

$$c = \sqrt{\frac{\kappa}{\rho}}$$

The compressibility, κ, is a measure of the resistance to compression of a material when pressure is applied. Since κ appears in the numerator of the formula, the higher the compressibility of a material, the higher the speed. On the other hand, the higher the density of the material the lower the speed. In everyday scanning we find that the more rigid the material, the greater the speed of sound.

The terms 'speed' and 'velocity' are used interchangeably in medical ultrasonics. Strictly speaking, speed is the magnitude of the rate of change of position, e.g. 50 mph, and velocity is the magnitude plus the direction of the rate of change of position, e.g. 50 mph due north. Speed is called a scalar quantity since no direction is associated with it, whereas velocity is a vector quantity. From the point of view of medical ultrasound, this distinction is a bit academic and will not be made in this text.

In diagnostic ultrasound, there are five situations in which a knowledge of the speed of sound is of some interest:

1. By far the most important is the conversion of echo-return time into depth of tissue. The manufacturer assumes an average for soft tissue when calibrating a machine. This is usually 1540 m/s.

2. Velocity of ultrasound can be used to calculate the acoustic impedance of tissue, ρc, which allows echo size to be estimated.

3. If the speed of ultrasound differs in two tissues, an ultrasonic beam may be deviated on crossing an interface between them. This is known as 'refraction'.

4. Motion within the body can be detected by noting the Doppler shift in the frequency of ultrasound on reflection from a moving surface. Knowledge of the velocity of sound allows the speed of the moving surface to be calculated from the observed frequency change.

5. As tissue alters as a result of disease, the change may influence the speed of sound in it. There is increasing interest in developing techniques to use the value of the speed to provide diagnostic information.

Of these five situations, only the first is important in routine studies. The operator should be aware of the velocity that has been used to set the time-to-distance conversion in the instrument.

Speed in tissues

The velocity of sound in tissue, like many of the physical properties of tissue, has not been measured extensively. In theory, velocity can be measured accurately in vitro, e.g. to an accuracy of better than 1%. In vivo techniques are still being developed, their performance depending very much on the site of the tissue in the body, but accuracies of 2 or 3% are being quoted for large organs like the liver. Measurements that have been made in different centres often show discrepancies, probably as a result of differences in technique, the state of the tissue specimens, or normal biological variation. As diagnostic ultrasound becomes widely used, the amount of high-quality data will, no doubt, increase. Fortunately, for most scanning applications, all that is required is a good estimate of the average value of the speed of ultrasound in soft tissue. When specific dimensions are to be measured accurately, it then becomes important to know the precise value of the velocity in the tissue of interest, for example, in assessing the size of chambers of the eye.

From Table 4.1, it can be seen that the velocity of sound in tissue is very high. We usually consider the velocity of sound in air to be high; the velocity in tissue is five times faster. It can also be seen that the assumption of 1540 m/s for soft tissue is very reasonable since many values are within 10% of this average. In general, as the collagen or water content of tissue increases, the speed of sound in it also increases, while an increase in fat lowers the speed.

The velocity of sound in water is of particular interest in a technique called 'immersion scanning', in which a large depth of water is interposed between the transducer and the patient. In addition, test models in water-baths are often used to check on instrument performance. At room temperature (20°C), the speed of sound in water is 1480 m/s. It can be increased to 1540 m/s by heating the water to 50°C.

As might be expected, since bone is one of the most rigid materials in the body, the velocity of sound in bone (3500 m/s) is much higher than in soft tissue. This high-velocity layer inside a struc-

Table 4.1 Speed of ultrasound and acoustic impedance in some common materials. Data from Wells (1969); Goss, Johnston, Dunn (1978); and Bamber (1986). The acoustic impedence cannot be calculated where the density of the material is not known.

Material	Speed (m/s)	Acoustic impedance (g/cm^{2}s)
Amniotic fluid	1510	————
Aqueous humour	1500	1.50×10^5
Air (NTP)	330	0.0004×10^5
Blood	1570	1.61×10^5
Bone	3500	7.80×10^5
Brain	1540	1.58×10^5
Cartilage	1660	————
Castor oil	1500	1.43×10^5
CSF	1510	————
Fat	1450	1.38×10^5
Kidney	1560	1.62×10^5
Lens of eye	1620	1.84×10^5
Liver	1550	1.65×10^5
Muscle	1580	1.70×10^5
Perspex	2680	3.20×10^5
Polythene	2000	1.84×10^5
Skin	1600	————
Soft tissue (average)	1540	1.63×10^5
Tendon	1750	————
Tooth	3600	————
Vitreous humour	1520	1.52×10^5
Water (20°C)	1480	1.48×10^5

ture of soft tissues may make it difficult to convert echo-return time into depth.

The unit m/s is normally employed in practice for speed. Since we are involved with ultrasound travelling short distances in short times, the unit mm/μs is probably more appropriate:

$$1540 \text{ m/s} = 1.54 \text{ mm/}\mu\text{s}$$

However, m/s is firmly established, and since the user of scanning equipment is usually only concerned with comparison of speeds in different tissues, it is probably not worth changing this commonly used unit.

Factors affecting velocity

Before leaving the topic of velocity, it is worthwhile to consider its dependence on quantities such as frequency or temperature. No change in the velocity in tissue is observed over the frequency range employed in diagnostic ultrasound. There is no need, therefore, to alter the range calibration when frequency is changed. When a physical quantity changes with frequency, it is said to exhibit dispersion. (The term 'dispersion' comes from optics, in which light of different frequencies, that is, different colours, is dispersed on passing through a prism.) In our case, velocity dispersion is unimportant. One exception to this may be bone, for which changes in speed of up to 12% have been quoted in going from 1 to 3 MHz.

The speed of ultrasound varies with temperature, as was pointed out for water. In a bath of water, a 5°C temperature drift causes a velocity change of 1%: a range calibration error of about 1 mm in 10 cm. This is not large and can readily be eliminated.

Finally, the condition of tissue, (e.g. whether dead or living) affects its mechanical properties and, hence, the velocity of sound. Care should, therefore, be taken in extrapolating in vitro results to investigations of living subjects; for instance, with regard to echo size and structure dimensions.

To produce B-scan images of structures, we must specify an average value for the velocity of sound in the examined tissues as a parameter of the machine, so that it can convert time into distance on the display screen. It is interesting to work out the errors that arise from using the

Table 4.2 Errors in range measurement as a result of assuming an average value, for c, of 1540 m/s or 1510 m/s in all tissues

Abdomen		Eye	
True depth	Depth using 1540 m/s	True depth	Depth using 1510 m/s
0———0		0———0	
Fat			
2 cm———2.13 cm			
Muscle		Saline	
3 cm———3.1 cm			
		60 mm———59.53 mm	
		Anterior chamber	
Fluid		64 mm———63.56 mm	
		Lens	
		67.5 mm———66.82 mm	
13 cm———13.23 cm		Vitreous body	
Muscle			
14 cm———14.2 cm		92.5 mm———91.66 mm	
Soft tissue		Fat	
20 cm———20.2 cm		102.5 mm———102.07 mm	
Error = 2 mm		Error = 0.43 mm	

average velocity rather than the exact velocity for each individual tissue. In abdominal scanning, the errors are typically 2 mm in a range of 20 cm, while for eye scanning, they are about 0.5 mm for a 10 cm range (Table 4.2). Although these errors represent a fairly fundamental limitation, they are not prohibitively large.

REFLECTION

Diagnosis from pulse-echo images is made essentially by interpreting the reflected and scattered ultrasound from tissue interfaces. We will first consider reflection in some detail and examine the size of echoes produced at large boundaries. Scattering occurs at small structures such as those of organ parenchyma or blood cells and is examined in the next section. Reflection is only relevant for large boundaries and may be regarded as a special case of scattering.

Acoustic impedance

An echo is generated at a tissue interface if the acoustic impedances of the tissues on either side are different. The acoustic impedance, Z, of a tissue is the ratio of the applied pressure, p, over the resultant particle velocity u; that is, $Z = p/u$. Making a few assumptions, such as the tissue being a weak absorber, we find that the acoustic impedance of a tissue is the product of the density, ρ, and the velocity of sound, c, that is, $Z = \rho c$. Echo size is dependent on the difference in the acoustic impedance of the two tissues forming the interface, i.e. on $\rho_1 c_1 - \rho_2 c_2$ (Fig. 4.1a). Note that it is the magnitude of the difference, not the actual value, that is most important. The terms 'characteristic acoustic impedance' and 'specific acoustic impedance' are sometimes encountered as equivalent or closely related to 'acoustic impedance'.

As shown previously, the velocity of sound, c, in a medium is related to its rigidity (compressibility). When the particles of one medium (1) strike those of a second medium (2) at an interface, the recoil energy might be expected to depend on the difference in their masses (densities) and on

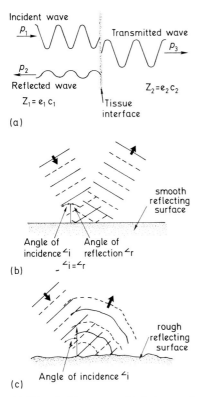

Fig. 4.1 (a) Wave incident perpendicularly on a flat surface, (b) wave incident at an angle to a flat surface, (c) wave incident at an angle to a rough surface.

how rigidly they are bound within their medium, that is, on ρ_1, ρ_2, c_1, and c_2. It is not surprising, therefore, that for tissue interfaces the difference, $\rho_1 c_1 - \rho_2 c_2$, plays an important part in determining echo size.

The ease with which any tissue mass, for example, a tumour, is detected in diagnostic ultrasound is highly dependent on its acoustic impedance relative to that of the surrounding tissue. Table 4.1 shows that the differences among the acoustic impedances of most tissues are not large. Air and bone, however, have impedance values that differ markedly from those of soft tissue. Very strong reflection occurs at air/soft-tissue or bone/soft-tissue interfaces.

The main point to note is that acoustic reflection depends on the change of acoustic impedance at a boundary. For a structure to be imaged, it must produce detectable echoes. Although large numbers of tissue interfaces within the body are detectable, some may not be if the acoustic impedances are well matched.

Another way in which structures are imaged relies on the echoes from within them being sufficiently different from those of the surrounding tissues. For example, many metastatic tumours in the liver are detected since they are 'echogenic' or 'echo-poor' but some are missed since their reflectivity is similar to that of the liver.

Reflection at boundaries

Let us now calculate the echo size owing to reflection at a particular interface. Take, for example, the idealized situation depicted in Figure 4.1a, in which an ultrasonic wave is incident at a right angle to a large reflecting surface. The quantity of greatest interest is the amplitude of the reflected wave, conveniently expressed as a ratio with the incident-wave amplitude. It is the pressure amplitude of the echo that the receiving transducer measures. The theory of wave reflection shows that the amplitude ratio is given by

$$\text{amplitude ratio} = \frac{p_2}{p_1} = \frac{\rho_1 c_1 - \rho_2 c_2}{\rho_1 c_1 + \rho_2 c_2}$$

By putting numeric values into this formula, echo size can be readily calculated, as, for example, at a muscle/blood interface:

(ρc) muscle $\quad = \rho_1 c_1 \quad = 1.70 \times 10^5$
(ρc) blood $\quad\quad = \rho_2 c_2 \quad = 1.61 \times 10^5$

$$\text{amplitude ratio} = \frac{1.70 \times 10^5 - 1.61 \times 10^5}{1.70 \times 10^5 + 1.61 \times 10^5}$$
$$= 0.027$$

The amplitude of the reflected echo is only 0.027 times that of the incident pulse.

Reflection in tissue

Idealized models for reflection as used above can give us an idea of the reflecting properties of tissue interfaces. Amplitude ratios for boundaries of interest are shown in Table 4.3 together with the percentage of the incident wave energy reflected. Note that the percentage of energy reflected from soft-tissue interfaces is small, allowing the beam to carry on largely undisturbed toward other interfaces. Several of the values in the table are of particular relevance. Typically, at soft-tissue boundaries the reflected wave amplitude is 0.05 times the incident wave amplitude. In contrast, between bone and soft tissue a very large echo is produced (0.65). This is so large that it greatly attenuates the transmitted beam and makes difficult the imaging of structures lying behind bone. Even more marked is the reflection at a gas/soft-tissue interface (0.9995). This virtually total reflection makes scanning through the lungs or gas in the bowel impossible. In practice, gas is regarded as an impenetrable barrier that gives rise to large echoes.

Often, ultrasonic vibrations are transmitted from the transducer through several centimetres of water to the skin of the patient. The percentage energy reflection at a water/tissue interface (0.23%) is low, allowing the ultrasound to penetrate the body without great loss in intensity. Techniques using water-baths are very successful in certain applications, for instance, in eye examinations.

A large acoustic mismatch exists between ceramic transducer crystals and soft tissue or water. Strong reflection occurs, therefore, at the crystal face and presents problems both in the transmission of ultrasound and in the detection of echoes. Some methods for attempting to reduce these difficulties are discussed in Chapter 27.

Since one often has to identify the sources of echoes or explain the dominance of some structures compared with others, it is worthwhile to acquire a knowledge of the reflection expected at different tissue interfaces.

Dependence of reflection on angle of incidence

So far, we have considered only waves that strike perpendicularly on surfaces. Note Figure 4.1b, where a beam strikes a perfectly smooth surface at an angle. The angle between the incident beam and the perpendicular direction to the surface is

Table 4.3 The ratio of the reflected wave to the incident wave amplitude and the percentage of energy reflected for perpendicular incidence

Reflecting interface	Ratio of reflected to incident-wave amplitude	Percentage energy reflected
Fat/muscle	0.10	1.08
Fat/kidney	0.08	0.64
Muscle/blood	0.03	0.07
Bone/fat	0.69	48.91
Bone/muscle	0.64	41.23
Lens/aqueous humour	0.10	1.04
Soft-tissue/water	0.05	0.23
Soft-tissue/air	0.9995	99.90
Soft-tissue/PZT crystal	0.89	80.00
Soft-tissue/PVDF plastic	0.47	22.1
Soft-tissue/castor oil	0.06	0.43

labelled the 'angle of incidence'. The corresponding angle for the reflected beam is the 'angle of reflection'. For a smooth surface, these angles are equal and opposite. This is analogous to the reflection of light from a polished surface and is termed 'specular reflection'.

For smooth surfaces, small deviations from perpendicular incidence, for example, 3°, reduce the detected signal by a large factor since only part of the echo strikes the transducer. Examples of surfaces that are most readily detected over a limited angular range are those in the eye chambers or the smooth muscle of the bladder.

The description of the production of echo signals in terms of reflections at smooth surfaces provides an indication of the magnitudes of signals to be expected from major tissue boundaries. It also shows that these echo magnitudes can be expected to vary with the angle of incidence of the ultrasound beam. Most tissue surfaces are not smooth, however, but have a degree of roughness. In addition, many interfaces are not large in extent compared to the ultrasound beam width. Small surface irregularities and small structures scatter ultrasound in many directions rather than reflect it as a beam (Fig. 4.1c). The resultant echoes at the transducer are weaker than those from perpendicular incidence on smooth-tissue boundaries. As instruments have been designed to handle a large range of echo amplitudes, scattered ultrasound has come to contribute the major portion of the echo information in images.

SCATTERING

For simple reflection to occur as described in the previous section, the dimensions of the reflecting surface must be greater than several wavelengths of the incident ultrasonic wave. Scattering of ultrasound occurs when an incident wave is reflected in many directions after interacting with a structure whose dimensions are similar to or less than the wavelength of the ultrasound. It is the change in acoustic impedance, i.e. the density or compressibility, at the structure which causes the scattering. Scattering in tissue has been explained using two theoretical models. In one, the scattering is considered to occur at randomly distributed, small-point scattering centres; in the other, the variations in density and compressibility are postulated to be of a more continuous nature. These two similar models give results which resemble the scattering observed in tissue. They therefore serve to increase our understanding of scattering in tissue.

When a wave of intensity I is incident on a target, say, a small volume of tissue, and the total scattered power is S, the ratio S/I is called the 'scattering cross section'. If scattering in a particular direction is considered, the ratio S/I is called the 'differential cross section'. In this case, the scattered power S is that passing into a specified angular range. Often the sound scattered back to the transducer (at 180° to the incident beam) is of interest since it is back-scattered ultrasound which is detected in most medical techniques. The cross section S (180°)/I is then referred to as the 'back-scatter cross section'.

The directions in which an ultrasound beam is scattered are very dependent on the size and arrangement of the tissue structures. The direction of scatter, i.e. the angular distribution of the scattered ultrasound, has been studied for a number of tissues and has been found to vary in a different, characteristic manner for each tissue. It is hoped that this may lead to a means of identifying tissues. A case of particular interest is one in which the dimensions of the structures are much smaller than the wavelength. Here scattering occurs equally in all directions; it is known as 'Rayleigh scattering' (Fig. 4.2).

Scattering is highly frequency-dependent. For example, in Rayleigh scattering, the amount of the scattered ultrasound varies with frequency to the fourth power, i.e. scattered power, S, is proportional to f^4. In other words, compared to scattering of 1 MHz ultrasound, 16 (i.e. 2^4) times as much will be scattered at 2 MHz and 81 (i.e. 3^4) times at 3 MHz. For slightly larger structures the power of the scattered sound varies less strongly with frequency, e.g. S is proportional to f^2 for structures of a few wavelengths in size.

The interaction of ultrasound in the 1–10 MHz frequency range with blood cells is an example of Rayleigh scattering in tissue. Within organs, many structures have dimensions of less than 1 mm and will, therefore, scatter ultrasound.

An interesting everyday analogy is the relatively

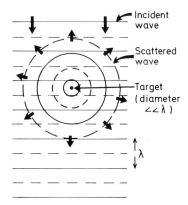

Incident wave

Scattered wave

Target (diameter $\ll \lambda$)

λ

Fig. 4.2 Part of the energy of an incident wave being scattered at a small target. Scattering at a target of a size that is very much smaller than the wavelength of the incident wave is known as Rayleigh scattering.

Table 4.4 Relative magnitudes of 2.5 MHz ultrasonic signals detected due to scattering in tissues

Tissue	Signal level (dB)	Signal level (fraction of reference)
Fat/muscle (reference level)	0	1.0
Placenta	−20	0.1
Liver	−30	0.032
Kidney	−40	0.01
Blood	−60	0.001

Reference level taken as signal magnitude from typical organ boundary.

strong scattering of the high-frequency blue component of sunlight as it crosses the atmosphere, creating the blue sky. The sun appears red at sunset since the blue components of the sunlight are removed by scattering in the long path to the observer through the atmosphere.

Scattering in tissue

Experimental measurements and theoretical analyses of scattering of ultrasound in tissue have been performed. It is a large and complex subject, and a great deal of hard data does not yet exist. Scattered ultrasound, however, provides much diagnostic information, both in imaging and in blood-flow measurement. It is, therefore, being more fully investigated at present. There is evidence that scattering increases with increasing fat in tissue, and decreases with increased water content. Collagen is also thought to contribute significantly to the level of scatter.

The magnitude of echo signals from 2.5 MHz ultrasound scattered from within organs is known to be only one-tenth to one-hundredth (−20 to −40 dB) of that received from organ boundaries. For scattering from blood cells, 2.5 MHz ultrasound produces signals one-thousandth of that from tissue boundaries (−60 dB). Table 4.4 presents data on the relative echo magnitudes produced in tissue structures of particular interest.

Scattering in lung tissue is a special case since it occurs at the air-filled alveoli and is extremely strong. Some attempts have been made to detect the presence of fluid in the lung by looking for a reduction in the level of this scattering.

In the previous section, we noted that large, smooth interfaces may be difficult to detect when they lie at an angle to the incident ultrasonic beam, since the reflected ultrasound is directed away from the transducer. In practice, many organ boundaries within the body are sufficiently rough to scatter sound back to the transducer even at fairly large angles of incidence, such as 45°. The detected echo is weak (e.g. one-hundredth of that for perpendicular incidence), but modern instruments are designed to preserve weak echo information. With a higher frequency, the scattering is stronger, and it is easier to visualize surfaces orientated at angles to the scanning beam.

Our picture of the means by which echoes are generated in diagnostic ultrasound from tissue boundaries has now become more complex than that described in Chapter 1. We now consider the ultrasound to be passing through densely packed scattering targets within organs and major tissue boundaries of varying degrees of roughness. The echo train received contains some signals from distinct tissue boundaries and other small signals resulting from a combination of overlapping echoes scattered at closely packed structures within organs (Fig. 4.3). Such echo trains still contain time and amplitude information from which images are created.

Scattering in blood

The scattering phenomenon in blood is of interest

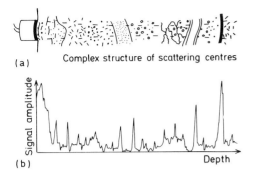

(a) Complex structure of scattering centres

(b) Depth

Fig. 4.3 (**a**) Representation of complex tissue consisting of discrete reflectors and scatterers, (**b**) typical echo pattern from complex tissue structures.

since it provides us with the signal which is examined for a Doppler shift to obtain information on the velocities of cells. Unlike other tissues, a reasonable amount of information exists on scattering in blood. There is also agreement between theory and experiment. The scattered signal from blood is due to the non-uniform distribution of the cells creating scattering centres, not to the individual cells. Back-scattering is about 6 dB (a factor of 2 in amplitude) stronger than that in the forward direction. The power of the scattered ultrasound increases with frequency rapidly as the ultrasonic frequency is increased. In fact, the scattered power is proportional to the fourth power of frequency, for example if 1 mW was scattered at 1 MHz, then 81 mW would be scattered at 3 MHz.

The power of the ultrasound scattered from blood depends on the haematocrit value. For low values of cell concentration, i.e. below 20%, scattering increases with haematocrit. Above 30%, the power of the scattered signal decreases.

An intriguing observation is that of echoes from blood which are sufficiently strong to be depicted in a real-time image. We noted above that the signals from blood are usually very weak and do not appear in echo images. The observed signals occur in slow venous flow and are thought to be caused by the formation of clusters of cells, i.e. rouleau formation.

REFRACTION

Refraction is the phenomenon whereby an ultrasonic beam is deviated when it strikes at an angle the interface between two tissues in which the velocity of ultrasound differs. When the beam strikes the interface perpendicularly, no deviation is experienced. Refraction is not of great importance in most diagnostic techniques as they stand at present, but it is a severe handicap in some applications.

Figure 4.4a shows an ultrasonic wave crossing a boundary from a tissue in which the velocity is c_1 to another tissue in which it is c_2 ($c_1 > c_2$). Beam bending occurs because the part of a wave front in the second tissue travels more slowly than that in the first. From the geometry of the situation,

$$\frac{\sin i}{\sin r} = \frac{c_1}{c_2} = \text{acoustic refractive index}$$

This is known as Snell's law. (In optics, it predicts the path of light waves through lenses and prisms.)

Refraction in tissue

Let us consider refraction at some specific tissue boundaries. Large beam deviations are to be expected where large changes in velocity occur. Figure 4.4b shows a beam being bent at a bone/soft-tissue interface. It can be seen that for an angle of incidence of 30°, the angle of refraction is 11°, that is, the beam is deviated by 19°. The reverse situation, when the beam passes from a low-velocity to a high-velocity medium, is interesting (Fig. 4.4c). For this example with an angle of incidence of 15°, the beam is deviated by 28° away from the perpendicular. At angles of incidence greater that 22°, the

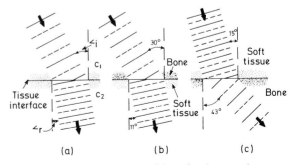

Fig. 4.4 Beam deviation caused by refraction at a tissue interface; (**a**) at interface where c_2 is less than c_1, (**b**) at bone/soft-tissue interface, in which velocity in soft tissue is less than velocity in bone, (**c**) at soft-tissue/bone interface.

angle of refraction, r, is larger than 90°, that is, the beam does not enter the bone, but is reflected back into the soft tissue; this is known as 'total internal reflection'. These examples illustrate the serious difficulties presented by bone because of refraction.

How much beam deviation is to be expected at an interface between two typical soft tissues? Putting some numeric values into the expression for Snell's law shows that deviations of 1 or 2° can be expected (Table 4.5). Such small deviations are not a serious problem, since they occur in different directions and so cancel each other, to some extent, as the beam passes through a series of tissue interfaces. A beam that remains off course for a large distance does create problems in imaging techniques. A beam deviated by 1.5° at the top interface of a full bladder could be displaced 3 mm from its intended position before it reaches the far side.

Table 4.5 Typical changes in beam directions due to refraction at tissue interfaces for an angle of incidence of 30°

Tissue interface	Deviation
Bone/soft tissue	19° 18′
Muscle/blood	0° 47′
Muscle/fat	2° 24′
Muscle/fluid	1° 4′
Lens of eye/aqueous humor	2°

Similarly, the shape of the lens of the eye usually causes a sound beam to be deviated away from the centre of the retina. Deviations of 3 or 4° can occur readily owing to refraction at both lens/fluid interfaces. As a result of this deviation, which neither the machine nor the operator can allow for, errors in location at the retina of around 1 mm arise.

At the wall of a cystic structure, refraction may contribute to the weakening of the beam and, hence, the production of a shadow. A wedge-shaped piece of muscle has been shown to act like a prism and deviate a beam. Finally, the low velocity of fat relative to other soft tissues results in beam deviation and degradation at many sites and is responsible for one of the main sources of image degradation.

To summarize, although, in most instances, refraction is not a major problem, there are some instances where it degrades the final image or significantly alters the direction of a Doppler beam.

ABSORPTION OF ULTRASOUND

When an ultrasonic transducer generates an ultrasonic wave in a medium, it imparts increased energy to the particles of the medium in the form of orderly vibrations. Absorption of ultrasound is the process by which this orderly vibrational energy is dissipated into other forms such as the random molecular motions of heat or internal molecular energy. Although the absorption of ultrasound is very strong in tissue, little is known of the many complex processes involved. Since absorption is capable of providing information on tissue state, it may receive more attention in future.

As an ultrasonic plane wave passes through an absorbing medium, its intensity and amplitude decrease (App. 7). The rate of fall of intensity is determined by the absorption coefficient, α, which is defined in Appendix 7. The larger the value of the coefficient, the more rapid the decrease in intensity. The magnitude of α is determined by the number and strengths of the absorbing processes involved at the frequency of ultrasound employed.

Absorption mechanisms

Absorption mechanisms for ultrasound are often explained as relaxation mechanisms. A relaxation process occurs in a material when a force applied within it causes energy flow that relaxes the stresses set up by the force. Consider a piece of material that stores energy in such different forms as internal molecular energy, structural energy, or energy of motion. Because the wave action compresses the material, the equilibrium between the energy stores is upset and energy flows. In particular, energy flows from the potential energy store as a result of applied compression to other energy stores. When the compressional wave action starts to decrease, some energy returns to the potential energy store. The wave action is reduced, however, since not all the energy returns, and some returns out of phase with the wave action.

The absorption of energy by a relaxation

mechanism in a medium is most effective near one particular frequency, known as the relaxation frequency of the mechanism. At much lower frequencies, there is sufficient time available for the transfer of energy so that on its return, it is not far out of phase with the wave-motion energy. At much higher frequencies, significant energy transfer does not occur in the time available.

Energy transferred to internal molecular energy and back is known as 'thermal relaxation'. If the transfer of energy takes the form of heat flowing from one region to another and back, it is called 'conductional relaxation'. Where the passage of energy is between two states of different physical structure, the process is known as 'structural relaxation'.

There are, of course, other mechanisms for absorbing ultrasound. For example, viscous liquids absorb ultrasound strongly as a result of friction between moving particles. Friction arises because the compressing action of the wave causes slight movement of some particles at right angles to the direction of wave propagation. Absorption caused by viscosity is sometimes termed a relaxation process, since it varies with frequency in a similar manner.

Ultrasonic absorption in solids exhibits most of the mechanisms described above, as well as some others caused by non-uniformities in structure.

This brief description of absorption mechanisms indicates how ultrasound can be absorbed. Too little is known of absorption in complex biological materials to allow us to identify the important mechanisms in tissue. Experiments are difficult to carry out accurately, mainly because of problems in preparing tissues, e.g. the problem of how to exclude gas bubbles. Results have been obtained by in-vitro measurement, but few in-vivo studies have been attempted. It is thought that absorption accounts for 80 to 90% of intensity reduction in soft tissue. In soft tissue, absorption appears to occur primarily in protein macromolecules.

Frequency dependence of absorption

Absorption increases with frequency in the materials and the frequency range met with in diagnosis. Since absorption has a frequency dependence, it is said to exhibit dispersion. The upper limit of the working frequency range (20 MHz) is a result of absorption processes becoming prohibitively strong.

Like velocity, absorption is influenced by temperature and tissue state. Absorption decreases with temperature in most tissues.

Absorption and its mechanisms are rarely considered in isolation in routine clinical techniques. Total attenuation, which includes a number of other factors as well, is a more relevant quantity. The term 'absorption' is often used loosely when 'attenuation' would be more correct.

TOTAL ATTENUATION OF ULTRASOUND IN TISSUE

As transmitted ultrasound and echoes pass through tissue, they are reduced in intensity. This reduction (or attenuation) is due to a number of processes such as reflection, scattering, refraction, absorption, and wave front divergence. The attenuation coefficient, μ, is defined in Appendix 7.

The increase in attenuation with frequency indicates that absorption is an important factor. The other phenomena can also be very significant. For example, an echo produced by a small target has a very divergent wave front, which contributes to its low amplitude at the transducer. One result of attenuation is that echoes from structures deep within the body are much weaker than those from superficial regions. In Chapter 2, we saw that the detecting system has to be manipulated to correct this imbalance.

In most situations, attenuation determines the frequency of ultrasound used, or the path along which the ultrasound beam is directed toward particular organs. Owing to attenuation, the working frequency range is typically 2–5 MHz for scanning the abdomen, heart, head, etc, and 5–15 MHz for the eyes and superficial blood vessels.

The measurement of attenuation in a tissue depends on accurate measurement of intensity, a measurement which is difficult because of the low levels used. The measurement of the ratio of one intensity to another, however, is easier since neither has to be measured absolutely. The ratio I_1/I_0 can be used as a measure of the intensity, I_1, if I_0 is a specified reference level. In diagnostic ultrasound, I_1, might be the intensity at a point of interest within the tissue and I_0 the intensity at the skin surface. In practice, it is $10 \log_{10} (I_1/I_0)$ which is used as a measure of I_1, and the unit is then defined as the decibel. The following is an example.

I_1/I_0 $\qquad = 100$
I_1 in decibel $\qquad = 10 \log (I_1/I_0) = 10 \log(100)$
(with I_0 as reference) $= 20$ dB

The decibel notation is discussed more fully in Appendix 3. For the moment, we note that intensity is often quoted in decibels and that this is not an absolute measure, but, instead, implies the specification of some reference level.

The attenuation coefficient, μ, is conveniently expressed as the rate of decrease of intensity in units of decibel per centimetre depth of tissue (dB/cm, App. 7). When measured thus, attenuation is found to increase linearly with frequency, for many tissues. On average, attenuation in soft tissue is given by the expression $0.7 \times f$ dB/cm, where f is the frequency in MHz. For example, at 5 MHz,

$$\text{attenuation} = \mu = 0.7 \times 5 = 3.5 \text{ dB/cm}$$

Attenuation in practice

To give some appreciation of the role of attenuation in practice, the thicknesses of tissues required to reduce intensity by half are listed in Table 4.6. Since attenuation is frequency-dependent, frequency must be quoted for each value of thickness. Available data are not as complete as might be desired. In some cases, the value in the table has been derived by assuming that attenuation in tissue varies linearly with frequency over the whole range of interest, that is, $\mu_f = \mu$ (at 1 MHz) $\times f$.

Some interesting points can be noted from the table and related to the practicalities of imaging tissue structures. First, many soft tissues have similar attenuating powers; for example, for brain and liver, the intensity of 2 MHz ultrasound is reduced by half in about 2 cm.

Blood, on the other hand, is less attenuating, which helps the visualization of cardiac structures. In general, liquids within the body absorb only weakly and are often referred to as 'transonic' or 'sonolucent'. Amniotic fluid, urine, aqueous humour, vitreous humour, and cystic fluid allow structures lying beyond them to be easily visual-

Table 4.6 Thickness of tissue required to attenuate the intensity of an ultrasonic beam by half (-3 dB)

	1 MHz	*2 MHz*	*5 MHz*	*10 MHz*	*20 MHz*
			Thickness (in cm) of material at		
Aqueous humour	—	—	6	3	1.5
Air (N.T.P.)	0.25	0.06	0.01	—	—
Blood	17	8.5	3	2	1
Bone	0.2	0.1	0.04	—	—
Brain	3.5	2	1	—	—
Castor oil	3	0.75	0.12	—	—
Fat	5	2.5	1	0.5	0.25
Kidney	3	1.5	0.5	—	—
Lens of eye	—	—	0.3	0.15	0.07
Liver	3	1.5	0.5	—	—
Muscle	1.5	0.75	0.3	0.15	—
Perspex	1.5	0.7	0.3	0.15	0.07
Polythene	0.6	0.3	0.12	0.6	0.03
Soft tissue (average)	4.3	2.1	0.86	0.43	0.21
Vitreous humour	—	—	6	3	1.5
Water	1360	340	54	14	3.4

ized. Indeed, a full bladder is a standard technique for obtaining a 'window' to the uterus.

Water itself is very useful because of its extremely low absorption; with 2 MHz frequency ultrasound, the half-value thickness is 340 cm. For most practical purposes, water can be considered to be unabsorbing and can therefore be used in immersion scanning. It is only at frequencies above 10 MHz, where the attenuation reaches 0.2 dB/cm, that any significant effect is noticed.

Muscle is of special note in that its properties are not isotropic. A difference of a factor of 2.5 has been reported between the attenuation across and that along its fibres. Well-developed musculature can degrade an ultrasonic beam and, hence, the image quality.

The high attenuation of adult bone, 20 times that of soft tissue, creates many problems for ultrasonic scanning. Scanning of the head is particularly difficult, and success has so far been mainly limited to examination of infants or the detection of blood flow by directing the beam through the temporal bone. Bone also limits viewing access to the heart, the abdomen, and the eye.

Gas bubbles in the lung cause high attenuation by extremely strong scattering of the ultrasound. For all practical purposes, it is impossible to penetrate a normal lung with diagnostic ultrasound. The lung, therefore, creates a problem in examination of the heart and much of the thorax.

A few non-biological materials also have noteworthy absorbing properties. Absorption of ultrasound in castor oil at low frequency is similar to that in soft tissue, so it is a convenient medium for constructing test and training phantoms.

Absorption in air is very high at diagnostic frequencies. Because of this high absorption and the low acoustic impedance, propagation of sound into air ceases to be practical above 0.5 MHz.

Little is known about the normal biological variation of the attenuating properties of tissue, e.g. variations with age, state, sex, or race. A few points of practical significance are worth noting. The neonatal brain exhibits around one-third the attenuation of the adult one. It is, therefore, much easier to image the infant brain than the adult brain even after the bone has been removed from the adult. Fatty infiltration increases attenuation,

for example, in the breast with age or in the liver, as more scattering occurs at the fatty/non-fatty interfaces. Contraction of muscle increases attenuation and may degrade images. The results quoted for the changes in tissue after death are variable, but it can be concluded that imaging of a cadaver may not produce results which are directly applicable to living tissue. Fixing of tissue with an agent such as formalin alters its ultrasonic properties, e.g. increasing its attenuation by 30% at 3 MHz.

Attenuation in liquids is almost 100% due to absorption mechanisms apart from the reduction in intensity caused by beam divergence. As the amount of structure in tissue increases, the attenuation also rises, e.g. in scar tissue, breast carcinoma, and myocardial infarcts. This is said to be due to the increased level of collagen resulting in more scattering of the ultrasound. Estimates of the contribution of scattering to the total attenuation vary, ranging up to 40%, but more typically it is put at 10%. These are rough estimates; a particular case depends on the tissue insonated and the frequency employed.

Numeric examples of the effect of attenuation

Finally, to relate attenuation to the practical case, Tables 4.7 and 4.8 illustrate typical situations: attenuation in the abdomen and the eye. At selected frequencies, the intensity at the tissue boundaries is expressed both in decibels with respect to the initial value I_0 and as fractions of I_0.

From these examples, it is possible to get an idea of the echo strength arriving back at the transducer in a typical situation. Suppose that the echo produced by the bottom surface in each figure has an intensity 30 dB below that of the pulse striking it. Note also that the echo suffers the same attenuation as the transmitted pulse. For the abdomen (frequency = 2 MHz), total intensity reduction = 20.52 + 30 + 20.52 dB = 71.04 dB. Therefore,

$$\text{returned intensity} \quad = \frac{I_0}{12\ 710\ 000}$$

$$\text{returned amplitude} \quad = \frac{A_0}{3565}$$

Table 4.7   Typical attenuation of an ultrasonic beam in the abdomen

Depth	Abdomen (2 MHz ultrasound) Decibel level	Intensity	Amplitude
0 cm——— Fat	0	I_0	A_0
2 cm——— Muscle	-2.52	$I_1 = I_0/1.786$	$A_1 = A_0/1.34$
3 cm——— Fluid	-5.12	$I_2 = I_0/3.251$	$A_2 = A_0/1.80$
13 cm——— Muscle	-7.12	$I_3 = I_0/5.152$	$A_3 = A_0/2.27$
14 cm——— Soft Tissue	-9.72	$I_4 = I_0/9.372$	$A_4 = A_0/3.06$
20 cm———	-20.52	$I_5 = I_0/112.7$	$A_5 = A_0/10.6$

Table 4.8   Typical attenuation of an ultrasonic beam in the eye

Depth	Eye (10 MHz ultrasound) Decibel level	Intensity	Amplitude
0 mm——— Saline	0	I_0	A_0
60 mm——— Anterior chamber	-1.32	$I_1 = I_0/1.4$	$A_1 = A_0/1.18$
64 mm——— Lens	-1.72	$I_2 = I_0/1.5$	$A_2 = A_0/1.22$
67.5 mm——— Vitreous body	-8.72	$I_3 = I_0/7.5$	$A_3 = A_0/2.7$
92.5 mm——— Fat	-11.22	$I_4 = I_0/13$	$A_4 = A_0/3.6$
102.5 mm———	-17.52	$I_5 = I_0/56$	$A_5 = A_0/7.5$

For the eye (frequency = 10 MHz), total intensity reduction = 17.52 + 30 + 17.52 dB = 65.04 dB. Therefore,

$$\text{returned intensity} = \frac{I_0}{3\ 192\ 000}$$

$$\text{returned amplitude} = \frac{A_0}{1786}$$

It is thus apparent that the echoes returning to the transducer are very much weaker than the transmitted pulse.

SUMMARY

It is essential to build up a knowledge of the ultrasonic properties of tissue since the interpretation of images depends on it. In this chapter we have seen that:

1. The speed of ultrasound in tissue is high. The values in soft tissue are close to 1540 m/s.

2. The speed is independent of frequency.

3. Most of the information used in pulse-echo imaging and Doppler techniques is obtained as a result of reflection or scattering.

4. The size of an echo signal generated at a tissue interface is determined to a large extent by the change in acoustic impedance. In pulse-echo images, it is the change of acoustic impedance at points in the scan plane which is presented on a display screen as the image information.

5. Boundaries between soft tissues reflect weakly; those involving gas or bone reflect strongly.

6. Scattering provides echo data from rough surfaces, organ parenchyma, and blood. It is very frequency-dependent.

7. Echoes produced by scattering are much weaker than those generated by reflection at organ boundaries.

8. Refraction deviates ultrasound beams, but it is not too limiting in soft tissues.

9. Absorption is one of the mechanisms of attenuation.

10. Attenuation in tissue is high and frequency-dependent. In many liquids of low viscosity, attenuation is low.

11. Equipment is designed to compensate for attenuation by amplifying echoes from deep structures more than those from superficial ones. The degree of amplification is governed by the TGC circuitry.

REFERENCES

Bamber J C 1986 Attenuation and absorption. In: Hill C R (ed) Physical principles of medical ultrasonics, Ch. 4. Ellis Horwood, Chichester, England

Bamber J C 1986 Speed of sound. In: Hill C R (ed) Physical principles of medical ultrasonics, Ch. 5. Ellis Horwood, Chichester, England

Chivers R C, Hill C R 1975 Ultrasonic attenuation in human tissues. Ultrasound Med Biol 2: 25–29

Dickinson R J 1986 Reflection and scattering. In: Hill C R (ed) Physical principles of medical ultrasonics, Ch. 6. Ellis Horwood, Chichester, England

Filly R A, Sommer F G, Minton M J 1980 Characterisation of biological fluids by ultrasound and computed tomography. Radiology 134: 167–171

Goss S A, Johnston R L, Dunn F 1978 Comprehensive compilation of empirical ultrasonic properties of mammalian tissues. J. Acoust Soc Am 64: 423–457

Gregg E C, Palagallo G L 1969 Acoustic impedance of tissue. Invest Radiol 4: 357–363

Kossoff G, Fry E K, Jellins J 1973 Average velocity of ultrasound in the human female breast. J Acoust Soc Am 53: 1730–1736

Lees S 1971 Ultrasonics in hard tissues. Int Dent J 21: 403–417

Shung K P, Sigelman R A, Schmer G 1975 Ultrasonic measurement of blood coagulation time. IEEE Trans Biomed Eng BME 22: 334–337

White D N, Curry G R 1975 Absorption of ultrasonic energy by the skull. In: White D N (ed) Ultrasound in medicine, Vol. 1. Plenum, New York

Wladimiroff J W, Craft I L, Talbert D G 1975 In vitro measurements of sound velocity in human fetal brain tissue. Ultrasound Med Biol 1: 377–382

5. Manipulation of ultrasonic waves

We have already seen that ultrasound can be generated in narrow fields and focused. We will now study the ideas and technology employed in the further manipulation of ultrasound. This will help in the understanding of established methods and recently introduced techniques.

INTERFERENCE OF WAVES

Thus far, we have usually considered one wave to be present in the propagating medium. If two waves are transmitted in the same direction into one medium so that they overlap, then the resultant particle motion at any point is obtained by adding the motion owing to one wave to that of the other. This phenomenon of waves adding together to give a resultant is called 'interference'. It occurs for both continuous and pulsed waves.

Waves of the same frequency

To see in more detail how the resultant-pressure waveform is produced, one must consider a line through the medium in the direction of wave travel and 'freeze' the waves temporarily. In addition, let the waves have the same frequency and be exactly in step, that is, in phase (Fig. 5.1a). The resultant waveform at this instant is obtained by adding the contribution from each wave at each point, as illustrated for point A in Figure 5.1a. For this addition, the signs of the pressure fluctuations at each point are taken into account, that is, whether they are positive or negative about the mean level. In the example shown, the resultant waveform has an increased amplitude. An increased intensity has, therefore, resulted from the interference of these two waves; this is called 'con-

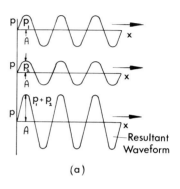

(a)

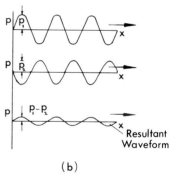

(b)

Fig. 5.1 (a) Increased wave amplitude caused by constructive interference, (b) reduced wave amplitude caused by destructive interference.

structive interference'. If the waves had been exactly out of step, or phase, the resultant amplitude would have been less than the larger amplitude of the two waves (Fig: 5.1b). This is known as 'destructive interference' and results in a decrease in intensity. The intermediate case when waves are neither completely in nor out of phase produces either an increase or a decrease in intensity, depending on the phase difference. That resultant waveforms can be obtained by adding contributions from each wave is known as the 'principle of superposition'.

In regions where waves are in phase, an increase in intensity results, and where they are out of phase, a decrease results. A complex distribution of intensity within a medium can be produced by interference.

Waves of different frequencies

The resultant waveform for waves of different frequency is again obtained by adding the contributions from each wave at each point and taking the signs of the pressures into account. Figure 5.2 shows a case where the frequency of one wave is double that of the other, and the waves have the same amplitude. Waves of different frequency will be of interest when we study pulsed sound and Doppler techniques.

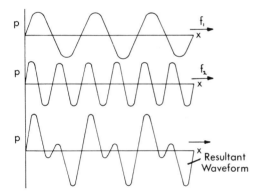

Fig. 5.2   Interference of waves of different frequencies.

Waves of neighbouring frequency

The result of waves of similar but not identical frequency interfering is shown in Figure 5.3. Along a line through the medium at any instant, the waves vary slowly in and out of phase. The result of this interference is a waveform whose amplitude exhibits slow variations or pulsations, which are called 'beats'. The frequency of the slow pulsation, that is, the beat frequency, is equal to the difference of the two frequencies $(f_1 - f_2)$. With Doppler techniques, a typical situation might be a wave of 2 MHz interfering with one of 1.997 MHz to produce beats of 0.003 MHz (3 kHz).

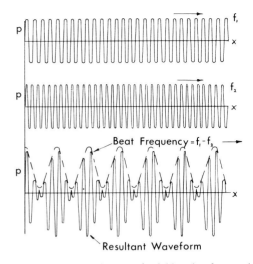

Fig. 5.3   Interference of waves of neighbouring frequencies.

STANDING WAVES

The phenomenon of standing waves, which is not used in diagnosis at present, occurs when two waves are propagated in the same medium, but in opposite directions. Again the resultant waveform at any instant is obtained by adding the wave pressures at each point (Fig. 5.4a). As an example, let us assume that the waves have equal amplitude and frequency. In this case, the resultant pressure varies with time in a cyclic manner at some points, for example, at point A, whereas, at others, the pressure fluctuations are constantly zero. The maximum limit of the fluctuations at each point along the paths of the waves is indicated by the broken curved line. The position of this curve remains stationary in the medium. Points at which the minimum pressure fluctuations occur are called 'nodes'; those with maximum fluctuations are known as 'antinodes'. Nodes are always the points of least pressure change, but have zero fluctuations only if the amplitudes of the waves are equal. What is most important is that standing waves give rise to regions of enhanced amplitudes, that is, higher intensities. Standing-wave patterns arise when waves travel past each other in opposite directions, for example, on reflecting a continuous wave at a flat surface. Standing waves are of less importance when pulsed ultrasound is used, since they only exist during the overlap time of the pulses. Steps should be taken to avoid setting up

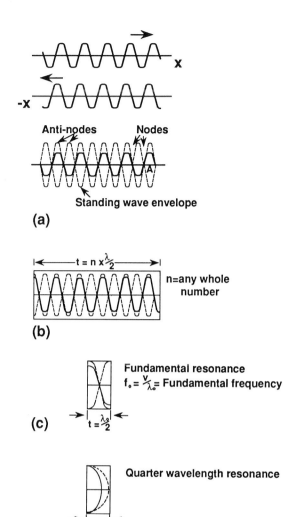

Fig. 5.4 (**a**) The formation of standing waves; (**b**) resonance due to the formation of standing waves in a slab of material of specific thickness, for example, $t = 11 \, (\lambda/2)$; (**c**) resonance at the fundamental frequency, f_0, corresponding to $\lambda_0 = 2t$; (**d**) quarter-wavelength resonance.

standing waves when ultrasonic intensity is being measured or during studies on the hazards of ultrasound. For example, care can be taken to ensure that the ultrasonic beam is not reflected back through the region of interest after the initial traverse.

RESONANCE

Consider the situation when waves are reflected back and forth between the two parallel reflecting surfaces of a slab of material. Because waves are passing each other in opposite directions, standing waves are generated. Resonance arises when the surfaces are separated by a distance equal to a complete number of half-wavelengths. Then the waves interfere constructively, and the pressure fluctuations are greatly enhanced (Fig. 5.4b).

If the frequency, f_0, of ultrasound is selected so that the thickness, t, of the slab equals one half-wavelength, $\lambda_0/2$, the pressure fluctuations are greatest (Fig. 5.4c). This is the 'fundamental resonance', that is, where $t = 1 \times \lambda_0/2$.

A second frequency f_1, chosen so that the thickness t is equal to $2 \times \lambda_1/2$, produces another resonance. The frequency f_1 is known as the first harmonic.

Similarly, for

$t = 3 \times \lambda_2/2$, f_2 is the second harmonic;
$t = 4 \times \lambda_3/2$, f_3 is the third harmonic;

and so on. As yet, harmonics are rarely employed in diagnostic ultrasound as a means of generating high-frequency ultrasound.

A transducer, containing a crystal piezoelectric element, is designed such that the crystal thickness is equal to half the wavelength corresponding to the required frequency of operation. During operation, therefore, the crystal resonates at its fundamental frequency, giving maximum efficiency in transmission and reception.

Resonance also occurs in material of thickness equal to one-quarter of a wavelength (Fig. 5.4d).

COMPARISON OF PULSED AND CONTINUOUS WAVES

An 'ideal' continuous wave has a fixed amplitude and one frequency, whereas a pulsed wave varies in amplitude throughout the pulse. What is less obvious is that each pulse contains a range of frequencies. This is a difficult concept that can be better understood by reference to Figure 5.3. The resultant from adding the two waves shown can be regarded as a train of closely spaced, high-frequency pulses of ultrasound. Thus, even in this very simple case, it is possible to generate pulse shapes and complex waveforms by adding continuous waves of different frequencies. It is possible to produce more distinct pulses by com-

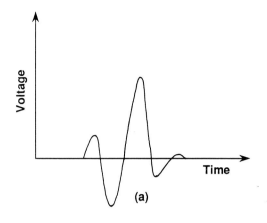

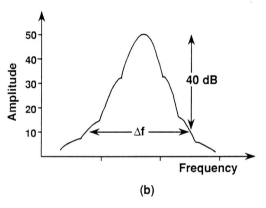

Fig. 5.5 A pulsed signal and its 40 dB frequency bandwidth.

phenomena such as interference are more complicated than for single-frequency continuous waves. It also means that, since during absorption in tissue the high-frequency components are absorbed preferentially, the pulse shape is altered in an unknown way as it propagates. Finally, the electronics of a scanning system must be able to handle the range of frequencies to preserve the pulse shape. Although all this may seem complicated, it often works to the advantage of diagnostic ultrasound. The many frequencies in a pulse result in a more uniform intensity distribution in its ultrasonic field.

MANIPULATION OF ULTRASONIC BEAMS

Until now we have assumed that transducers emit highly directional beams similar to those of miniature searchlights. We will now study beam shapes in more detail and consider ways of manipulating them.

Ultrasonic beam shape

In the great majority of imaging techniques, the transducer operates both as a transmitter and a receiver. It transmits ultrasound into the transmission field and receives echoes from a similarly shaped reception zone (Fig. 5.7a). For single-element transducers, reception is the converse process of transmission, so the field and zone shapes are identical. Later in this chapter, we will study electronic focusing during transmission and reception with array transducers, in which case the field and zone shapes are usually different (Fig. 5.7b).

In order for us to have an accurate understanding of ultrasonic imaging techniques, we should bear in mind that both transmission and reception contribute toward the narrowness of the scanning-beam shape. For example, if a target is situated away from the central axis of the beam, the ultrasonic pulse striking it is of low intensity, resulting in a weak echo. The signal produced by this echo at the transducer is further reduced because the target is situated at the edge of the reception zone. A target placed on the central axis, on the other hand, is in a good position to produce a strong signal since both the transmitted intensity

bining many waves with different frequencies and phases. A single pulse can be generated from a very large number of frequencies, but only those in a particular frequency range are important (Fig. 5.5). This range is called the 'frequency bandwidth of the pulse'. The frequencies in this bandwidth are often called the 'Fourier components' or 'frequency spectrum' of the pulse.

As the pulse becomes shorter, then the range of frequencies it contains becomes greater; that is, the greater is its bandwidth. For example, a 2.5 MHz pulse of length 7 cycles has a bandwidth of about 1 MHz, whereas a 2.5 MHz pulse of 3 cycles has a bandwidth of about 2 MHz (Fig. 5.6). Calling a pulse '2.5 MHz' in scanning refers to the central frequency in its bandwidth.

In practice, the fact that a pulse has a number of frequency components means that wave

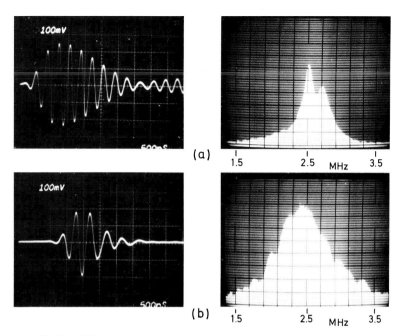

Fig. 5.6 The shorter pulse has the larger bandwidth (courtesy of Pye D).

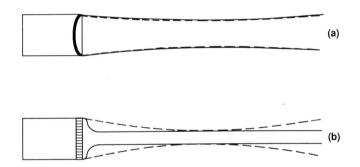

Fig. 5.7 (a) The transmission field and reception zone for a single-element transducer, (b) the transmission field (broken line) and reception zone (solid line) for an array transducer. Electronic focusing with an array usually produces different shapes of field and zone.

and the reception sensitivity are high, close to the axis. The signals from targets close to the central axis are therefore enhanced relative to those from targets off-axis because of the combined effect of the transmission and reception zones (Fig. 1.2).

In Chapter 12, we will see that the idea of the beam shape depending on both the transmission field and the reception zone has important practical consequences in achieving high-resolution images. These consequences arise since the effec-

tive widths of these fields and zones can be altered by varying the instrument controls that govern the sensitivity.

In a few situations, for instance, where the transmitted intensity distribution is being studied, we are concerned only with the transmission field. Quite often, in this type of work, the transmission field is referred to as the 'beam'. The above considerations show that it is best to distinguish the transmission field from the scanning beam, since the latter depends on both transmission and reception.

Basic single piezoelectric element transducer

It is somewhat surprising that a transducer can generate a directional field of sound waves. The directionality of the field can be explained by the following theoretical approach. The element surface is considered to be divided into a large number of small elements of diameter around one wavelength of the transmitted ultrasound (Fig. 5.8a). Each element is then considered to act as a vibrating source generating a spherical wave front (Fig. 5.8b). The resultant pressure amplitude from the interference of these wave fronts can be calculated for any point in the propagating medium. It is found that the interference effects are such that most of the ultrasonic energy is transmitted along a main central region. The pressure fluctuations are very small at the side of this region. In one or two lobes at the side (side-lobes), the pressure amplitude may be one tenth (-20 dB) that on the central axis (Fig. 5.9). The above approach may be applied to any shape of source, for either pulsed- or continuous-wave ultrasound. It gives insight into the origin of ultrasonic field shapes.

Reception side-lobes, down about one tenth in sensitivity (-20 dB), also exist (Fig. 5.9). The

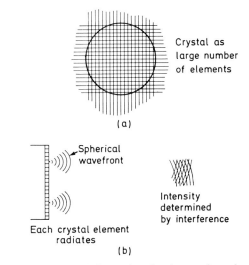

Fig. 5.8 Model depicting a piezoelectric crystal as a large number of small sources for prediction of field shape.

combined effect of the transmission and reception means that a target in a side-lobe produces an echo of amplitude one hundredth (-40 dB) of that from a similar target in the central beam.

The transmission-field and reception-zone shapes for array transducers can be calculated in the same way as that indicated above. The elements are considered to be subdivided into small sources generating spherical waves. In the case of arrays, the side-lobes are called 'grating-lobes'.

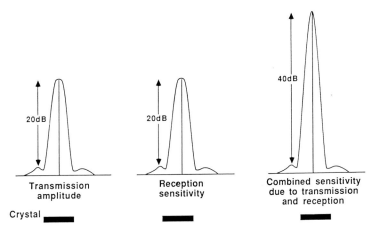

Profiles across beam with significant side lobes

Fig. 5.9 Side-lobes in a transmission field and a reception zone. The enhanced on-axis sensitivity owing to the combination of transmission and reception is also illustrated.

Grating-lobes in early arrays were quite large, resulting in beam shapes which were not ideal. Techniques have been developed which improve the beams from arrays.

Focusing

Normally, when we think of a lens focusing light or ultrasound, we think in terms of rays being refracted at the lens surfaces and then converging on the focal region (Fig. 5.10a). A more accurate description, however, is to consider the wave front as passing through the lens and to observe the delays which occur for each small element of the wave front. Figure 5.10b illustrates a plane wave front of ultrasound striking a plastic lens. The velocity of ultrasound in plastic is higher than that in water. Beyond the lens, the central elements of the wave front are delayed relative to those toward the side. The subsequent spreading out of ultrasound from each element and interference produce a high intensity region, referred to as the 'focus'. Note that focusing has been achieved by introducing delays, that is, phase shifts, across the wave front. Generating an ultrasonic field from a concave source results in similar focusing. Here it is obvious, from the moment of generation, that the central elements in the wave front are delayed behind the others (Fig. 5.10c). Since reception is the converse of transmission, the reception zone is also focused and the greatest sensitivity of detection is at the focus.

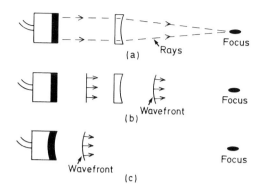

Fig. 5.10 Focusing of an ultrasound beam. (a) Ray representation, (**b**) wave front representation of focusing by a lens, (**c**) wave front representation of focusing by a curved element.

The focal point is the point at which the beam is narrowest. The width of the beam is defined as the distance across the beam between the points where the echo signal from a small target is a specified number of dB below the on-axis value, e.g. -40 dB (Fig. 5.11b). In ultrasonic imaging, it is desirable to have a beam which is narrow over an extended region, the focal depth. The focal depth may be defined as the length along the axis near the focus for which the width of the beam is less than twice the width at the focus (Fig. 5.11).

It may appear that focusing the transmitted ultrasound will result in tissue being irradiated at higher intensity. However, since focusing produces larger echoes, it is then possible to reduce the level of the transmitted ultrasound and

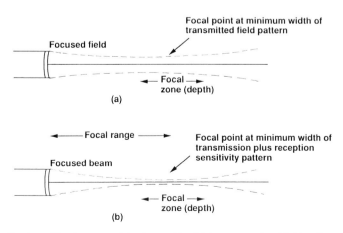

Fig. 5.11 Specification of focal range and focal zone (depth) for a transmitted field and an ultrasonic beam.

still obtain adequate echoes. Focusing on reception results in larger echo signals, permitting a further reduction in the transmitted intensity.

Electronic focusing (swept focusing, dynamic focusing)

Focusing, by introducing delays into portions of a wave front, can be achieved electronically. For example, a transducer consisting of five strip elements can be activated with slight time delays between the excitation pulses applied to each element. These delays can be arranged such that the contributions from the elements arrive in phase at one particular point, and, hence, interference produces a high-intensity focus. With no delays at the instant of transmission, there is never compensation for the different path length travelled by each contribution to a point on the beam axis; hence, they are out of phase, and there is no focusing. To achieve focusing with an array of elements in practice, we excite the outer elements ahead of the inner ones (Fig. 5.12a). The position of the focal region can be changed by altering the pattern of delays of the excitation signals.

To focus the reception zone, we apply electronic delays to the echo signals at each element (Fig. 5.12b). Again, the focal point can be moved by changing the set of applied delays. Indeed, the focal point can be altered very rapidly by changing the delays during the reception of echoes. In this way, the reception-zone focus can be made to sweep along the beam axis such that it always coincides with the depth of the reflectors that produced the echoes being received at that instant. This is obviously a very attractive feature, since it results in focusing being applied over a considerable length of the range of penetration.

In the above description of electronic focusing during transmission, one should note that once the pulses have been emitted they are no longer under the control of the electronics, and the transmission-field focus cannot, therefore, be swept. However, at consecutive transmissions, the focus can be stepped along the beam axis to provide an extended focal region (Fig. 5.13). Since the beam then dwells longer in each position, the frame rate is reduced.

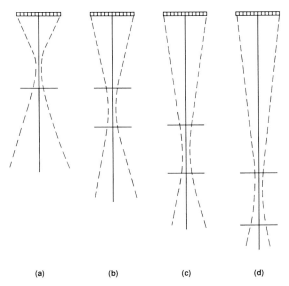

Fig. 5.13 Stepped focusing by an array at successive cycles of transmission and reception.

In both linear and phased arrays, the number of strip elements can be large, e.g. 32, 64, or 128. Large transducers using 128 elements provide a very sharp focus (Fig. 5.14). The larger the width (i.e. aperture – see later discussion) of a transducer relative to the wavelength of ultrasound, the sharper the focus. Large

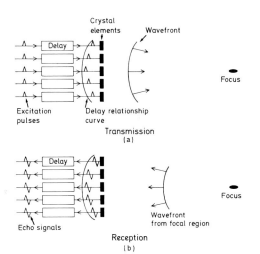

Fig. 5.12 Electronic focusing. (**a**) Focusing in tramission, (**b**) focusing on reception.

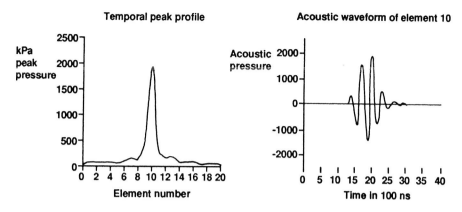

Fig. 5.14 Field profile and transmitted pulse shape at the focus of a large array. The total width of the horizontal axis is 20 mm. There are 20 small elements placed side by side in the measuring hydrophone.

transducers are particularly important for achieving focusing at the greater depths in the field of view. Transducers with 128 elements have proved to be successful where the tissues do not distort the beam; for example, in obstetrics.

Electronic focusing by strip elements, as found in linear and phased arrays, makes the beam narrower in the direction at right angles to the length of the strips (the in-plane direction). With these devices, focusing does not occur in the direction parallel to the strips (the out-of-plane direction). In other words, the thickness of the slice of tissue interrogated by the beam is not reduced. Electronic focusing truly about the central axis of the beam requires a transducer that consists of an-

nular elements or a two-dimensional array of small elements (Fig. 5.15).

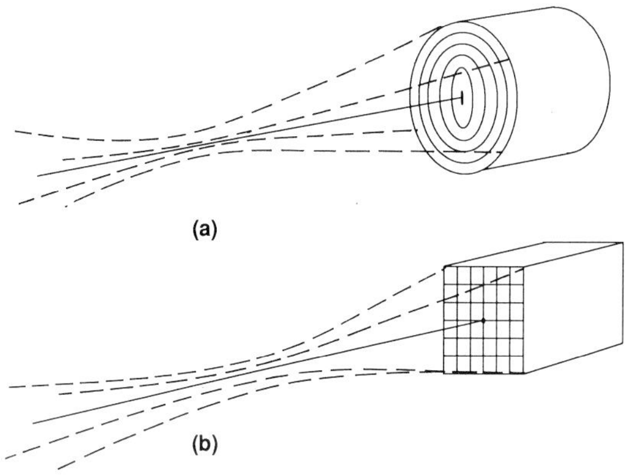

Basic theory shows that annular arrays can produce reasonable focusing with about 7 annular elements. As more flexible ways of driving these transducers are developed, the number of elements may increase, as happened with linear and phased arrays. An example of flexible operation is the variable-aperture technique discussed below. The principles of electronic focusing also apply to annular arrays. Just as has been described for linear and phased arrays, the transmit focus of an annular array is at a fixed range, or may be stepped at successive transmissions, whereas the reception focus is swept along the beam axis.

Electronic beam-steering

If the elements of a transducer consisting of strips are excited simultaneously, the resultant field is along the central axis (Fig. 5.16a). This is analogous to a single, flat-faced element transducer. If the excitation pulses, however, are delayed, by constant amounts, from one strip to the next across the transducer, the contributions from each element interfere, producing a field at an angle to the central axis (Fig. 5.16b). The reception zone is made to coincide with the transmission field by similarly delaying the received echo signals. Rapid alteration in the beam direction can be achieved between each cycle of transmission and reception by altering the delay

Fig. 5.15 True axial electronic focusing made possible by two-dimensional arrays.

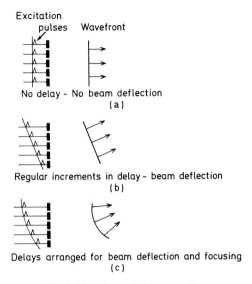

Excitation
pulses   Wavefront

No delay - No beam deflection
(a)

Regular increments in delay - beam deflection
(b)

Delays arranged for beam deflection and focusing
(c)

Fig. 5.16   Electronic beam-steering.

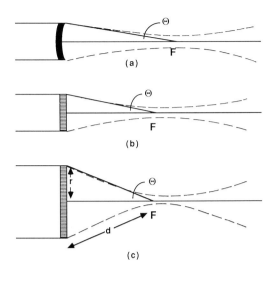

Numerical aperture = sin Θ = $\frac{r}{d}$

Fig. 5.17   Definition of numerical aperture.

magnitudes. It is thus possible to perform a real-time, sector-scanning action. This is the technique employed in electronic sector-scanners (phased arrays). Sector angles of 90° are achieved while the transducer remains stationary. Electronic beam-steering is not possible with annular arrays; they are incorporated into mechanical scanners.

Electronic beam-steering plus focusing occurs when the appropriate delay patterns are combined (Fig. 5.16c). The focusing pattern (increasing delay from the outside to the centre) is combined with the steering pattern (regular changes in delay across the array).

Variable aperture

The aperture of a transducer is defined as the sine of the half angle which the transducer subtends at its focal point (Fig. 5.17a and b). To generate a sharply focused beam, the transducer should subtend a large angle at the focus (Fig. 5.17c). It is easy to appreciate that for a point at long range, a large transducer is required to give a large aperture and, hence, sharp focusing. For short-range focusing, a small transducer can provide a large aperture. With array transducers, it is possible to have the same aperture value, and therefore similar focusing, for each focal depth by increasing the number of elements in use as the focal depth

is increased. This can be done with both linear and annular arrays by using a few elements for short range and all of the elements at long range. Variable-aperture operation is a common feature of array transducers.

When one group of elements is used to transmit and a different group to receive, it is possible to arrange that the side-lobes or grating-lobes for transmission do not coincide with those for reception, while retaining a focused main beam. As a result, echoes caused by the lobes are reduced in size. The beam shape and the size of lobes can also be altered by adjusting the relative contributions from the elements. For example, the contributions from the outside elements, during both transmission and reception, may be reduced. Adjusting the contributions is known as 'apodization'. These types of manipulation illustrate the flexibility introduced in transducers by array technology.

WAVEGUIDES

Ultrasound will pass readily along a wire or metal tube of dimensions similar to or less than its wavelength. This propagation along a cylindrical structure occurs for certain modes (patterns) of vibration (Fig. 5.18). A few modes may occur for compressional waves in which the pattern of vibra-

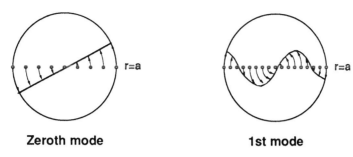

Zeroth mode   **1st mode**

Fig. 5.18   An example of the complex motion of the particles in a waveguide.

tion across the cylinder is different; for example, maximum amplitude of motion at the centre in one mode and maximum amplitude at the outside edge in another. In addition to longitudinal (compressional) waves, flexural and torsional waves are possible. Wires or tubes used in this manner to conduct ultrasound are known as waveguides. Biopsy needles, stylets, and catheters act as waveguides when sound enters them from a scanning beam. By mounting a crystal on the outside end of a needle or catheter, it is possible to detect when the scanning beam is striking the tip. Fine wire probes have also been described for plotting beam-intensity patterns. Surgical devices have been reported in which high-power ultrasound is conducted into the body to destroy tissue at specific points.

Waveguide techniques are widely applied with radio waves and in very fine, optical fibres.

SUMMARY

In this chapter we noted that a continuous sine wave has only one frequency component, whereas a pulsed wave has a band of frequency components. We noted also the following ways in which waves may be manipulated:

1. When waves overlap, interference occurs which may give rise to complex intensity patterns or to directional ultrasound beams.

2. Waves passing one another in opposite directions may produce standing waves. These are to be avoided in studies of bio-effects and in the measurement of field parameters such as intensity, but they are not a problem in diagnostic techniques.

3. Resonance occurs in structures of dimensions related simply to the wavelength of the ultrasound. It is due to the contributions from reflected waves adding up constructively. Resonance can give rise to high local intensities and pressure amplitudes.

4. The narrow beam produced by a flat-faced transducer can be made even narrower by focusing, using methods analogous to those of optics, or by electronic techniques.

5. Electronic focusing during reception can be swept over much of the depth of penetration. Focusing during transmission is at a fixed range. To extend the transmission focus for a particular beam direction, we move the focal region between successive transmission pulses. This reduces the frame rate, but it is a widely used and worthwhile facility.

6. Electronic beam-steering is fundamental to the operation of phased arrays.

7. The versatility of array transducers (linear, phased, and annular) was illustrated by apodization, side-lobe reduction, and variable-aperture processing.

8. Waveguides were described briefly.

REFERENCE

Nicholson N C, McDicken W N, Anderson T 1989
    Waveguides in medical ultrasonics: an experimental study
    of mode propagation. Ultrasonics 27: 101–106

6. Manipulation of ultrasonic signals

When the received ultrasound is converted into an electrical signal, it can be processed in many ways to extract information. In analogue processing, an electrical signal is treated while still in a form in which the varying voltage is analogous to the varying pressure of the ultrasound.

In digital processing the signal voltage is sampled at short intervals along its length (Fig. 6.1). Each sample voltage is converted into a series of pulses, digits, which can be stored in a computer memory. The arrangement of these digits is directly related to the magnitude of the sample voltage. A signal stored as a series of digitized samples can then be readily manipulated in a computer. Digitization of signals is discussed further in Chapter 10, in which storage of the echo signals of images in electronic memory is considered. There are advantages in analogue processing since the circuitry can often be made simple, but

it is prone to drifting of set voltage values. More and more digital processing is used since it is stable and exceedingly flexible.

It is not necessary for the user of ultrasonic equipment to know the details of each sort of signal processing, but a familiarity with the terminology removes the mystique.

SIMPLE ARITHMETIC PROCESSING

Once two signals (Fig. 6.2a) have been stored as a series of digital samples, arithmetic procedures can be undertaken. For example, the signals may be added by simply adding the samples which occur at the same instant (Fig. 6.2b). Subtraction is similar, the corresponding samples being subtracted (Fig. 6.2c). Figures 6.2d and 6.2e illustrate multiplication and division. Again, the corresponding pairs of samples are multiplied and divided.

FILTERING

A common processing technique is to put the signal through an electronic filter, which passes only some of the frequency components in the spectrum of the signal. Figure 6.3 presents the characteristic response curves of some typical filters. Figure 6.3a shows a high-pass filter in which frequency components greater than about 200 Hz are passed. This type of filter is found in Doppler units, in which it is desirable to cut out low-frequency Doppler shifts corresponding to slowly moving tissue. Figure 6.3b is a low-pass filter that is found in pulsed-Doppler units to remove unwanted high frequencies. Figure 6.3c is a band-pass filter that passes frequencies in a specified range; it is found

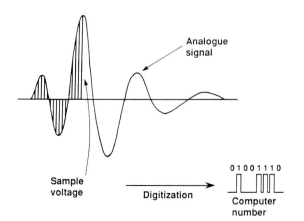

Fig. 6.1 Digitizing an analogue signal to produce digital samples. Each sample is stored as a computer number.

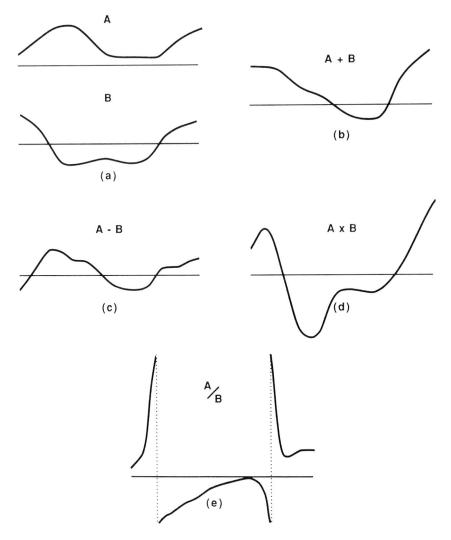

Fig. 6.2 Arithmetic processes performed on two signals. Samples at corresponding times are added, subtracted, multiplied, and divided.

in some devices that analyse the frequency content of a signal.

Note that the transition from pass to stop occurs over a significant frequency range. There are technical problems associated with the design of very sharp filters. Note also that in the stop-frequency range, the components are not blocked completely, but are severely attenuated. A significant fraction of a very large component in the stop range may still be present after filtering.

Figure 6.4 illustrates the effect of passing a signal through a low-pass or a high-pass filter.

FREQUENCY ANALYSIS (FOURIER ANALYSIS, FFT ANALYSIS)

We have seen that the shape of a signal provides information, for instance, from its amplitude or rate of decay. The spectrum of a signal is also often examined to identify useful characteristics such as its high-frequency content.

Frequency analysis has been an extremely powerful tool in other fields such as X-ray CT imaging and electronic engineering. It often presents data from signals in a way in which the signal

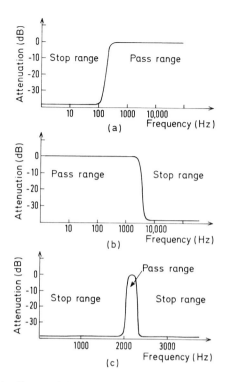

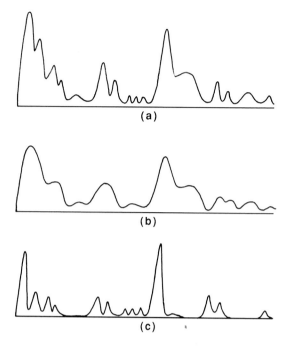

Fig. 6.3 Characteristic response curves of common types of filter: (**a**) high-pass filter, (**b**) low-pass filter, (**c**) band-pass filter.

Fig. 6.4 Effect of filtering on an ultrasonic signal: (**a**) unfiltered signal (**b**) low-pass filtering, (**c**) high-pass filtering.

characteristics can be more readily appreciated, or in which the data can be processed mathematically. It is possible, after processing the spectrum, to reconstruct a modified version of the original signal by the converse of analysis, that is, synthesis. Frequency analysis is widely discussed in the research literature on ultrasound, but, apart from its widespread use in Doppler blood-flow studies and instrument design, it has still to be proven of value in the field of diagnostic imaging.

To perform frequency analysis on a signal, the operator passes the signal to one of several types of frequency analyser. In one type, the signal is fed repetitively into a narrow band-pass filter that systematically moves through the expected frequency range and passes the amplitude of each frequency component present in the signal to the output display (Fig. 6.5a). This is a useful, but rather slow, approach.

Another type of analyser employs a bank of fixed filters of which each is designed to pass components in a specific part of the frequency range

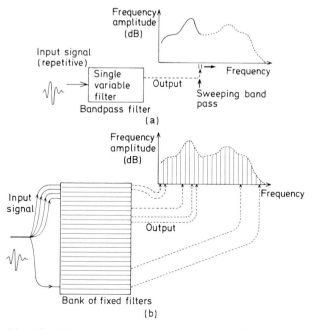

Fig. 6.5 (**a**) Frequency analysis by sweeping a band-pass filter, (**b**) frequency analysis by a bank of filters.

examined. The ultrasonic signal is fed simultaneously to all the filters, and the spectrum is obtained immediately (Fig. 6.5b). This is called 'real-time' frequency analysis.

Digital computational techniques are most commonly employed to analyse signals. The signal is captured by a device that rapidly samples the amplitude at regular time intervals along the waveform, for example, 5 samples per cycle (Fig. 6.6). The samples are stored as numbers in the computer memory. A program then acts on this data and mathematically derives the frequency spectrum. High-speed programs and silicon computer chips have been designed to carry out frequency analysis in milliseconds. The name 'Fast Fourier Transform', or 'FFT', analysis is applied to these programs. These techniques are particularly valuable in studies of blood flow in which the results are obtained in real-time.

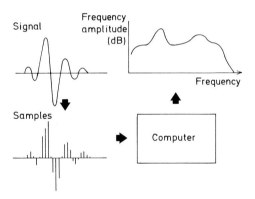

Fig. 6.6 Frequency analysis by making measurements on a signal at regular intervals to obtain samples for processing in a computer.

We have seen that, as ultrasound is propagated in tissue, a number of frequency-dependent phenomena occur; scattering, absorption, etc. Some research projects involving frequency analysis are aimed at quantifying the effect of such phenomena on the frequency spectra of ultrasonic signals and, hence, finding out more about the characteristics of tissue. For example, different tissues may scatter or absorb the frequency components of a pulse by different amounts. One of the main problems in this field is to separate the effects of overlying tissues from those of the tissue of interest.

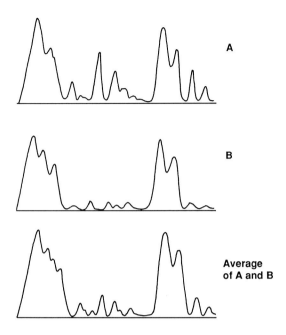

Fig. 6.7 Averaging of two signals by averaging the samples at corresponding times.

AVERAGING

If a signal is almost obscured by noise, there are considerable benefits in collecting the signals several times and then adding them together to calculate the average value of the signal (Fig. 6.7). The reason for this is that the signal voltages add together directly and so increase in strength, but the noise voltages fluctuate both positively and negatively, and, thus, the noise level builds up more slowly than the signal level. If N collections are made, the signal will become N times larger, but the noise will only increase by $\sqrt{N}$. So for 16 collections the signal is 16 times bigger, but the noise is increased by a factor of 4. The main drawback of averaging is that it obviously takes longer than a single collection. Averaging is used to improve the signal-to-noise ratio (S/N) in images and Doppler spectra.

INTERPOLATION

Interpolation is the generation of new artificial 'samples' from existing samples. Suppose two signal samples exist, then a third 'sample' may be artificially produced by taking the average of the

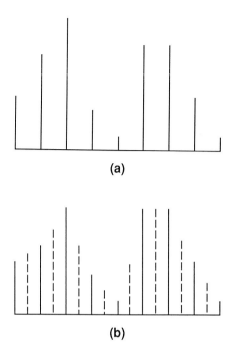

Fig. 6.8 Interpolation of sample values in (a) to produce additional values in (b).

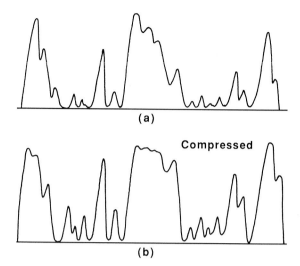

Fig. 6.9 Compression of the large amplitudes in a signal to give more emphasis to small amplitudes.

two genuine ones. If this average is now placed between the two originals, the stream of sample values will appear to change more smoothly (Fig. 6.8). A common application of interpolation is the generation of additional artificial echo values in imaging. This is employed to increase artificially the number of displayed lines in an image. Although this is essentially a cosmetic operation, it does improve the appearance of some images.

COMPRESSION

Electronic circuitry and display screens can only accommodate a limited range of signal magnitudes; this range is called their 'dynamic range'. Signals which are too large saturate and have their tops flattened, or all appear at the same maximum brightness on a screen. Signals which are too small are rejected. Rather than allow these effects to happen by chance, it is common to compress the range of signals electronically prior to passing them to the circuitry or display screen (Fig. 6.9). In this way, the most important signals are preserved, e.g. the weak echoes from organ parenchyma or blood.

MODULATION AND DEMODULATION

Modulation and demodulation are techniques for the manipulation of waveforms. They are not widely used in diagnostic ultrasound, although they are common in other fields, such as radio engineering, and they could find application in medical ultrasound.

The description of waves in terms of amplitude, frequency, and phase was noted in Chapter 3. If any of these parameters of a continuous wave is made to vary in time in a manner determined by a second signal, the continuous wave is said to be modulated by that second signal. This is illustrated in Figure 6.10, in which the amplitude of the continuous wave, termed the 'carrier wave', is varied by a modulating signal; this is called 'amplitude modulation'. The modulated carrier wave now carries information about the modulating signal. In the reverse process (demodulation or detection), the modulating signal is extracted from the modulated carrier wave. Note that modulation is not the same as interference of waves; that is, the two signals are not added as in interference, but are, in fact, multiplied.

Frequency modulation and phase modulation are similar and are the processes by which the frequency or phase of the continuous wave is altered by the modulating signal (Fig. 6.11). Here, too,

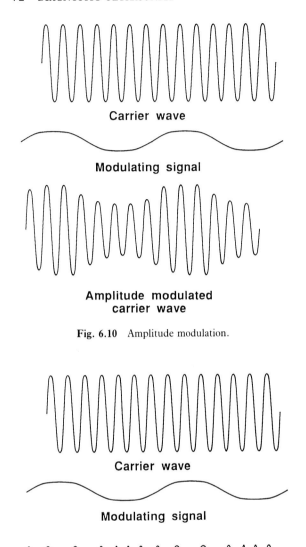

Carrier wave

Modulating signal

Amplitude modulated carrier wave

Fig. 6.10 Amplitude modulation.

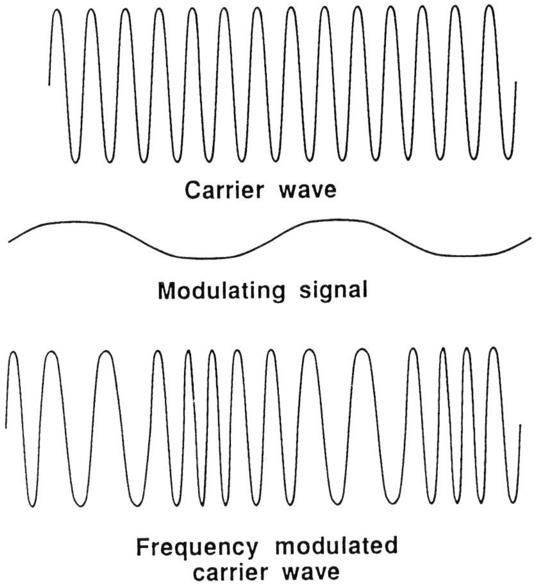

Carrier wave

Modulating signal

Frequency modulated carrier wave

Fig. 6.11 Frequency or phase modulation.

the modulating signals can be recovered by demodulating the modulated carrier wave.

The term 'demodulation' occasionally arises in diagnostic ultrasound when the oscillatory nature of echoes is smoothed out to make them more suitable for display purposes. The train of short oscillatory pulses is thus regarded as equivalent to very strong amplitude modulation of a carrier wave. Demodulation occurs extensively in Doppler instruments when the low-frequency Doppler shift signal is extracted from the ultrasonic carrier signal.

Amplitude modulation (AM) and frequency modulation (FM) are commonly associated with radio and television. In radio transmission, a carrier radio wave of a particular frequency is modulated by the microphone signal. The receiving radio is tuned to the frequency of the carrier wave, which is picked up and demodulated to recover the microphone signal. In television transmission, picture and sound information are contained in the modulated carrier wave.

IMAGE PROCESSING

Once the echo signals have been formed into a two-dimensional array of pixel values which constitute the image (Ch. 10), further processing of the signals may be carried out, with a view to improving the image. Typically, processing is aimed at reducing speckle noise, and so improving the detectability of small contrast changes, or at sharpening the edges in an image to increase measurement accuracy.

A simple way of reducing noise is to average each pixel value with those of its immediate neighbours. Unfortunately, although this reduces speckle noise, it blurs the tissue boundaries. More sophisticated techniques are therefore being sought; techniques which, for example, act only on parenchymal signals while leaving the boundary signals sharp. Terms such as 'smoothing', 'adaptive filtering', and 'post-processing' are applied to this manipulation of image signals. Some processing techniques are incorporated into present-day scan-converters; others are still being developed. Image processing is discussed further in Chapters 10 and 28.

AUTOCORRELATION

Autocorrelation processing provides a plot, or function, related to how a signal changes with time. This plot can clarify periodic fluctuations in the signal; in other words, it can reveal informa-

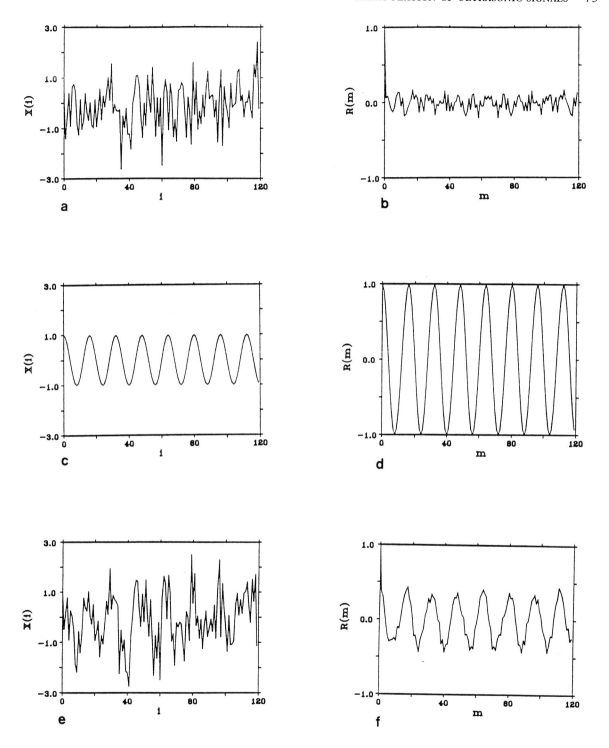

Fig. 6.12 Autocorrelation. No evidence of cyclic variations in the random noise signal (**a**) is detected by producing its autocorrelation function (**b**). The cyclic variation of the signal in (**c**) is clearly detected by its autocorrelation function in (**d**). Cyclic variations in the noise-corrupted signal in (**e**) are clearly detected by its autocorrelation function in (**f**) (courtesy of T Loupas).

tion about the frequency content of the signal. The processing is carried out by multiplying the original signal by a version of itself which has been delayed by a time, t (Multiplication – see above). One point in the plot is produced by first multiplying the corresponding sample pairs in the original and delayed signals. The value for this point in the plot is then obtained by adding the results of the multiplications of the sample pairs. Further points in the plot are generated by repeating this process for more combinations of the original signal and versions subject to different values of delay.

Examples of autocorrelation plots, or functions, are illustrated in Figure 6.12. The first shows the function generated for a noise signal (Fig. 6.12a). In this case, the original signal is obviously random, and this is reflected in its autocorrelation function, which fluctuates close to zero (Fig. 6.12b). Figures 6.12c and d present a sine-wave signal and its function. Since the sine wave signal is periodic, its autocorrelation function is also periodic. The signal in Figure 6.12e is a sine signal corrupted by noise. Although the sine-wave component is not very evident in the original signal, it is clearly demonstrated by the autocorrelation function (Fig. 6.12f).

In Chapter 20, we will see that once the autocorrelation function for a Doppler blood-flow signal is derived, further processing of the function gives the mean velocity of the blood cells and also a measure of the spread of velocities about the mean, i.e. the variance of the velocity values. The direction of flow can also be ascertained from the autocorrelation function. All of this processing can be carried out very rapidly, and it allows colour-flow imaging to be carried out in real-time.

QUADRATURE PHASE-SHIFTING

If a signal is subject to a delay as it passes through electronic circuitry, it appears to have suffered a phase change when it is examined at the output. This change in phase is most easily seen by comparing the output signal to an unprocessed reference version of the signal (Fig. 6.13). The components of the delay circuit can be chosen to introduce any desired phase change.

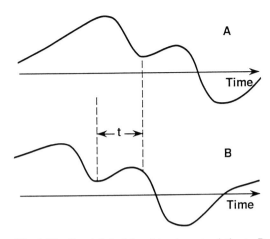

Fig. 6.13 Signal A is delayed by time, t, relative to B.

If a signal is delayed by a 90°-phase shift relative to an unprocessed version of it, the two signals are said to comprise a quadrature pair. Quadrature phase-shifting performed on a Doppler signal is found as part of a technique of detecting direction of blood flow (Chs 18 and 19). The name 'quadrature' arises since 90° is one quadrant of a full cycle of 360°.

HETERODYNE FREQUENCY SHIFTING

It is possible to shift the frequency of a signal by multiplying it by a second signal whose frequency is equal to the desired shift. For example, a 12 kHz signal may be shifted to 15 kHz by multiplying it by a 3 kHz signal. The multiplication process would actually produce a difference frequency at 9 kHz and a summation one at 15 kHz. The 9 kHz component is then removed by filtering. Frequency shifting by multiplication can be easily demonstrated experimentally or mathematically. Heterodyne frequency-shifting is found in Doppler devices in which it is desired to move a signal to a different frequency range for ease of display.

SUMMARY

Methods of processing electronic signals have been briefly studied in this chapter. The aim has been to familiarize the reader with the techniques encountered in diagnostic ultrasound and to emphasize the fact that the underlying ideas are often essentially simple. The list of processes mentioned here is very far from exhaustive; indeed, signal processing is a major field of electronic engineering. Implementation of signal processing can often be difficult.

1. Recall the basic idea of each of the processing methods discussed.

2. Recall where you might expect to find them in diagnostic ultrasonics.

7. Controls of equipment for pulsed-echo imaging

MANIPULATION OF CONTROLS

So far, we have studied in detail the properties of ultrasound. In the following chapters, we will consider further the various techniques for putting ultrasound to work. Most diagnostic techniques using pulsed ultrasound for imaging of tissue structures collect data about tissue in a similar way. They differ primarily in the manner used to present the data for interpretation. We will, therefore, begin by studying techniques to produce and process the basic ultrasonic data. Having studied in Chapter 2 the principles of pulsed-echo imaging, we can see how ultrasonic signals are manipulated by examining the controls of machines. Similar controls are found on real-time, A-, B-, and M-scan instruments.

On first sight, the controls of an ultrasonic scanner may seem very complicated. For particular examinations, however, baseline settings for the controls can be established. Once the baselines have been established, it is necessary to manipulate only one or two controls as the scans are being performed. The introduction of grey-scale imaging and scan converters has greatly increased the ease of producing images. This improved ease of operation, however, has been accompanied by the desire to interpret fine detail in the image: for example, in the identification of liver metastases or in the examination of structure in the fetal spine. It remains worthwhile to obtain a good knowledge of the effect of each control and how to use it most effectively.

Controls can be grouped under four headings:

1. Operational controls
2. Sensitivity controls
3. Scan-converter processing controls
4. Display and recording controls

We shall leave the discussion of scan converter controls until Chapter 10.

OPERATIONAL CONTROLS

Operational controls determine the mode of operation of a machine. They vary from unit to unit and may be made to function by permanently labelled control knobs, or via a keyboard terminal. Their use is straightforward and causes the operator little concern. A well-written user's manual is an essential accessory for most machines. This may seem obvious, but it is surprising how often such manuals are difficult to obtain.

Examples of the types of control that fall into the operational category are mode selection (real-time sector/linear; A-, B-, and M-scan; and Doppler scan) and grey-shade test routines. Motorized control of scanning gantries on some specialized machines also fall into this group.

Examples of operational controls that influence the image are transducer selection, field-of-view size, focal depth, frame rate, and frame freeze.

It is almost impossible to damage most machines by misuse of controls. A few points that are worth watching include:

1. Very bright spots or lines on a display screen can burn the phosphor.
2. Frequent switching on and off of a display tube reduces the life of the electron-gun filament.
3. Mechanical real-time scanners left running for unnecessarily long periods show wear of some of the moving parts.

SENSITIVITY CONTROLS

The sensitivity controls as listed below alter the basic signals, making them suitable for passing to a display system or a scan-converter storage unit.

1. The 'frequency' of ultrasound is selected at the start of an examination. From the point of view of sensitivity, it is reasonable to regard frequency as a control.

2. The ultrasonic 'power' or 'intensity' governs the amount of ultrasonic energy per pulse transmitted into the patient and, hence, the size of the echoes.

3. The 'amplification' of the received echoes depends on the settings of the gain and time-gain compensation (TGC).

4. The 'suppression' level can be employed to remove the weakest echo signals should they be considered to detract from the image.

5. Dynamic range — this control is not commonly available. It is discussed at the end of the chapter.

Frequency selection

In diagnostic ultrasound, the frequency range used is 0.5–20 MHz. Choice of frequency is based on the principle that the greater the penetration required, the lower the frequency employed. Note that penetration and depth are not necessarily equivalent: a thin piece of bone is difficult to penetrate. A good working rule is to use the highest frequency that will give the necessary penetration, and to change to a lower value only when the gain and intensity controls have reached a maximum. Most abdominal scanning can be performed at 3 MHz, but it may be necessary to use 2 MHz to see some deep structures. Care must be exercised when studying echo free regions at a depth that the ultrasound beam may have difficulty in reaching. As we will see later, the reason for selecting high frequencies is that they give the greatest detail in an ultrasonic image.

Commercial instruments usually offer a range of operating frequencies, for example, 2, 3, 5, 7, and 10 MHz. The appropriate transducer is selected and the instrument is tuned to function at that frequency; in most instruments, tuning is automatic when the transducer is plugged in.

Since the range of frequency components in a pulse alters as it passes through tissue, owing to dispersive attenuation and non-linear propagation, a few machines alter the range of frequencies accepted as echoes from deeper and deeper structures are detected. Matching the range of frequencies to the pulse components reduces the noise in the image.

A choice of transducer at the selected frequency may be available. The size and type of the transducer may be important with regard to coupling to the patient.

Output power and intensity

Many instruments allow the intensity or power of the transmitted ultrasonic pulse to be varied. This is achieved by varying the size of the excitation voltage applied to the piezoelectric element of the transducer. The switch control that changes the voltage is often called an 'attenuator'. An attenuator usually reduces the applied voltage from maximum in a series of discrete steps. Obviously, this electronic attenuation should not be confused with the attenuation of the ultrasonic pulse in tissue because of absorption, scattering, etc.

Ideally, the output from a machine would be labelled as intensity in watt/cm^2 or power in watt units. Unfortunately, it is fairly difficult to calibrate instruments absolutely, since intensity or power levels are low and vary from one transducer to another. Absolute calibration is now being supplied for a few machines. It is more customary, however, to label output-control settings using the decibel notation (dB notation). A dB label on a control setting is not an absolute calibration, but it is a measure of that output relative to a specified reference level. The decibel notation is described in Appendix 3.

The electronic methods used in diagnostic ultrasound have evolved from those of radio engineering, radar, and audible acoustics, in all of which decibel units are in wide use. In many circumstances, however, it is unfortunate that the absolute output powers are not quoted. This would allow the operator to have a better knowledge of the dose given to the patient and make it easier to compare the work of different investigators.

The specified reference level is usually either the maximum or minimum output of the machine. If it is the minimum, all other levels are greater, and the decibels are labelled positively, for example, +20 dB. When the reference is the maximum, the other levels are lower, and the decibels are labelled negatively, for example, −31 dB.

The relationship between decibels and absolute-intensity calibrations may give the impression that conversion from one to the other is a troublesome process. In practice, however, such conversion is unnecessary. The operator need only develop an appreciation of the results obtained for the possible settings of the control knobs.

Gain (amplification, overall gain)

The voltages appearing on a transducer element as a result of echoes from tissue boundaries are small. These voltage pulses are in the microvolt and millivolt range and must be amplified to volts for processing, display, and recording purposes. The gain control governs the amplification that the echoes receive. In any study, the investigator may need to manipulate the gain control to obtain a suitable number of echoes of convenient size on the display. When the amplifier gain is too high, it will overload the display and make it uninterpretable by presenting the large echoes very strongly and allowing many small echoes to be overemphasized. Conversely, too low a gain may result in very few echoes being displayed.

The decibel notation is used to label the gain control of linear amplifiers, i.e. those in which the same amplification is applied to large and small echoes. For example, consider an amplifier that takes an input signal V_1 and produces an output signal V_2 for a particular setting of the gain control. The gain is therefore the ratio V_2/V_1. The gain expressed in decibels is

$$\text{gain} = 20 \log_{10} \left(\frac{V_2}{V_1} \right)$$

which is still a measure of the increase in signal size (App. 3).

As with intensity-decibel labelling of controls, it is not necessary, in practice, to convert from voltage ratios to decibels, but rather to know the performance of the instrument at various decibel settings.

A problem in diagnostic instruments is the range of echo magnitudes to be handled. With a linear amplifier; the large echoes may begin to saturate even if the gain is not high enough to register the weak echoes. For this reason, amplifiers are often used which have a logarithmic response and, therefore, amplify weak echo signals more than strong ones (Fig. 7.1).

Logarithmic amplifiers are difficult to calibrate since different signal levels are amplified by different amounts. Again, in practice, it is only necessary to appreciate the performance of the instrument at each position of any control associated with the logarithmic amplifier.

In this section, we have noted how the gain influences all echo signals. Because of attenuation in

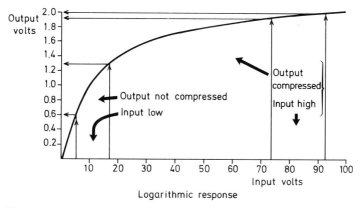

Fig. 7.1 Response of a logarithmic amplifier. The large signals are compressed into a smaller voltage range.

tissue, however, the echoes received from superficial structures are much larger than those from interfaces deep within the body. To compensate, we must amplify deep echoes more than superficial ones. This is done by adding swept-gain or time gain compensation as described in the next section.

A few machines have electronic attenuators, which are devices for changing voltage levels by calibrated amounts. In ultrasonic instruments, such devices are used both to adjust the voltage level applied to excite the transducer, and to alter the size of the echo signals between the transducer and the receiving amplifier. They therefore perform the function of changing the output power or of altering the gain of the receiving system by decibel increments. Some attenuators offer changes over a range, in steps such as 1, 2, 5, or 10 dB. An attenuator may be built into the ultrasonic scanner as the intensity or gain control. They are also available as separate add-on units.

Time gain compensation (TGC)

Alternative terms for TGC are swept-gain, depth-gain compensation (DGC), distance-attenuation compensation, time-gain control, sensitivity-time control, near-and-far-gain, and depth-varied gain.

In Chapter 4, the numerous phenomena that attenuate ultrasound as it passes through tissue were considered. The result of this strong attenuation is that both the transmitted and reflected ultrasound are reduced in amplitude as they pass through the body. The thickness of absorbing tissue through which the ultrasound passes is, thus, an important factor in determining the size of echo received from a surface.

In the light of the effect of attenuation, it is obviously not desirable to apply the same amplification to all echoes. Additional circuitry is therefore included to reduce the amplification from the level set by the overall gain control when echoes from superficial structures are being received. The controls associated with this additional circuitry are known as the TGC controls. There are, thus, two sets of controls for the receiving amplifier: the overall gain control, which affects all echoes equally, and the TGC controls, which modify the performance of the amplifier

during a selected period after the instant of transmission.

The way the TGC of the amplifier is made to vary with time after the instant of transmission is called the TGC function. On most instruments, there are at least two controls with which the operator can govern the characteristics of this function (Fig. 7.2a). The two most important controls determine the starting level of the TGC and fix the rate of increase of gain, that is, the slope. A third control, TGC delay, delays the starting point of the slope by any desired time after the instant of transmission. This third control is not present on all machines.

More complex TGC functions than those just discussed can also be employed. For example, it may be advantageous to have high gain at some depths and low gain at others. To accomplish this, we subdivide the depth range, for example, into 2 cm divisions, and a separate control governs the gain in each division. With slider controls, the operator is provided with a visual representation of the gain applied at each depth (Fig. 7.2b). This type of TGC is most commonly found in practice.

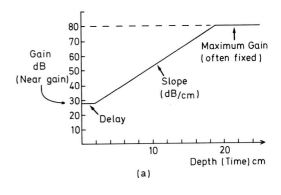

(a)

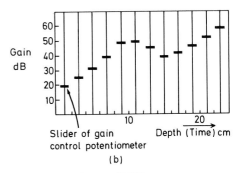

(b)

Fig. 7.2 Types of TGC systems.

It is particularly common in cardiac instruments where it is advantageous to apply high gain for weak echoes from valves and low gain for heart-wall echoes.

The way in which amplification is made to vary with time, that is, the shape of TGC function, depends on the clinical examination. The operator must fully understand the effect of the controls that determine the compensation. It is helpful to the operator if the TGC function is displayed in some way on a TV screen or on the control panel of the instrument. A useful exercise is to observe a typical A-scan display of echoes from tissue structures and to note the effect of adjusting the TGC controls by known amounts.

Manufacturers have a variety of techniques for displaying TGC. The most common method is to present the function or a related controlling voltage on a display (Fig. 7.3). This display reveals the initial gain, the delay before the amplification is made to start increasing, the rate of increase, and the depth at which the overall gain level is reached. The baseline setting for each sort of clinical study can thus be determined. From patient to patient, small changes from these baselines will be required to achieve optimal results.

TGC can also be shown by precisely labelled and calibrated controls or by presentation of data on the display screen; for example, initial gain, delay, slope, and maximum gain. With these calibrations, the operator can readily adjust and record the function.

It is normally possible to adjust the TGC function through many shapes, for example, from a completely flat shape (zero TGC) to one in which the initial gain reduction is very severe, for example, -80 dB. Setting up the TGC is best done in conjunction with he other sensitivity controls; it is discussed below. For the moment, we will consider some typical functions and the underlying considerations.

Earlier it was noted that the attenuation in tissue is very frequency-dependent. The optimum shape of the function, and, in particular, the slope, depends, therefore, on the frequency of ultrasound used. There are other, less well quantified considerations that influence the variation of the echo size with depth; for example, the changing transmitted-field shape and the divergence of the echo wave front. With a frequency of ultrasound of f MHz, the slope of the TGC function must usually be around $2f$ dB/cm. For instance, in ab-

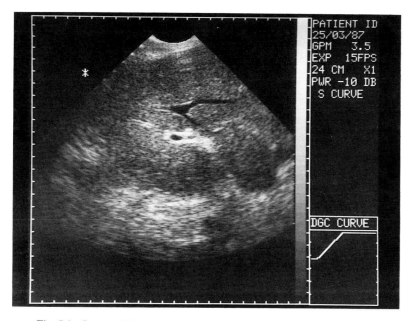

Fig. 7.3 Bottom right corner of display presents the TGC (DGC) function.

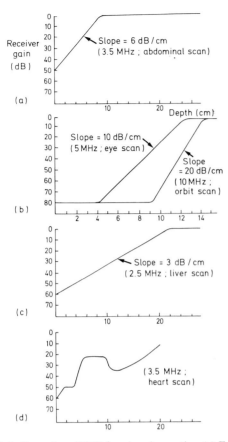

Fig. 7.4 Examples of TGC functions in practice. (**a**) For general abdominal scanning, (**b**) for water-bath scanning of the eye, (**c**) for liver scanning, (**d**) for heart scanning.

dominal scanning at 3.5 MHz, a slope of 6 dB/cm is satisfactory (Fig. 7.4a).

Figure 7.4b shows examples of functions employed successfully in eye scanning with a water-bath of depth 6 cm. The example for 10 MHz ultrasound brings out the point that, in some situations, it may be desirable to apply the total available increase in gain accurately in a tissue layer of particular interest, especially if echo sizes are to be interpreted. Here the total available range of TGC is 80 dB, so a rate of 20 dB/cm is applied in the 4 cm of tissue behind the bulb of the eye.

The liver is an example of an homogeneous structure in which the ability to assess the reflecting powers of the tissue interfaces is advantageous. To compensate for uniform attenuation in the liver, researchers have found a uniformly rising TGC to be satisfactory (Fig. 7.4c).

A TGC function for heart scanning is illustrated in Figure 7.4d. Initially, the gain is held low to prevent the large anterior echoes from merging. In the range of 5 to 10 cm, the gain is increased by about 20 dB to help in the detection of echoes from the fast-moving mitral valve. Beyond this, the gain is reduced to allow the deeper walls to be depicted clearly. Note that heart scanning is an unusual case in two respects. Firstly, the echoes from moving structures alter in amplitude as the surfaces change their orientation to the ultrasonic beam, and, secondly, the heart is a mixture of low-attenuation, blood-filled chambers and muscle that is a more typical soft tissue.

When employing water-bath scanning, the absorption in water can be neglected. The rise in gain is delayed, therefore, for a time corresponding to a distance roughly equal to the depth of water. The TGC then compensates for the distances that the ultrasonic pulses actually travel in tissue. Should the skin surface be at varying distances from the transducer during the scan, its echo can be made to trigger the start of the rise in amplification. Subsequent echoes, following that from the skin surface, receive amplification related to their path length in tissue. Examples of first-echo triggered TGC are found in breast scanners.

The large selection of possible TGC settings emphasizes the need to establish baseline positions for the controls for each type of application. Note also that, although TGC controls are versatile, they will never be exactly correct because the nature of the tissues being scanned is not known in advance, and different tissue structures are encountered as the beam alters its direction.

Suppression (reject, threshold)

It may not be desirable to present the very weakest echoes on the display. For instance, if the weakest signals are artefacts arising from multiple reflections, they may make difficult the identification of fluid-filled vessels. One way to reduce the number of echoes is to reject all below a certain adjustable level. In practice, the operator adjusts the suppression-level control until a suitable number of echoes is displayed. There are a number of electronic circuits for performing suppression. The best remove the small echoes and have little effect on the large ones. In some instruments, however, the suppressor also reduces the large echoes and may appear to be similar to gain. It is worthwhile to distinguish gain and suppression, since the suppression control usually has a much more marked effect on small echoes. We will see below that it is better to leave the suppression control at a low level, if possible, since small echoes often contain valuable information.

Setting up sensitivity controls

The controls discussed above (ultrasonic power, gain, time-gain compensation, frequency, and suppression) govern an instrument's ability to detect tissue interfaces. It is advisable, before using an ultrasonic machine, to identify these sensitivity controls. They may be readily observed control knobs or keys on a computer terminal, with numeric values for each control appearing on the display screen. If they are used in a logical and related fashion, high-quality results are more likely to be obtained. The following procedure is one way for the operator to use the controls effectively:

1. Select the most suitable frequency and transducer for the application. This is usually fairly well established during the development of a technique (Ch. 13).
2. Adjust the suppression to its lowest position so that the weakest echoes are displayed.
3. Set the initial gain reduction of the TGC so that it is reducing only a few echo signals from superficial structures; that is, so that it is in a position where it is having little or no effect.
4. Adjust either the overall gain or the ultrasonic power to make the echoes from deep interfaces a suitable size on the display, that is, neither too small nor too strongly saturated.
5. Now adjust the starting level of the TGC (the initial gain reduction) to present echoes from the superficial structures satisfactorily. Introducing a small amount of delay may help to achieve this.
6. Turning your attention to the middle-range echoes, choose a slope to show well the interfaces of interest. As noted earlier, a suitable slope will

often be about $2f$ dB/cm where f is the ultrasonic frequency in MHz.
7. If it is not possible to remove unwanted small echoes by a slight reduction in the overall gain or power without influencing echoes of interest, the suppression level can be increased. Otherwise, it is best left in a low position.

Another procedure is employed when the TGC is adjusted by a series of potentiometers, each of which governs the gain in a particular range of depth.

1. Select the most suitable ultrasonic frequency.
2. Set any suppression control at a low level so the weak signals are displayed.
3. Set the gain or transmitter power at a reasonably high level.
4. Move the potentiometer controls back and forth by large amounts to obtain an appreciation of the depth range which each influences.
5. Adjust the potentiometers to present the echoes at each depth satisfactorily. The reduction in gain set by the potentiometers should increase toward the transducer to compensate for the increased strength of the received echoes when uniform tissues are scanned. When less uniform tissues are examined, the optimum position of the potentiometers will exhibit more variation. Usually, fine adjustments are required to avoid bands across the image corresponding to non-optimum TGC settings.
6. If it is not possible to remove unwanted small echoes by a slight reduction in the gain or power, increase the level of the suppression control.

These techniques should allow baseline settings for the sensitivity controls to be established for particular applications. During the ultrasonic examination, the operator will probably need to manipulate only the overall gain or power and perhaps the starting level of the TGC. For instance, if the overall gain or ultrasonic power is increased to show more echoes at depth, a reduction in the initial gain level, that is, near gain, will keep the superficial echo signals at a suitable level. In Chapter 13, a series of images will be presented to illustrate the effects of the sensitivity controls.

A feature of some computer-controlled scanners is that it is possible to store the baseline settings for each type of examination in memory. The sensitivity is then quickly set up by picking the appropriate baseline setting from the list presented to the operator on demand. In the light of experience, the user can alter or extend this list of stored settings.

DYNAMIC RANGE

Dynamic range is a term that appears in discussions of seemingly unrelated topics, for example, tissue, transducers, or displays. It is a most useful concept for assessing the performance of the individual parts of an ultrasonic system. Dynamic range is a measure of the range in signal magnitudes that are generated or can be handled by the portion of the system under study. An amplifier that can handle a maximum-to-minimum input signal amplitude ratio of 100 to 1 without degradation is said to have a dynamic range of 100:1 (40 dB).

If, after the application of TGC to allow for attenuation, the echo range from a tissue structure is 60 to 1, the dynamic range of the tissue would then be quoted as 30 dB.

Good transducers are designed to reduce the size of echo signals generated by side-lobes to less than one-hundredth of those produced by the central beam. Such transducers have dynamic ranges of 40 dB or more. A typical scan-converter storage memory may store echo amplitudes in the ratio 128 to 1 (42 dB).

Finally, the dynamic range of the display is of obvious relevance. Values of dynamic range of 20 (10:1) to 30 dB (32:1) are encountered in grey-tone imaging. It is the dynamic range of the display, the recording medium, or our ability to appreciate grey shades that reduces the image dynamic range to about 24 dB (16:1). This is not quite as serious as it looks, since the weaker echo amplitudes carrying the diagnostic information can often be accommodated by this range. The ideal system preserves the amplitude information at least as far as the scan converter store, and this allows processing of the data in a variety of ways (Fig. 7.5).

A few machines offer a dynamic range control, often in place of suppression. This control alters the dynamic range of the amplifier; for example, continuously from 20 to 40 dB. The underlying idea of this approach is that the dynamic range of the amplifier can be matched to that of the tissue. The input tissue signals are then spread over the full maximum-to-minimum pulse-voltage levels that the amplifier can handle. In practice, the operator can usually adjust the dynamic range control to a maximum value and leave it there.

ADAPTIVE GAIN CONTROL (AUTOMATIC TGC, AUTOMATIC GAIN CONTROL, AUTOMATIC SENSITIVITY CONTROL)

Although time-gain compensation is applied successfully in pulse-echo instruments, it has a number of limitations, and its effectiveness should not be overestimated. It provides average compensation that may be far from the ideal for any specific beam path. Consider, for example, the tissue paths encountered by an ultrasonic beam sweeping through the pregnant uterus. Consecu-

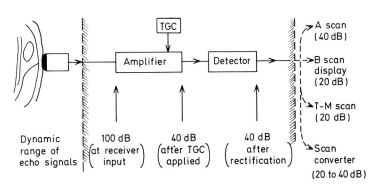

Fig. 7.5 Dynamic range of echo signals at points throughout a basic electronic system.

tive dominant structures in the beam paths might include the fluid-filled bladder, the fetal head, amniotic fluid plus trunk, and fundal placenta. Alteration of the plane of scan results in another variety of beam paths. A similar situation exists in cardiac studies, where the problem is compounded by the motion of the tissues. Another limitation of TGC is that the operator is required to judge the optimum settings, and, hence, the final image is operator-dependent. Obviously, a more desirable state of affairs would be one in which, for each scan, the same reproducible image is obtained from a particular section, and in which the operator is concerned more with the clinical problem than with manipulating machine controls. These are two of the goals of development in the field of automatic sensitivity control.

Automatic sensitivity control is achieved by using the echo-amplitude information that has just been received to control one of the sensitivity factors, such as gain, suppression, or intensity. Normally, because gain is influenced, the technique is labelled AGC (adaptive gain compensation) or ATGC (adaptive time-gain compensation). A simple approach to AGC is to receive one set of echoes from a first transmission with no compensation or fixed TGC applied. From the echo information, the rate at which the echo amplitude is decreasing with depth can be noted and a compensating voltage function derived and stored in a memory. During the next transmission–reception cycle, a TGC function derived from the stored data is applied to the amplifier to provide compensation matched to the attenuation experienced for that beam direction. This example illustrates the idea of one approach to AGC. Unfortunately, this approach is too simplistic to be generally useful since, for example, the echoes from the first transmission may come from a large cystic structure and, in that case, would not indicate a true rate of attenuation for the tissue.

An AGC technique applied, in practice, to real-time scanners is illustrated in Figure 7.6. The field of view is divided into sections at regular increments of depth, for example, 0–2 cm, 2–4 cm . . . 18–20 cm. The average echo amplitude from each range is detected and used to generate an appropriate compensation function. Since for each range the entire width of the field of view is

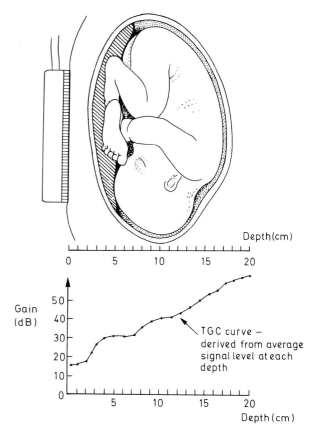

Fig. 7.6 Simple automatic gain control in real-time B-scanning.

used to obtain the average echo amplitude, the system is not greatly influenced by large echo variations in a small region. Refinements can be built into this approach, such as maintaining a smooth transition in the ATGC function from one range to the next. With this type of AGC, images are obtained of a quality as good as those of an experienced operator employing manual TGC controls (Fig. 7.7).

More sophisticated AGC has been developed in which the compensation is better suited to each beam direction. Such systems respond to changing echo patterns more quickly than is possible for an operator using manual controls. Automatic or adaptive techniques are still not widely utilized, but their value is being recognized as their performance is proven in clinical application (Fig. 7.8).

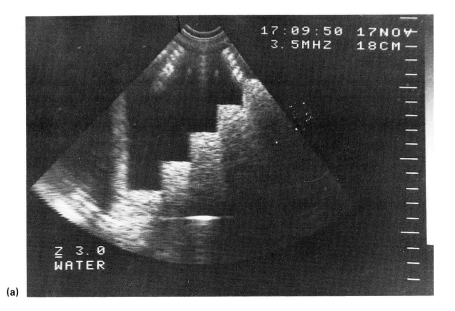

(a)

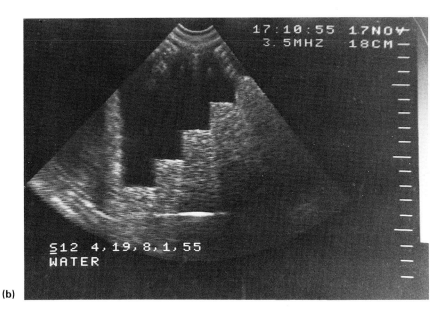

(b)

Fig. 7.7 (**a**) Manual TGC; (**b**) automatic TGC. In the bottom image, saturation is avoided beyond the low attenuation layers of the tissue-mimicking phantom (courtesy of Pye S D).

DISPLAY CONTROLS

We will now consider controls that influence the way in which echoes are presented on a display screen. The operator sets most of these controls at the beginning of an examination. They then need little adjustment. Although display controls are less important than sensitivity controls, they should not be neglected, because they can have a great bearing on the quality of the final results.

Brilliance (intensity of display)

The brilliance of the echo spots on a display screen

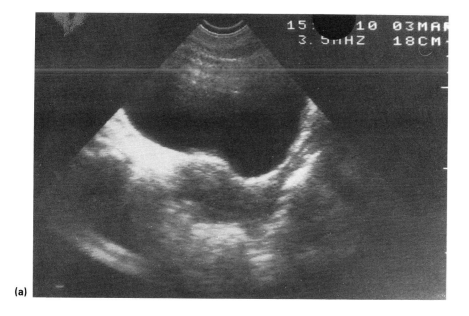

(a)

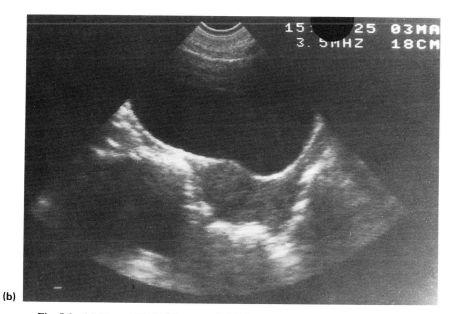

(b)

Fig. 7.8   (a) Manual TGC; (b) automatic TGC (courtesy of Pye S O and Wild S R).

is determined by the size of the electron-beam current in the TV cathode-ray tube. When adjusting the brilliance control, the operator should take care to ensure that it is set neither too high nor too low. Too high a brilliance blots out image detail, whereas weak echoes are not recorded when it is too low. In short, the brilliance control plays a large part in determining the quality of the final image.

Contrast

The contrast control determines the range of brilliance from the weakest to the strongest echo. In a television display, brilliance and contrast are interactive and can present difficulties in the setting-up procedure. They are also usually poorly calibrated, which creates further difficulties. Some displays and most multiformat, film-recording systems have their controls numerically calibrated.

Focus

The electronic focus is best manipulated while echoes are being observed. It should be adjusted to the setting that produces the sharpest trace or the smallest spots. As instruments heat up during use, the focus control may require a final adjustment. In TV-monitor displays, manipulation of the focus may not be feasible by the user and may require the service engineer. In addition to studying the echo presentation, the crispness with which characters are written on the screen is a test of sharpness of focus.

Astigmatism

Some instruments have an astigmatism control that governs the shape of the spot and the uniformity of focus over the whole display screen. Setting up of the astigmatism control involves the optimizing of echo spot sizes in different areas of the display screen. This control normally requires little attention once it has been checked.

Display scale (range selection, time-base)

Display screens used for ultrasonic images are of a variety of dimensions, for example, 4×2 cm to 40×30 cm. On average they are around 20×20 cm. The operator should display the echo information of interest on a scale that allows it to fill the screen. Unnecessarily small images can result in a loss of detail as a result of the finite size of the echo spots.

Normally, for A-scanning, one or two controls allow a large range in the scale of presentation to be selected, for example, from 2 to 50 cm filling the screen. In imaging, the picture can usually be made to expand in a series of discrete steps, for example, 1/4, 2/4, and 4/4 times full life size or even twice or 10 times life size for ophthalmic

applications. Scan-converter units also permit a region in the image of any size to be selected and then enlarged to fill the display screen. This is known as the 'zoom facility'. In some versions of zoom expansion, the selected region is rescanned with a higher line density to give higher resolution.

The terms 'sweep speed' and 'time-base' are sometimes used in connection with the picture scale of old instruments. They relate to the fact that the scale of the presentation is determined by the rate at which the electron beam of the CRT is made to sweep across the screen.

Calibration

To both identify structures and measure their dimensions, the operator must know the scale of the echo patterns. On A-mode, this can be achieved by putting electronic markers at 1-cm tissue intervals on the A-scan trace. Markers separated by intervals of 1 mm are also found. A second way of calibrating an A-scan trace is to superimpose on it two bright spots that can be moved and have their separation altered. The distance between these spots appears on a numeric display. The device designed to do this is called a calliper, since, by placing the spots on the leading edges of two echoes, the thickness of tissue between the echo-producing surfaces can be read from the numeric display.

To calibrate images, one can also use a calliper to locate two movable bright markers at any points on the display screen. A calliper enables accurate measurements to be made. Alternatively, a line of regularly spaced marks at the side of the image is a very convenient way of presenting the scale. Other techniques for the measurement of the length of curved surfaces and cross-sectional areas are described in Chapter 13. During measurement of dimensions from a photographically recorded image, care should be taken to check for any change of image size introduced by the camera.

Rectified and unrectified A-scan display

When the pressure fluctuations of an echo interact with the transducer, a fluctuating voltage appears across the piezoelectric element. If this voltage is amplified and presented on an A-scan display, the trace appears as in Figure 7.9a; this is known as an 'unrectified display'. Such displays are not used much in practice, but are useful for examining echo signals in detail and for making accurate range measurements. In biometry of the eye, accurate measurements can be made by using the same point on each unrectified pulse; for example, where the trace crosses the baseline after the largest amplitude in the pulse.

It is much more common, however, to smooth out the unrectified signal and present an A-scan as a rectified trace (Fig. 7.9b). This can be done by electronically removing the negative parts of the fluctuating voltage, and then smoothing out the larger positive peaks that manage to pass the threshold level of the suppressor. Some instruments allow either rectified or unrectified traces to be displayed.

B-scope display

For a basic B-scope presentation of echo spots, the echo signals are normally rectified and passed

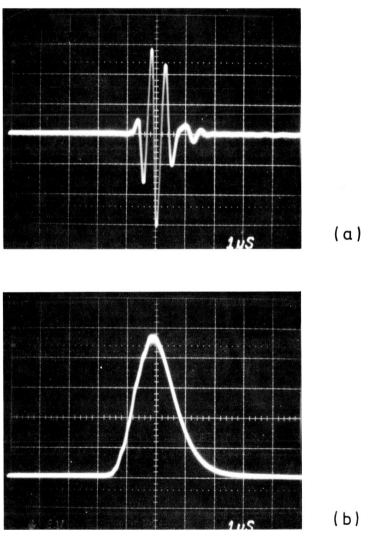

(a)

(b)

Fig. 7.9   (a) Unrectified echo signal, (b) rectified echo signal.

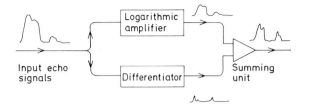

Fig. 7.10 Electronic processing to provide grey shades and emphasize leading edges of signals.

through a video amplifier, which compresses their range of magnitudes to make it suitable for storage and display, as, for example, with a logarithmic amplifier. This is a simple and successful approach. More elaborate processing is also to be found in machines. Figure 7.10 illustrates a technique designed to produce grey shades and emphasize the leading edges of echo signals. The signal is made to pass along two paths. One performs logarithmic compression, and the other performs differentiation; that is, it produces pulses whose heights are a measure of the slope of the signal edges. The two paths are then recombined to give an echo signal with enhanced edges. Full details of the signal processing employed in instruments are rarely revealed by the manufacturers.

Not all scanners store the echo signals after they are rectified and passed through the video amplifier. Some store them as unrectified waveforms (RF signals) or, to be more exact, samples related to the RF waveforms (Ch. 10). All these processing techniques result from the constant striving by manufacturers to improve image quality.

Setting up display controls

Unlike the sensitivity controls, the display controls function independently for the most part. Some attention should be paid to the collective optimization of brilliance, contrast, focus, and camera settings.

The brilliance and contrast of a television display are to some extent interrelated and are, therefore, difficult to optimize exactly. One approach is to turn the controls to a minimum, fully counterclockwise. The brilliance is then increased

until a very faint image appears on the screen. The contrast is then turned up to produce an image with grey tones from bright white to dull grey or black.

Having established the brilliance and contrast levels, the operator should check the focus. Note that alteration of the brilliance or contrast may affect the focus. If the focus cannot be made satisfactorily sharp by adjusting a control the unit should be serviced.

The display from which images are to be recorded may be set up in a similar manner. To obtain the correct exposure of the photographic images, we systematically alter the exposure time, and the most suitable is picked. It is often necessary to vary systematically the brilliance, contrast, and exposure time to find the best combination. The recording of images is further discussed in Chapter 26.

SUMMARY

The operator soon masters the controls of a scanner, which can look daunting at first. There is a strong similarity among the controls of different machines.

1. Controls may be classified into four groups: operational, sensitivity, processing, and display.
2. The sensitivity controls are central to the acquisition of good-quality images. They are frequency, power, overall gain, time-gain compensation (TGC), and suppression. These controls must be used as a related group rather than in isolation.
3. ATGC (adaptive time gain control) was described in several forms.
4. The term 'dynamic range' was defined, and its application to a range of subjects was explained.
5. The decibel notation was introduced for labelling gain, TGC, and power controls. It is merely a convenient way of labelling.
6. Display controls are largely self-explanatory, but their large impact on image quality should always be borne in mind.

Machines are used more profitably if the operator develops an appreciation of how the controls influence the echo signals in their passage through the system.

8. The safety factor in diagnostic ultrasonics

Safety is obviously an important topic for the user of ultrasonic equipment. However, this chapter could be read later if your prime concern is to become familiar with the technical aspects of machines.

INTRODUCTION

We have seen in earlier chapters that tissue is stretched and compressed as an ultrasonic wave passes through it. We have also been very aware of absorption of ultrasonic energy. Since tissue is influenced by the passage and deposition of wave energy, the possibility of harmful effects must be considered. In this chapter, biological effects and safety will be studied from the point of view of the user of imaging and Doppler instruments. Several excellent reviews and books on the whole subject are listed in the reference section at the end of the chapter.

SUMMARY OF ULTRASONIC-OUTPUT PARAMETERS

Many parameters can be employed to specify the transmitted field of a transducer. Indeed, the situation can be somewhat confusing. Fortunately, the users of diagnostic equipment need concern themselves with only about four parameters. This number is unlikely to increase much in the future. One particular quantity which may be introduced is the temperature rise that the field can produce in specific tissues. Temperature rise as an indicator of safety is still under assessment. Figure 8.1 is a representation of an ultrasonic field supplied to aid the understanding of the following definitions of output parameters.

1. The power of an ultrasonic field is the rate of flow of energy through the whole cross-sectional area of the field. It is usually measured in water close to the transducer face. The unit of power is the watt.

2. The intensity at a point in an ultrasonic field is the rate of flow of energy through unit area placed at that point. The unit of intensity is the watt/cm^2.

3. The peak positive-pressure amplitude $(p+)$ is the maximum positive-pressure fluctuation in the wave. The unit of pressure is the pascal.

4. The peak negative-pressure amplitude $(p-)$ is the maximum negative-pressure fluctuation in the wave.

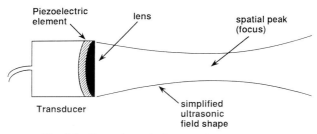

Fig. 8.1 Very schematic diagram of ultrasonic field.

For a continuous wave field, the intensity measured at the spatial peak is commonly quoted; it is labelled 'Isp'. If the intensity at a specified distance from the transducer is averaged across the field, it is called the spatial average intensity (Isa):

Isp — the intensity at the spatial peak.

Isa — the intensity at the specified distance averaged across the cross section of the field.

With pulsed ultrasound, the above definition of intensity still holds, but we must also state whether the instantaneous intensity is being considered or if it is averaged over the time between the pulses. This gives rise to several intensity parameters:

Isptp — the intensity at the spatial peak at the instant when the peak pressure in the pulse passes the point.

Ispta — the intensity at the spatial peak averaged over time.

Isata — the intensity averaged over the cross section of the field and averaged over time.

Isatp — the intensity averaged over the cross section of the field at the instant when the peak pressure in the pulse passes the point.

The most commonly quoted quantities, for example, in safety statements, are Isp for CW ultrasound and Ispta for PW ultrasound. These two quantities are equivalent.

The methods for measuring these quantities should help relate them to physical reality (App. 4). Some typical values are given in Table 8.1. The values for echo-imaging instruments relate to M-scanners and to real-time B-scanners of the mechanical-sector, linear-array, and phased-array types.

Most of these values have been measured and recorded in the literature. Those marked with an asterisk are not available and have been calculated from other related outputs, taking into account the mode of operation of the instruments. The two parameters most appropriate in studies of hazards include:

1. Peak pressure — related to non-thermal effects.

Table 8.1 Pressure, intensity, and power output of diagnostic ultrasonic instruments: pressure (MPa), intensity (mW/cm^2), power (mW). In real-time B-scanning and colour-flow imaging, the beam is moving. Colour-flow imaging values are estimated from PW Doppler values.

	Typical value	Example of high value
Real-time B-scan		
Spatial peak temporal peak positive pressure (Psptp)	3	7
Spatial peak temporal average intensity (Ispta)	20	50
Power	10	80
M-Scan		
Spatial peak temporal peak positive pressure (Psptp)	3	7
Spatial peak temporal average intensity (Ispta)	130	600
Power	5	40
CW Doppler		
Spatial peak pressure(Psp)	0.07	0.12
Spatial peak intensity (Isp)	50	455
Power	10	84
PW Doppler		
Spatial peak temporal peak positive pressure (Psptp)	1	6.5
Spatial peak temporal average intensity (Ispta)	200	1200
Power	20	84
Colour-flow Imaging★		
Spatial peak temporal peak positive pressure (Psptp)	1	6.5
Spatial peak temporal average intensity (Ispta)	10	60
Power	20	84

★Estimated

2. Ispta — related to heating at the focus on the beam axis. The exact relationship between Ispta and temperature is not simple, and factors such as beam width and pulse distortion by non-linear propagation need to be taken into account.

As knowledge is built up of non-thermal effects, the values of peak pressure in diagnostic fields will require to be carefully compared to those which produce bio-effects.

A further complication in the measurement of Ispta is the contribution from neighbouring fields during the scan sweep. In fact, this can more than double the intensity measured as compared to that for a single isolated beam. The accurate measurement of ultrasonic intensity is not a simple matter.

The output levels quoted in Table 8.1 raise some important points. It can be seen that some machines produce intensities (Ispta) above 100 mW/cm^2, a level which for several years has been regarded as a safety threshold, and below which no significant biological effects have been observed. Safety specifications as propounded by several organizations are discussed in more detail later in this chapter. The high outputs of pulsed Doppler units are of particular concern. These outputs are probably due to bad design and to the use of imaging transducers in the Doppler mode for which the transducers lack sensitivity as a result of the damping effect of the backing material. It is known that PW-Doppler units can be made to operate satisfactorily at intensities below 100 mW/cm^2 except, perhaps, in adult cardiological and neurological applications.

THE INTERACTION OF ULTRASOUND AND TISSUE

Ultrasound interacts with tissue in a number of ways which are outlined below. The importance of each of these interaction mechanisms, from the point of view of hazard, has not been established by researchers in the field. Discussions on hazards are often somewhat clouded by a lack of precise knowledge of the mechanisms involved. On the positive side, the lack of knowledge promotes work in a wide range of topics e.g. chromosome damage, blood-coagulation rates, cell-surface behaviour, the immunological system, and the nervous system. In the long run, this is probably desirable in the search for deleterious effects, but, in the short term, it has given rise to a large number of unrelated and often unconfirmed reports. At present, the mechanisms most cited as explanations of bio-effects are heating and cavitation. A few investigations show results which are not thought to be attributable to either of these two, but which are said to result from some direct interaction between the ultrasonic pressure fluctuations and the tissue.

One attractive feature of ultrasound is that repeated low-intensity insonations are not cumulative in their effect, provided that the intensity is below the threshold of possible damage mechanisms. This contrasts with ionizing radiation such as X-rays, of which even low intensities produce some damage and, hence, repeated doses may accumulate significant damage.

Compression and rarefaction

We have seen that as an ultrasonic wave passes through tissue, the material at each point experiences compression and stretching. Atoms are moved distances comparable to their dimensions. This basic wave motion is not often cited as an explanation of a bio-effect; however, it may be one of the 'direct' mechanisms invoked to explain results not attributable to heating or cavitation. Compression and rarefaction have been postulated to give rise to small voltages in bone as a result of the piezoelectric effect. This is a theory offered to explain the healing of bone fractures by ultrasound. Membranes of cells may also be influenced by direct wave action.

Non-linear propagation (shock waves)

In Chapter 3, we studied non-linear propagation of ultrasound and saw that it leads to the pressure waveform becoming distorted and possibly developing a spiked form known as a shock wave. Shock-wave formation readily occurs in liquids, such as water, which exhibit low attenuation. A 3 MHz continuous wave of initial pressure amplitude 1MPa shows a shock waveform after passing through 5 cm of water. Urine in the bladder and amniotic fluid are obviously suitable media for the formation of shock waves. An awareness of the relevance of this phenomenon in diagnostic ultrasound has grown in recent years. The phenomenon may also be present when tissue samples are irradiated through liquid in laboratory experiments. To date, it has not been referred to as a bio-effect mechanism.

Heating

The phenomenon we call 'heat' is the random vibration of atoms and molecules. The heating effect of ultrasound is a consequence of the conversion of the orderly vibrational wave energy into random vibrations. At a relatively high intensity, say, 5 W/cm^2, and at a frequency of 3 MHz, the temperature of tissue can be raised through several degrees Celsius in 2 or 3 minutes. Indeed, similar levels of intensity are used to produce deep heat in therapeutic applications of ultrasound. For many of the intensities used in diagnosis the rises in temperature are, at most, around 1°C and are not thought to produce hazardous effects. Tissues are well able to accommodate temperature variations of these magnitudes. Computational techniques are being developed which may allow us in the future to ascertain the rise in tissue temperature associated with a particular application.

Electrical heating of the transducer has been shown to be large in some instruments and could cause patient discomfort or even injury. This is not an effect of ultrasound on tissue and can easily be checked.

Cavitation

There are two types of cavitation: normal (transient) cavitation and stable cavitation. Normal cavitation occurs readily in liquids when ultrasound of high intensity and low frequency is present; for example, 10 W/cm^2 at 30 kHz. Normal cavitation is a phenomenon in which very small bubbles form at points experiencing the low-pressure half of the wave cycle. The word 'pressure' is not very apt here since the particles of the medium are actually subject to tension resulting from the forces associated with the wave motion pulling them in opposite directions. The very small bubbles which form are located at nu-

clei, i.e. discontinuities in the container or particles in the liquid. During the next half of the wave cycle, the pressure rises, causing the bubbles to collapse and release large amounts of energy. At high frequencies, high intensities are required to produce cavitation; for example, 100 W/cm^2 at 1 MHz. In theory, normal cavitation could be generated by some of the higher intensity pulses used in diagnostic imaging. This has caused increased interest in cavitation as a possible damage mechanism which may act directly or indirectly by generating free chemical radicals in the tissue.

Stable cavitation occurs when small bubbles, which already exist in the medium, grow and resonate as a result of the pressure fluctuations of a wave. A process called 'rectified diffusion' makes them grow more in the low-pressure half of the cycle than they shrink in the high-pressure half. This form of cavitation is not thought to occur with pulsed ultrasound as used in imaging and Doppler beams, since there is not sufficient time for the bubbles to grow. However, it is feasible for it to be produced by a continuous-wave Doppler beam. An exposure duration of at least 2 or 3 ms is considered necessary to create stable cavitation. Its presence in tissue has not been demonstrated for Doppler beams, but there are reports of it being detected in therapeutic beams of 680 mW/cm^2 at 0.75 MHz.

Streaming

Fluid streaming results from the absorption or reflection of ultrasound in complex liquids. When some of the energy of the wave is taken up by absorption in the liquid, the corresponding amount of momentum is also transferred to the liquid. This results in flow of the liquid in the direction of the beam. An equivalent way of looking at this process is that associated with the absorption of energy at a point where there is a change of momentum, which produces a force acting on the liquid at that point. This force, called the 'radiation force' or 'radiation pressure', causes the liquid to flow. Streaming of liquid also commonly accompanies stable cavitation. The flow of liquid can cause shear stresses in molecules and cells, from which damage ensues. However, streaming has not been identified as a source of hazardous effects in the conditions encountered in diagnostic ultrasound.

INTENSITY VERSUS EXPOSURE-TIME

A bio-effect in tissue can often be related to the energy which is deposited in the tissue or passes through it and to the duration of the irradiation. It is, therefore, appropriate to study the combinations of intensity and exposure-time which can produce effects. This can be done by using a diagram of intensity versus exposure-time to show which combinations of values produce effects. Such a plot has been made for tissue from our knowledge of bio-effects (Fig. 8.2). The area defined as the hazard zone corresponds to the higher values of intensity and exposure-time, whereas the safe zone is associated with lower values. The division between these zones is not sharply drawn, but the plot does serve as a guide to acceptable outputs from machines and examination times. It can be seen from the plot that if the intensity (Ispta) is less than 100 mW/cm^2, then there is no reason, apart from prudent practice, to limit the exposure-time.

Recently, it has been shown that some machine outputs have been above the 100 mW/cm^2 level (broken line box). Although this is not a rigidly defined level, it has been recommended by several research workers and scientific organizations. It is possible to design real-time B-scan, A-mode, M-mode, and CW Doppler instruments with output intensities well below the hazard zone. In the case of pulsed Doppler, intensities are often higher and may exceed the 100 mW/cm^2 level, since high PRF values are required. This can be justified only if there is a proven benefit to the patient from a result that cannot be obtained at lower intensity. Further discussion of the output limits recommended by standards organizations is presented later in this chapter.

The above plot has been derived from experiments in which heating is the main agent of effects. We did note, however, that non-thermal effects are of interest at diagnostic levels. Non-thermal effects are likely to relate to the pressure amplitude of the ultrasonic wave. Appropriate plots, in this case, might be pressure amplitude versus exposure-time, or pressure amplitude versus number of pulses. Sufficient data are not yet available to allow such plots to be constructed for non-thermal effects.

STUDIES OF BIO-EFFECTS

There is a large body of literature on the bio-effects of ultrasound. The effect of ultrasound on matter has been studied at a molecular, sub-cel-

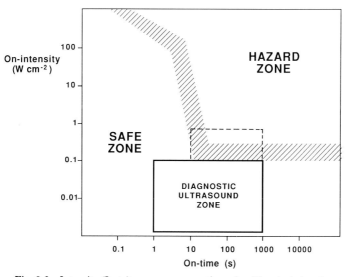

Fig. 8.2 Intensity (Ispta) versus exposure-time plot. The shaded region indicates the lack of a well-defined boundary between the hazard zone and the safe zone.

lular and cellular level. Cells, tissues, and whole animals have been studied in terms of biochemistry, morphology, function, physiology, behaviour, genetics, and epidemiology. It might, therefore, be expected that a reasonable amount of information on possible biological effects of diagnostic ultrasound could be gleaned from these studies. However, most of the work, particularly the high-quality work in which the results have been confirmed, has been carried out at therapeutic energy levels. There is a paucity of results at diagnostic levels. The situation is doubly unfortunate since with ultrasound it is not valid to extrapolate the results obtained at high-intensity levels to low levels. High-energy ultrasonic waves produce more and different effects than do low-energy ones. This contrasts with ionizing radiation, like X-rays, in which the intensity of a beam can be raised by increasing the number of X-ray photons without altering the energy of each individual photon. The biological effects of the photons are therefore not altered.

When one is considering a publication on bio-effects, several questions should be asked to ascertain its relevance and validity:

1. How accurate is the dosimetry?
2. Have the results been confirmed by workers in another centre?
3. How experienced are the workers in the field of bio-effects?
4. Can an unusual result be explained merely by the statistical spread to be expected in the results?
5. Is the ultrasonic exposure similar to that encountered in diagnostic examinations?

Bio-effects of special interest

Among the plethora of bio-effects, a few have assumed particular prominence in the field of hazards. These are chromosome damage, sister chromatid exchange, growth retardation, and abnormalities in the fetus. Sister chromatid exchange (SCE) is the interchange of small equivalent parts in a chromosome in a cell. SCEs occur, to some extent, spontaneously and their significance is not fully understood. Some chemicals can be used to cause SCEs in a controlled way, but, surprisingly, ionizing radiations such as X-rays are not particularly effective.

In the 1970s, chromosome damage was used as an indicator in the search for an effect of ultrasound. Eventually, it was generally concluded that diagnostic intensities did not cause chromosome damage. In the late 1970s, the sister-chromatid-exchange phenomenon was applied to the search for effects. This test is said to be about 100 times more sensitive than the chromosome-damage indicator. Growth retardation and abnormalities have been used for several decades and continue to be used.

At present, there is interest in the possibility that ultrasound causes an increase in the rate of sister chromatid exchanges. Around 20 studies report negative results, that is, no effect due to ultrasound, while about three publications have described a small, but statistically significant, increase. It is worth noting that these investigations have not all been carried out with the same type of cells, and that some workers have used continuous-wave ultrasound while others have used pulsed wave. It is also worth remembering that when a group of negative experimental results are interpreted statistically, a small number (e.g. 1 in 20) will be deduced to be positive owing to the spread in the data. This emphasizes the importance of scientific results being repeated before too much credence is put on them. More work is required on SCEs and their relation to diagnostic ultrasound in vivo. Some workers regard the SCE test as too variable, both within and among laboratories, and that it is less useful than had formerly been supposed.

With therapeutic intensities, growth retardation has been demonstrated in fetal mice and rats, as has the induction of abnormalities. It has also been possible to establish the dependence of fetal weight reduction on exposure for these levels of ultrasound. Extrapolation of this dependence to diagnostic levels shows that the fetal weight reduction would be expected to be low at intensities below 100 mW/cm^2 and perhaps not significant. Although around 80 reports exist for this aspect of bio-effects, many of them are incomplete, and further work is required to clarify the results and extend them to the diagnostic field.

Epidemiological reports

The acid test for the safety of ultrasound is to survey the population for effects. Unfortunately, this is very difficult to do since matched groups of people are required for comparisons. These groups should be matched for age, health status, social class, etc. Since the application of diagnostic ultrasound is so widespread, it is becoming increasingly difficult to arrange patients in groups, one of which is a control group not exposed to ultrasound.

The second main difficulty is the problem of detecting a small increase in the rate of an effect which already occurs spontaneously without irradiation by ultrasound. To detect such an increase, one must examine fairly large numbers of patients. For example, if an effect occurred naturally at a rate of 4% (i.e. 4 per 100 normals) and ultrasound increased it to 5%, just over 1000 patients would need to be studied to detect this increase. If ultrasound increased the rate to only 4.5%, about 4500 patients would be required. All of the early surveys lacked sufficient patient numbers, and the results are therefore questionable from a statistical point of view.

Larger surveys are now being attempted and initial findings are being published. They have not revealed any deleterious effects of diagnostic ultrasound. It is to be hoped that it is not too late to find unexposed control groups and that randomized clinical trials of adequate size can be arranged. The random allocation of patients into the exposed and unexposed groups is essential if the results are not to be hopelessly biased. This bias arises because patients with problems or a difficult obstetrical history inevitably end up in the exposed group. Several workers in the field doubt if it is still possible to carry out a large-scale trial on the safety of ultrasound.

A third problem is deciding what effects to look for. Obviously an effect may be missed if it is not considered, or if it is very subtle. Likewise, it may be missed if it is delayed and takes years to manifest itself.

A fourth difficulty is associated with the rapid change of ultrasonic techniques. Results gathered over several years are likely to be related to different types of scanning machine. The dosimetry of earlier years is also likely to be inadequate.

We can be sure that diagnostic ultrasound does not cause gross effects since such effects have a low natural rate of occurrence, and any increase due to ultrasound would have been detected by some of the surveys carried out.

Conclusions on bio-effects field

A number of conclusions can be drawn from the work carried out so far in the field of bio-effects.

1. The most relevant experiments from the point of view of diagnostic application are those performed in vivo, preferably on mammals.

2. In-vitro studies are only indicators for future in-vivo investigations and do not provide direct evidence of hazard. This is due to the fact that some interaction mechanisms can occur much more readily in vitro than in vivo; cavitation, streaming, and non-linear propagation are all more likely if cells or tissue are suspended in liquid.

3. Studies at intensities higher than those used in diagnosis are also only indicators for future research.

4. Very little information exists on intensity or duration thresholds for interaction mechanisms.

5. Non-thermal effects are of particular interest for diagnostic ultrasound.

6. The selection of subjects for bio-effect research seems to be almost random. More concentration on the embryo and fetus is highly desirable.

7. The pitfalls and complexities of interpretation in biology and the difficulties of ultrasonic dosimetry mean that work should be attempted only in well-equipped laboratories by experienced scientists.

8. Users of equipment need pay attention only to results which have been confirmed in other laboratories.

9. If possible, more work should be done on the epidemiology of ultrasound.

A few references and textbooks on this subject are listed at the end of the chapter.

SURVEYS OF THE HAZARDS LITERATURE

In recent years many organizations have conducted surveys of the literature on hazards and issued reports and statements on the subject. Concern about hazards has been worldwide, as witnessed by the range of organizations involved, namely the World Health Organization, the Japanese Society of Ultrasonics in Medicine, the American Institute of Ultrasound in Medicine, the National Institute of Health, the Royal College of Obstetricians and Gynaecologists, the National Council on Radiation Protection and Measurements, the European Federation of Societies for Ultrasound in Medicine and Biology, the US Food and Drug Administration, and others. Some excellent reviews have also been produced by individuals and research groups. Each body has approached the subject from its own particular point of view. However, they have largely come to the same conclusions. The main conclusions may be summarized as follows:

1. There have been no confirmed deleterious effects on mammalian tissue from ultrasound as used in diagnosis.

2. Ultrasonic techniques should be used where there is indication of benefit to the patient. Most, but not all, organizations advise against routine scanning of all patients since some unconfirmed laboratory studies of animals suggest the possibility of reduced birth weight caused by ultrasound.

3. There is a need for more work on potential hazards with ultrasonic exposures as found in diagnostic applications. Unfortunately, it has become almost impossible to carry out epidemiological studies as a result of the difficulty of finding unexposed control populations. Only a handful of such studies have been attempted, and they almost all suffer from insufficient patient numbers, a defect which makes them statistically inadequate.

4. Operators should be trained to use the lowest exposure which will provide a diagnosis.

5. Demonstrations on volunteers are not recommended by some reports.

6. Manufacturers should give information on machine outputs.

7. Studies should be undertaken to establish the benefits of ultrasonic techniques.

References for these reports are quoted at the end of this chapter.

From time to time, the American Institute for Ultrasound in Medicine (AIUM) has issued statements on aspects of safety, the most central, which is quoted below, was approved in 1987.

'In the low megahertz frequency range there have been (as of this date) no independently confirmed significant biological effects in mammalian tissues exposed in vivo to unfocused ultrasound with intensities[*] below $100 mW/cm^2$, or to focused[**] ultrasound with intensities below $1 W/cm^2$. Furthermore, for exposures times[***] greater than 1 second and less than 500 seconds for unfocused ultrasound or 50 seconds for focused ultrasound, such effects have not been demonstrated even at higher intensities, when the product of intensity and exposure-time is less than 50 joules/cm^2.'

It is worth bearing in mind that this statement is based mostly on data that relates to other mammals rather than to man, and to continuous rather than pulsed ultrasound. The statement is not intended to imply complete safety for every possible application. In addition, the data used to prepare the statement did not necessarily show minimum levels which can produce effects. As more sensitive tests are developed, it may be necessary to reduce the values quoted in the statement. The 6 dB beam width of less than 4 wavelengths represents quite a high degree of focusing, e.g. 2 mm at 3 MHz, which is not achieved by all pulsed-Doppler or echo-imaging instruments. Higher intensities are permitted with strong focusing since heat passes more quickly from the small focal region.

From the above, it can be seen that continuous-

---

[*]Free-field spatial peak, temporal average (SPTA) for continuous wave exposures, and for pulsed-mode exposures with pulses repeated at a frequency greater than 100 Hz.
[**]Quarter-power (-6 db) beam width smaller than four wavelengths or 4 mm, whichever is less at the exposure frequency.
[***]Total time including off-time as well as on-time for repeated pulse exposures.

wave Doppler units, the fields of which are not normally highly focused, should be designed to have an output intensity as far below 100 mW/cm² as is compatible with good performance. Similarly, pulsed-Doppler and echo-imaging instruments which are not highly focused should have an intensity below this value. A glance at Table 8.2 will show that, at present, this is sadly not the case, as many manufacturers have utilized increased intensity as a means of improving performance.

We can see from Table 8.1 that a real-time B-scanner with its beam moving is likely to have an intensity (Ispta) well below 100 mW/cm². However, when the beam is stopped in M-mode, this is not necessarily the case. The slower scanning action of static B-scanners means that the intensity levels have to be considered carefully. There have been several instances of B-scanner outputs exceeding the recommended Ispta.

The AIUM statement also refers to a lack of observed effects at higher intensities, provided the exposure-time is between 1 and 500 seconds, and the product of the intensity and exposure-time is less than 50 joules/cm²; i.e.

intensity (Ispta) × exposure-time <50 joules/cm²

This actually allows high intensities to be employed, provided the exposure-time is kept short. For example 2 W/cm² could be employed for up to 25 s since the product of these two quantities would remain below 50 joules/cm² for such a range of exposure-times.

The 1 second lower exposure-time mentioned in the statement is included, since if a very short time was used in the intensity–exposure–time product, it would appear that it is safe to use a very high intensity since the product could be below 50 joules/cm². This is obviously not the case, since then cavitation might occur.

In 1985, the US Food and Drug Administration drew up a guide which allows the supply of equipment with output intensities above the 100 mW/cm² limit. The permitted level depends on the application (Table 8.2). These new levels allow for the attenuation in tissue and specify the permitted *in situ* (also called 'derated') intensity levels at typical depths for each application. The equivalent 'in water' values, which are the more

Table 8.2 Provisional values of intensity (mW/cm²) quoted by the US Food and Drug Administration. The *in situ* ('derated') values allow for typical attenuation in the applications quoted. The corresponding values in water assume no attenuation.

Use	Ispta (*in situ*)	Ispta (in water)
Cardiac	430	730
Peripheral vessel	720	1500
Ophthalmic	17	68
Fetal imaging and other★	94	180

★Abdominal, intra-operative, paediatric, small organ (breast, thyroid, testes), neonatal cephalic, adult cephalic.

common way of specifying outputs, are seen to be greater than 100 mW/cm². Another consideration behind the new FDA limits is that no new machine should have an output greater than those in use prior to 28 May 1976, the 'pre-enactment date'. A fairly simple calculation allows the *in situ* values to be obtained from the 'in water' measurements. This guidance has been the subject of much debate and is now being reconsidered. It may well be that new guidance will be forthcoming based on the ALARA principle which is widely used for ionizing radiations. ALARA is an abbreviation for 'as low as reasonably achievable'. With this approach, the operator can use the output intensity or pressure amplitude that will enable a clinical diagnosis to be made.

The British Medical Ultrasound Society favours the retention of the 100 mW/cm² limit, since equipment can be designed within this limit for most applications except, perhaps, cardiac and neurological examinations in adults. This approach probably also preserves a separation between diagnostic intensities and those at which significant bio-effects occur. Because of the increasing interest in cavitation as a possible damage mechanism, this society has put forward provisional limits on the wave-pressure amplitude, positive and negative, of 4 MPa. This limit may be more exactly justified or altered in the future, but, at present, it is based on the fact that machines of good performance can operate within this limit.

The European Federation of Societies for Ultrasound in Medicine and Biology has a Radiation Safety Committee which constantly scrutinizes the scientific literature. Safety statements are issued annually. To date, no deleterious effects have been reported with diagnostic ultrasound.

REDUCTION OF PATIENT EXPOSURE

Role of the operator

By judicious use of a scanner, the operator can greatly reduce the total amount of ultrasonic energy transmitted into the patient.

1. Check that the instrument transmits acceptable intensities below those currently recommended as upper limits by standards organizations.

2. Use the lowest transmitted power possible. If a choice is available, high gain rather than high power should be employed to achieve high sensitivity. Some machines are designed with the receiving amplifier fixed at high gain and with a variable ultrasonic power output.

3. Use the minimum duration of examination.

4. With a pulsed-Doppler unit, use, if possible, the lowest PRF which will measure the highest velocity of interest at the selected depth. In many units, the PRF is related automatically to the depth selected for the sample volume, so the operator has little control over it.

5. With M-mode, use the lowest PRF which will allow fast edges on the trace to be recorded.

6. Use a low frame rate, provided this does not increase the line density.

7. Do not leave the transducer resting on the patient.

8. Check to see that the transducer ceases transmission when the image is frozen.

With these guidelines, it is feasible to reduce the average intensity by a factor as large as 1000 from that which is possible as a result of careless practice. The peak pulse pressure can typically be reduced by a factor of 20.

Role of the equipment designer

The designer plays a very large part in determining the power transmitted into the patient. A recent survey of echo-imaging instruments showed a range of beam intensity from 0.02 to 440 mW/cm^2 (Ispta). For pulsed-Doppler units the range was 40 to 4000 mW/cm^2. The purchaser should remember that high output levels may be the result of poor design.

Role of the quality controller

Obviously, a well-maintained machine will give results more quickly and, hence, reduce the duration of the examination. It is not uncommon for the performance of a machine to decrease with age. This may be unconsciously compensated for by the use of higher power.

Selection of scanner and technique

The intensities of fields from mechanical-sector, linear-array, and phased-array, real-time scanners are very similar. As regards safety, there is no benefit to be gained from choosing among them.

In static B-scanning, the transmitted pulse rate, i.e. the PRF, is about one-fifth that of a real-time B-scanner. The average intensity of ultrasound in the patient is, therefore, also about one-fifth. However, in B-scanning the scan action is less smooth, and some tissues are irradiated more than others. The examination times are also longer in B-scanning. From the point of view of safety, there is little to chose between the two techniques.

When an M-mode scan is selected, the beam is held fixed in one direction. The PRF in that direction may be 20 times that of the real-time scan, so the average intensity is 20 times higher. A machine should not be left transmitting an M-mode beam into a patient for longer than is necessary.

The output intensities of CW-Doppler instruments are low, and any possible hazard is likely to arise from the duration of the irradiation rather than the intensity. Stable cavitation is an example of a tissue-interaction mechanism which normally requires a continuous irradiation of at least several milliseconds to get established.

Pulsed-Doppler techniques in which the beam is placed in one direction have high average intensities. Their duration should be limited to that required to obtain the clinical data. The blood flowing through the beam spends less time in it than the static tissue.

PW-Doppler flow-imaging machines alter their beam direction at a uniform rate and, therefore, in any one direction have average intensities about 1/20 of that of the corresponding PW fixed-beam instruments. Flow-imaging machines are not of major concern from the point of view of hazard.

QUESTIONS AND ANSWERS ON SAFETY

Q1. Is the technique safe for the patient?

A1. If the output intensity, pressure amplitude, and exposure-time are within guidelines provided by several national organizations, then diagnostic ultrasound is a safe technique.

Q2. Is the technique safe for the operator?

A2. Yes.

Q3. If there is a possibility of hazard, for example, when it is considered necessary to use high-intensity or insonate sensitive tissue, how can the risk be minimized?

A3. Minimize the exposure-time and use CW- rather than PW-Doppler if it will give a result.

Q4. From present knowledge, what output intensities are acceptable?

A4. If possible, use less than 100 mW/cm^2 (Ispta) measured in water. Otherwise, keep within the guidelines laid down by the FDA and the AIUM. Little consideration has been given to pressure amplitude in safety documents. It appears that the pressure amplitudes should be less than 4 MPa.

Q5. What duration of examination is acceptable?

A5. This depends on the examination, but the British Medical Ultrasound Society has suggested the times presented in Table 8.3 as reasonable for obstetric scanning.

Q6. When studying hazard literature, what results are directly relevant to safety?

A6. In-vivo results relating to diagnostic intensities, pressure amplitudes, exposure-times, frequencies, and pulse lengths. Results obtained using regimes which do not closely resemble conditions encountered in diagnosis can be regarded only as indicators for future studies.

Q7. Has each new technique been optimized for safety?

Table 8.3 Maximum examination times recommended by the British Medical Ultrasound Society for obstetrics scanning.

Single fetal measurement	5 minutes
Routine antenatal scan to confirm viable intra-uterine pregnancy, assess gestational age, detect early pregnancy failure, detect twins, image fetal abnormalities	10 minutes
Fetal anatomy survey	15 minutes

A7. This is not always the case, but most can be adjusted to bring the exposures within guidelines.

Q8. Are Doppler techniques as safe as pulsed-echo imaging?

A8. The high intensities caused by the high PRF values of some PW-Doppler units can give cause for concern with regard to heating of tissue. The high-pressure amplitudes in focused beams from some instruments require further study. Within the published guidelines, both techniques appear to be safe.

Q9. Can I justify the use of high intensity?

A9. If the product of intensity and exposure-time is less than 50 joules/cm^2 and the exposure-time is in the range 1–500 seconds for unfocused, or 1–50 seconds for focused, it can be justified. Otherwise, a very clear benefit to the patient or a good lawyer are required.

SUMMARY

1. Parameters which describe CW and PW fields were presented. The best parameters for the specification of safe usage have still not been categorically identified, since all possible hazard mechanisms are not known.

2. The user of an ultrasonic instrument should know the maximum intensity produced by the transducer selected. Isp should be known for a CW unit and Ispta for a pulsed one.

3. If possible, the peak positive and negative pressure amplitudes should be known (Psp for CW, Psptp for PW).

4. In the future, induced temperature rises in tissue for each instrument may become available.

5. A working knowledge of the outputs of different types of machine should be acquired.

6. Five ways in which ultrasound interacts with tissue were discussed.

7. Examination of an 'intensity versus exposure-time' plot, derived from the limited data available, showed that 100 mW/cm^2 is a desirable upper limit for output intensity (Isp or Ispta).

8. The reader should keep up with current opinion on bio-effects.

9. Epidemiological studies are most relevant to the question of safety. Unfortunately, they are becoming difficult to undertake.

10. Several organizations throughout the world put out safety statements at regular intervals.

11. The exposure of the patient may be substantially reduced by prudent use of the technique.

REFERENCES

American Institute of Ultrasound in Medicine 1988 Bioeffects considerations for the safety of diagnostic ultrasound. J Ultrasound Med 7: No 9 (suppl)

British Institute of Radiology 1987 The safety of diagnostic ultrasound. Brit J Radiol No 20 (suppl)

British Medical Ultrasound Society 1988 Prudent use of diagnostic ultrasound. Bulletin No 50, London

Lyons E A 1986 Human epidemiological studies. Ultrasound Med Biol 12: 689–691

National Council on Radiation Protection and Measurements 1983 Biological effects of ultrasound: Mechanisms and clinical implications. Report No 74, Bethesda, Md.

Nyborg W L and Ziskin M C (eds) 1985 Biological effects of ultrasound. Churchill Livingstone, New York

Royal College of Obstetricians and Gynaecologists 1984 Report of the RCOG Working Party on routine ultrasound examination in pregnancy. London

ter Haar G R 1986 Assessment of possible hazard in use. In: Hill C K (ed) Physical principles of medical ultrasonics, Ch. 14. Ellis Horwood, Chichester, England

Williams A R 1983 Ultrasound: Biological effects and potential hazards. Academic Press, London

9. A-scan instruments performance and use

Clinical interest in the A-scan mode is very limited. This mode can be used in anatomy when the tissue boundaries are clearly defined; for example, in the detection of midline shifts in the brain and for ophthalmologic examinations. The A-scan mode is also of some interest as the only presentation in which we see echo signals in an almost unprocessed form. It can therefore give us an appreciation of the reflecting powers of tissue boundaries, and it can also illustrate the way echo signals are handled in any pulse-echo instrument such as a basic real-time B-scanner or M-scan unit.

The A-scan facility is encountered either as a stand-alone instrument or as a mode of operation of an imaging machine.

FEATURES OF A-SCAN INSTRUMENTS

The basic instrumentation for performing A-scanning includes one or two hand-held transducers, an electronic processing-and-display unit, and a camera. A photograph of an A-scan instrument for locating the midline of the brain is shown in Figure 9.1a. An instrument designed for eye work is shown in Figure 9.1b. Such instruments are used in ophthalmology for measuring the dimensions of the ocular structures and assessing the nature of tissue masses.

Two transducers are normally supplied with A-scan instruments for head scanning using the transmission mode. Transmission-mode scanning is a procedure in which one transducer on one side of the head transmits an ultrasonic pulse, and a second transducer, coupled to the other side, detects this pulse on completion of a transit through the head. This allows the direction of the

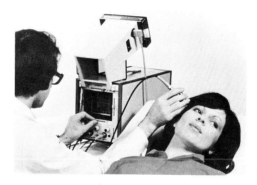

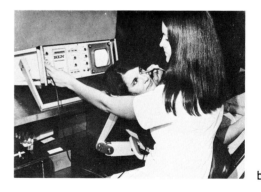

Fig. 9.1 (a) A-scan instrument for head examination, (b) A-scan instrument for eye examination (courtesy of Kretz).

ultrasound beam through the head to be ascertained. For adult-head studies, two transducers, similar to that shown in Figure 1.3 and operating at a frequency of 1.5 MHz, are suitable. For examining the infant head, where the attenuation caused by bone is less, two transducers of about 2.5 MHz frequency are used. Transducers for eye work operate at high frequencies, 7 to 15 MHz; they have been constructed in a variety of forms.

COMPONENT PARTS OF A-SCAN INSTRUMENTS

Let us now briefly consider the functions of the component parts of an A-scan instrument. Figure 9.2 is a block diagram of a basic A-scan unit. It is worth considering the production of echo data by an A-scan unit, since the same technique is employed by real-time B-scan and M-mode instruments.

The start-pulse generator triggers off the system by producing an electronic pulse that is fed simultaneously to the high-voltage pulse generator and the TGC generator. This pulse causes each of these units to perform its specific function. The high-voltage pulse generator applies an excitation pulse to the transducer element; for example, one of 300 V amplitude and 0.5 μs duration. This shocks the piezoelectric element into a short burst of mechanical vibration. An ultrasonic pulse is thus generated and is propagated into the body.

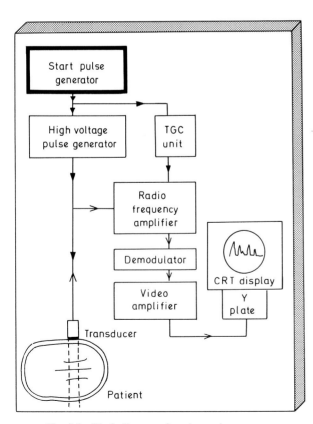

Fig. 9.2   Block diagram of an A-scan instrument.

Echoes returned to the transducer cause small fluctuating voltages to appear across the element. Since these voltages are typically of the order of millivolts or less, they must be amplified so that they will register on a display system. The first stage of amplification is performed by a radio-frequency (RF) amplifier, which is capable of handling frequencies in the MHz range. The output of this amplifier is typically a few volts. We noted in the discussions of TGC, however, that it is not desirable to amplify all echo signals equally. The output of the TGC generator, which is triggered by the start pulse, is applied to the amplifier to hold its gain low initially, and then to allow the gain to rise later when echoes from greater depths are being received.

The amplified echo signals pass to the demodulator, where the echo signals are rectified and smoothed to produce voltage pulses of a non-oscillatory shape. Small echo signals may be suppressed at this stage. Finally, the echoes are amplified to tens of volts by the video amplifier to make them suitable for application to the Y-plates of the display CRT.

A third course taken by the start pulse is to the time-base, where it causes a steadily rising voltage to be produced. This voltage is applied to the X-plates of the display tube, causing the electron beam to sweep across the phosphor of the display screen. The rate of sweep of the spot across the screen can be varied by altering the rate of rise of the time-base voltage. On moving across the screen, the spot is deflected temporarily from its baseline when echo signals are received and applied to the Y-plates.

An A-scan trace is, thus, the result of a number of units functioning simultaneously. The complete process is performed in less than 1 ms and is repeated at the rate of generation of the start pulses, the pulse-repetition frequency (PRF) of the instrument.

RECORDING A-SCANS

A-scans are normally recorded with a Polaroid camera but occasionally a 35 mm film camera is used. A suitable camera has a large lens aperture and a range of exposure times from 1/125 to 1 s. A hood attachment that allows viewing of the screen while the photograph is being taken is also desirable.

Exposure settings

Since the operator can manipulate the brilliance of the displayed pattern, it is not possible to specify particular settings that give optimum results. The brilliance and the camera settings that give the best results are ascertained by trial and error. For example, with Polaroid film and a low brilliance, an aperture of f3.5 and an exposure time of 0.1 s should produce a good-quality result. Increasing the brilliance would require a reduction in the aperture, for example, to f8, or a shorter exposure time. It is difficult, in practice, to obtain a clear record of both the leading edges of echo signals in an A-scan trace and the baseline. They appear with different brilliances on the display screen, since the spot is being rapidly deflected at leading edges. Many display screens also have a fixed graticule in front that can be illuminated to superimpose a measuring grid on to the photographic print.

Camera focus

To check the focus, the operator can insert a ground-glass screen, supplied for this purpose, into the back of the camera where the Polaroid film is normally situated. With the lens shutter open, a faint image of the echo pattern is observed on this screen. Adjustment of the focus is achieved by releasing the locking screws on the camera-supporting structure and moving the lens and film holder with respect to the CRT screen. With a typical oscilloscope camera, sharp focusing is obtained for a range of movement of about 0.5 cm when the lens aperture is wide open.

Cameras for 35 mm film are usually supplied with focusing instructions that permit them to be focused *in situ* while loaded with film. Failing that, the operator can use a ground-glass screen technique.

Photographic film

Good-quality ultrasonic images are obtained using Polaroid film packs that fit into a special holder on the oscilloscope camera. The pack gives 8 black-and-white prints (7.25 × 9.5 cm) on high-speed (3000 ASA), high-contrast film. Mishaps can occur in Polaroid photography, but are easily avoided if their cause is recognized (see Ch. 26). A suitable 35 mm film speed is around 400 ASA. The 35 mm film is economical and convenient for recording a large number of images, but it takes time to develop.

AUTOMATIC MIDLINE-SHIFT DETECTOR

Operator bias is not easily removed from an A-scan determination of the midline of the brain. In an attempt to remove operator bias and to ensure that a series of measurements is made, fully automatic, midline-shift detectors have been developed. The operator of such an instrument does not observe echo patterns on a CRT screen but, instead, carries out a set procedure several times. From each individual procedure, one data point is obtained for a histogram, which ultimately builds up to indicate the position of the midline. It is only at this point that a decision is made about the possibility of a midline shift.

This type of instrument may run into difficulties when midbrain structures have been altered. The spread then obtained in the histogram alerts the operator to this possibility. When injury hinders readings from both sides of the head, acceptable histograms can still be obtained. The midline can be usually located to within 4 mm.

A-SCAN PROCEDURE

The procedure for A-scanning has much in common with other ultrasonic imaging modes. The operator selects a transducer of suitable size, frequency, and beam pattern, and sets the sensitivity controls at familiar baseline positions. The display scale is next adjusted to present the whole range of interest, with attention paid to the scale calibration because mistakes might occur if the scale of display is not fully appreciated. A quick check of the display controls, that is, brilliance and focus, and of the camera settings is also worthwhile at this stage.

It is important to remember that echoes of many sizes are incident on the transducer crystal. As discussed in Chapter 7, an acceptable echo pattern is obtained by closely observing the display screen and manipulating one or two controls. With practice, the operator can soon predict the changes resulting from specific control adjustments.

One factor, which has not, so far, been mentioned and which plays an important part in obtaining good results is the amount of searching for and interpreting of echo patterns that is necessary to direct the beam through the specific tissues to be studied. We will see that this necessity occurs in many ultrasonic scanning techniques. The operator is involved in manipulating the instrument and simultaneously relating the results to the tissue anatomy.

Later in this chapter, we will discuss techniques for measuring both the distance between echoes and their magnitudes. Care must be taken in making deductions from A-scan traces, and artefacts associated with the technique must be clearly understood.

RESOLUTION IN A-SCANNING

In A-scanning, the aim is to detect surfaces that lie one behind another. The fundamental question therefore arises: 'What is the minimum separation of two surfaces that gives rise to two identifiable echo signals?' In other words, we are interested in the resolution attainable.

Resolution is determined as follows. Imagine two surfaces lying one behind the other and producing echoes as illustrated in Figure 9.3a. Each produces an echo of finite length, and, because the surfaces are far apart, the displayed signals are widely separated. When the two surfaces are moved closer together, there comes a point when the displayed signals merge, and it is difficult to know if there are two echoes or a single large one (Fig. 9.3b). The separation, d, of the surfaces for which two echoes can just be identified is called the 'resolution' of the system. As the distances involved are in a direction along the ultrasonic beam, this resolution is called the 'axial', 'range', or 'linear' resolution of the system.

The A-scan illustrates clearly that axial resolution thus depends on the ultrasonic pulse length. In theory, it is equal to half the pulse length. From Figure 9.3, it is evident that if the echo pulses are

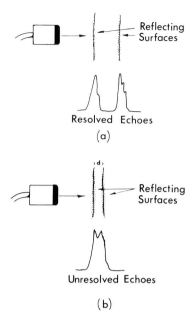

Fig. 9.3 Resolution in A-scanning.

long, the displayed echoes will merge for larger values of d. To have good axial resolution, it is therefore necessary to generate short pulses. Pulse length, in fact, depends on the design of the transducer and the frequency of the ultrasound. In routine practice, only the frequency can readily be altered. The higher the frequency, the easier it is to make the pulse length short and, hence, the better the axial resolution. Table 9.1 gives the typical values of axial resolution that can be achieved in practice, and, therefore, an appreciation of the minimum separation of surfaces for which echo signals can be resolved.

Another relevant point is that as displayed echoes increase in height they also increase in length, as the tail portions become more significant. For optimum axial resolution, the highest

Table 9.1 Typical values of resolution achievable in practice with A-scanning

Frequency (MHz)	Axial resolution (mm)
1	4.6
2	2.3
5	0.9
10	0.5
15	0.3
25	0.2

frequency that will give the necessary penetration should be employed, and the sensitivity settings adjusted so that the echo signals are not unduly large.

Note that although the distance of a small reflector from the transducer face can be ascertained fairly accurately, its distance from the central axis of the beam is not so well specified. For any measured range from the transducer, the reflector may be laterally situated anywhere in the cross section of the beam.

MEASUREMENT OF DISTANCE FROM AN A-SCAN TRACE

Time-to-distance conversion

Dimensions of tissues can be most accurately measured using an A-scan display, since individual echoes are clearly presented and the pattern of signals corresponds to one direction through the structures.

Earlier, we noted that the echo go–return time is converted into distance by assuming a velocity of ultrasound in tissue (Ch. 1). Most measurements are made assuming an average velocity of sound in tissue close to 1540 m/s. For greater accuracy in specific tissues, more exact values of velocity are used for the conversion. When measuring eye length, the times are measured between the echoes from each interface. The length of each component part of the eye, such as the anterior and vitreous chambers or the lens, is calculated using the appropriate velocity of sound for each medium.

Accuracy of measurement

Measurements from A-scan traces are made from the leading edge of the first pulse to the leading edge of the second. The leading edges are chosen since they are well-defined parts of the pulse. The leading edge of the transmission pulse corresponds to the front face of the crystal, and measurement of depth is made from that point.

The unrectified signal is a more accurate representation of the echo signal than is the rectified video signal, and it is used in precise measurement. Examples of suitable points in the pulse

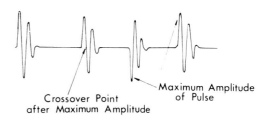

Fig. 9.4   Measurement points on an unrectified trace.

from which to measure are the position of the largest amplitude in the pulse, or the point where the oscillatory signal crosses the baseline on either side of the largest amplitude (Fig. 9.4). Note that in selecting the largest amplitude, only the magnitude matters, not whether it is positive or negative. A large positive amplitude can be changed to a large negative amplitude on reflection at a tissue interface, or vice versa. This occurs when a pulse travelling in a medium of a particular acoustic impedance is reflected at an interface with a medium of lower acoustic impedance. Unrectified displays of A-scan traces are not widely used except in ophthalmology.

The question of the best accuracy that can be achieved with ultrasonic techniques has no easy answer. With an unrectified display and a perfectly flat surface, measurement can be made to within a fraction of a wavelength, for example, $\lambda/20$, if the beam strikes the surface perpendicularly. Such accuracy only arises, in practice, in a few highly specialized experimental systems; normally, measurements made to within plus or minus one wavelength would be considered very accurate. Table 9.2 gives the wavelength of frequencies commonly used in soft tissue. Measurements of eye structures can be made to 0.05 mm, and those of the biparietal diameter of

Table 9.2   Wavelengths and related frequencies in soft tissue

Frequency (MHz)	Wavelength (mm)
1	1.54
2	0.77
5	0.31
10	0.15
15	0.10
25	0.06

fetal heads to 1 mm. However, note that the main factors that usually limit accuracy are those associated with the practicalities of making the measurements, not those connected with the basic physics.

MEASUREMENT OF ECHO SIZE

Factors that determine the size of echo signal on an A-scan display or in an image are:

1. The change in acoustic impedance at the tissue interface
2. The shape of the target
3. The position of the target in the beam
4. The attenuation of the transmitted and reflected pulse
5. The electronic processing of the echo signal

It is therefore difficult, but, nevertheless, possible, to get information regarding the nature of the reflector from its echo size. In certain applications, tissues can be differentiated by accurately measuring echo size. Probably the most successful field of application is in identifying tissue masses in the ocular system; for example, cysts, haemorrhages, and tumours. In liver scanning, the mean echo height has been studied as a source of diagnostic information. Finally, the change produced in an echo pattern for a specific change in the sensitivity controls can provide information. Attempts have also been made to use this technique to study tissue lesions, such as those of the breast.

For the operator to make deductions from echo magnitudes, a standardized technique for adjusting the sensitivity controls is essential. One method is to fix most of the sensitivity controls at a well-defined baseline for the particular examination and to use just one, for example, the gain, as a variable. The gain setting noted is that required to make the echo from a surface at a particular tissue depth appear as a specified size on the display screen. This value of gain is a measure of the reflecting power of the interface. For example, a weakly reflecting surface near the retina of the eye may require 90 dB of gain to produce a signal of the specified height on the display, whereas a strongly reflecting interface may need only 50 dB to be presented at the same height.

In attempts to make results independent of the type of instrument used, several investigators compare the echoes from tissue with those from a standard reflecting interface. A popular reflector is a flat glass plate placed in oil or water at a fixed distance from the transducer. Care is taken to ensure that the beam strikes the plate perpendicularly in order to give the maximum echo signal. The gain setting required to make this standard echo signal a particular size on the display is compared with that required to make a tissue echo of the same size.

LIMITATIONS OF A-SCANNING

One-dimensional nature

One of the main limitations of A-scanning is that only echoes from surfaces lying on one line through the body are displayed simultaneously. This can be partly overcome by systematically examining a number of directions and thus accumulating knowledge of the anatomy.

Identification of reflecting surfaces

As might be expected with such a limited scanning technique, it is difficult to establish the precise relationship of the echoes with their associated tissue interfaces.

Specular reflection of ultrasound

Some A-scan techniques depend on detecting clear and strong echoes from dominant structures. Since the scan is only along one line, not all the surfaces to be recorded may intersect the ultrasonic beam at a suitable angle.

ARTEFACTS IN A-SCANNING

Like other imaging techniques, ultrasonic scanning can produce erroneous results from artefacts. While artefacts are not a major problem, it is as well to be aware that they can affect the echo pattern. Artefacts are discussed at length in Chapter 15. The following are pertinent to A-scanning and can be studied in Chapter 15:

1. Refraction
2. Multiple reflection (reverberation)

3. Shadowing
4. Converse of shadowing (echo enhancement)
5. High- or low-velocity layers
6. Beam-width artefact
7. Transducer-defect artefacts
8. Electronic-processing artefacts
9. Lack of coupling medium

SUMMARY

The A-scan mode is used in only a limited number of clinical applications. However, it does demonstrate the basic process of echo collection. The following features were discussed:

1. The component parts of the A-scan instrument — transducer, electronic transmitter and receiver, CRT display, camera.

2. The concept of axial resolution was introduced and shown to depend on pulse length. We shall meet this component of resolution in imaging techniques.

3. Measurement with an A-scan device was shown to be accurate if the dimension to be measured is selected with certainty.

4. The main factors which influence the size of an echo were listed.

5. Limitations and artefacts were noted. These are often also found in ultrasonic images.

10. Scan converters and computers in grey-shade imaging

The merits of good grey-tone tone images are well known from the fields of conventional photography and X-ray imaging. A full appreciation of the importance of grey-tone imaging and of the role of weak echoes in images has greatly increased the power of diagnostic ultrasound.

Digital scan converters are computers that can accept image information, store it electronically, process it, and put it out to display units. The name arises because the device typically accepts information in one scan mode, for example, scan line by scan line from a sector scanner, and sends it to the display unit in a second scan pattern, for example, as a series of horizontal television-raster lines.

In the 1970s, scan converters made a large impact in the field of ultrasonic imaging because they enabled bright grey-scale images to be displayed. The echo information can also be manipulated while it is stored in the electronic memory of the scan converter.

Digital scan converters and auxiliary computers are the central hub of modern scanners. The auxiliary computer carries out functions such as interacting with the operator via instruction menus, performing internal tests, and identifying faults.

Analogue scan converters store image information as an electric-charge distribution on a silicon wafer. They suffer from instability and are now essentially obsolete.

GREY-SHADE IMAGES

We noted earlier that after TGC has been applied to an echo train, the dynamic range of echoes may be about 40 dB (100–1). The range of echo amplitudes arises from several sources:

1. Differences in acoustic impedance changes at reflecting and scattering targets
2. Size and shape of reflectors and scatterers
3. Dependence of the magnitude of the returned signal on the angle of beam incidence at reflecting and scattering targets
4. Spatial variations in intensity in the ultrasonic beam
5. Interference producing a speckle pattern
6. Inexact TGC

Figure 10.1 presents data on types of tissues and the echo magnitudes received from them. Taking fat and muscle to be a typical example of an interface that delineates major boundaries, we can

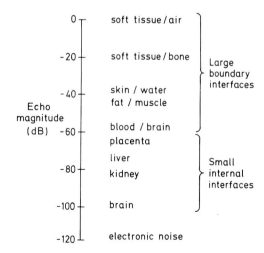

Fig. 10.1 Magnitudes of echo signals from tissues (courtesy of Kossoff G, Garrett W S, Carpenter D A et al 1976).

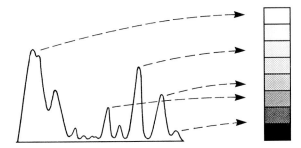

Fig. 10.2   Allocation of signal levels to shades of grey.

see that signals from within organs, for example, the liver and kidneys, are 30–40 dB down on those from major boundaries. Very strong echoes, such as those from a soft-tissue/bone interface, are allowed to saturate on the display, whereas those from very weak reflectors, such as blood, are normally not depicted.

In grey-tone imaging, different echo magnitudes are presented as different shades of grey (Fig.10.2). Unfortunately, the human eye cannot appreciate 100 different shades of grey in a pattern, so the signal range has to be compressed, typically to 10–1 (20 dB). This is not as big a loss as it seems, since echo magnitudes cannot be interpreted too exactly. In addition, the compression is carried out in a manner designed to preserve the information in weak echoes.

Our ability to distinguish shades of grey depends on the way in which they are presented. It is possible to distinguish about 16 levels in a parallel grey bar pattern on X-ray film, 12 on a television screen, and 8 on a print. If an irregular pattern is viewed, the number of identifiable levels appears to be almost halved; however, it is then much more difficult to assess just how many levels are contributing to the overall image quality. Systems are, therefore, designed to present images with more levels than might be indicated from the above figures. For example, the echo amplitude range might be compressed to only 20 to 1 (26 dB).

The interpretation of grey shades in an image depends, to some extent, on the way in which the data have been gathered and processed. If possible, it is worth acquiring some knowledge of how the data are processed in the scan converter. A more common approach is to hope that the desig-

ner has done a good job and to build up experience of the performance through usage. Since the designer's decisions are somewhat arbitrary, it is essential to scrutinize the grey shade performance of a machine before purchase.

DIGITAL SCAN CONVERTER

Pixels

It is convenient when implementing computer storage and processing of images to consider the image to be composed of a large number of small picture cells, referred to as 'pixels'. For example, an ultrasonic image of area 25×20 cm may be considered to consist of a matrix of square cells, each of area 1 mm^2. The matrix is therefore of size 250×200, making a total number of 50 000 pixels. Associated with each pixel of the image there is a brightness level corresponding to the ultrasonic signal level in that small part of the image.

The computer memory required in digital scan converters is constructed as a large number of individual storage locations. When an image is stored in such a memory, each pixel is allocated a particular storage location and the signal level at the pixel is stored as a number in that location (Fig. 10.3). As an ultrasonic scan is being performed, the pixel position for each echo is calculated. Voltage signals from the beam direction measuring system of the scanner and the echo return time are used in this determination of the appropriate pixel for each echo. Each echo signal amplitude is converted to a number by a unit called a 'digitizer'. Two quantities are therefore derived for each echo signal; namely its storage location (pixel position) and a numerical value for its amplitude.

The process of allocating the pixel for each ultrasonic echo is very fast. For example, an echo can be stored in a location in memory in less than 1 μs. Retrieval from the memory is also rapid; a complete image is reproduced on a television screen in about 40 ms. The retrieval process does not alter the stored data, so it can be repeated 20 to 30 times per second to provide a flicker-free image.

Memories found in digital scan converters can

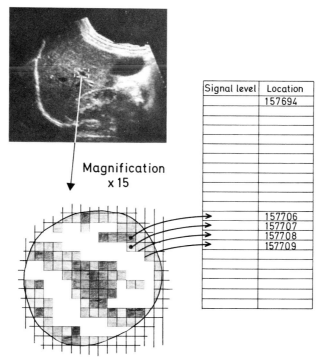

Signal level	Location
	157694
	157706
	157707
	157708
	157709

Magnification
x 15

Fig. 10.3 Allocation of pixels of the image to storage locations in the electronic memory.

be larger than those indicated in the above discussion. The matrix size could be 640 × 512. For a life-size image of 30 × 25 cm subdivided into this pixel arrangement, the lengths of the sides of the pixel correspond to 0.5 mm of range in tissue. It is obviously desirable to make the pixel dimensions less than those of the smallest structure in the image. If the image is recorded on a greater-than-life-size scale, the pixel dimensions correspond to an even smaller tissue range, for example, 0.1 mm, but in this situation the area of tissue presented on the display is reduced. When a selected area is to be imaged in more detail, some scanners implement a high-resolution mode in which the area is rescanned with an increased line density.

Digital storage

In the previous section, we noted that the echo amplitudes are digitized and stored in memory as numbers. The signals from the beam-direction-measurement electronics and the echo-return time are also converted to numbers to allow computer calculation of echo locations. A fuller under-standing of this process gives a feeling for the operation of a digital scan converter.

In our everyday activities, we use the decimal number system in which numbers are based on 10 digits, 0, 1, 2, 3, 4, 5, 6, 7, 8, 9. We tend to forget that other number systems are also possible. For example, if man had eight fingers, we would, no doubt, use the octal system, which has eight digits, 0, 1, 2, 3, 4, 5, 6, 7. Computers use the binary system of two digits, 0, 1. A specific number of items may be equivalently expressed in these number systems; for example, 19 (in decimal) = 23 (in octal) = 10 011 (in binary). In diagnostic ultrasound, we do not need to be concerned with the conversion from one number system to another; we just need to appreciate that voltage levels are processed as binary numbers in digital equipment.

The binary system is popular in computers, since the two digits, 0 and 1, can be equated to two states of an electronic device. An electronic device switched on can be regarded as 1, and switched off as 0. Within a computer or its memory, the six-digit binary number 100 111

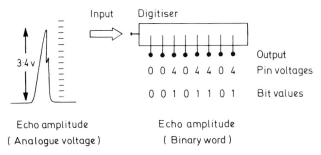

Fig. 10.4   Analogue-to-digital conversion of an echo signal.

could be stored by six sets of transistor circuitry, four of which are switched on and two off. In effect, the number is stored as six voltage levels, four at + 5 volts (on-state), and two at 0 volts (off-state).

Figure 10.4 illustrates the conversion of an echo signal of +3.4 volt amplitude to a binary word, which is then stored in memory. The process of conversion from an analogue voltage to a binary number is called 'digitization', because the analogue signal is then represented by the binary digits, 0 and 1. The word 'bit' is a commonly used abbreviation for binary digit. In the above example, the signal is said to be stored as a six-bit word. The largest number stored by a six-bit word is 111 111, that is, 63 (in decimal); the smallest is 000 000, that is, 0 (in decimal). This six-bit word can therefore store 64 levels of echo magnitude. Table 10.1 presents other word lengths encountered in ultrasonic systems. Eight-bit words are commonly used in computing and are known as 'bytes'. Several bytes linked together are used to specify large numbers and, hence, allow the computer to calculate to great accuracy. The byte is very common in computer technology; in scan converters, 7 bits are often used to store 128 signal levels, and if necessary 1 bit to store the signal

level sign (+ or −). By coincidence the eight bit byte can readily store the typical 100–1 range of echo levels encountered in imaging.

Pixel size and the accuracy with which echo amplitudes are digitized have a very marked effect on the appearance of an image (Fig. 10.5).

Sampling

When echo signals are passed to a digital scan converter, the process of digitization is carried out at very short intervals along the echo train. In most scanners, the echo train is rectified prior to digitization; however, in a few, the oscillatory RF signal is used. A train of 3.5 MHz ultrasonic echoes may be digitized at 0.1 mm intervals, a binary word or sample being produced at each position (Fig.10.6). Several samples are obtained within each pixel, but not all of them are used. Instead, the samples corresponding to each pixel are examined by the controlling computer, and a selection criterion is applied. For instance, the largest value sample, the average value, or that from the centre of the pixel may be selected for storage.

Figure 10.7 is a schematic diagram of a digital scan converter reduced to a series of functional blocks. For the remainder of this discussion, we will consider this example. The details of the systems vary from manufacturer to manufacturer.

Preprocessing

Computer memory is inexpensive, and it is possible to digitize echoes to 7 or 8 bits and transfer the samples directly into the scan converter. However, echoes are sometimes digitized to more bits

Table 10.1   Binary word lengths as encountered in ultrasonic systems

Bits	Number of levels
3	8
4	16
5	32
6	64
7	128
8	256

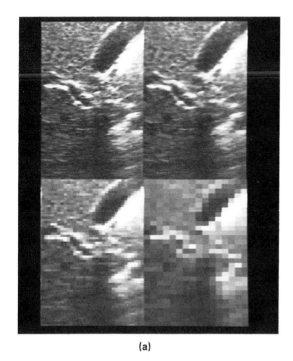

(a)

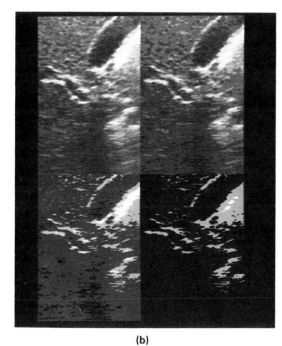

(b)

Fig. 10.5 (a) The effect on the quality of an image of reducing the number of pixels (Array sizes 128 × 256, 64 × 128, 32 × 64, 16 × 32). (**b**) the effect of altering the number of levels of digitization (Number of levels 32, 16, 8, 4) (courtesy of T Loupas).

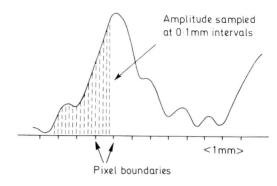

Fig. 10.6 Sampling of echo signals at closely spaced intervals.

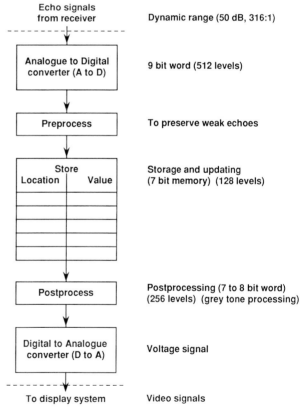

Fig. 10.7 Block diagram of a typical scan converter

than the scan converter can handle. This allows preprocessing of the echoes in the manner considered best to preserve the diagnostic information. Typically, the operator is given four preprocessing options to choose from in order to optimize the image for each application. By and large, preprocessing options have not proven useful and may, therefore, not be present in a scanner.

Storage and updating

In the above paragraphs, the storing of echo data into previously cleared pixel locations has been described. It could be that echo magnitudes, such as those from the preceding sweep of the beam, are already stored in some of the locations. The question then arises of how the new echo data should be used to update that already stored. A number of options (update computer programs called 'algorithms') may exist, from which the operator can select.

The simplest approach is to replace the old with the new. This results in a very useful 'search' or 'survey' mode of scanning, in which the image is continually refreshed as the ultrasound beam is swept through the tissue of interest. The high-writing speed of digital scan converters allows this scanning action to be performed smoothly and quickly.

Other updating algorithms could be applied, such as replacing the old pixel value with the average of the old and the new. This may produce a better estimate of the reflectivities of the tissues in the image.

Further criteria can be applied by the computer to the updating process. For example, the computer can subdivide each pixel into a 4×4 element array and calculate whether the scan line of the echoes passes through the centre or edge of the pixel. The computer can then be programmed to add less to the old pixel value when the scan line passes through the edge than it does when the line passes through the centre. If the scan line misses a pixel completely, say, at a depth in a sector scan where the lines are spread out, the computer inserts a value derived from neighbouring pixels. This avoids black holes in the image.

This discussion has explored some examples of updating algorithms. The search mode and average writing mode are of known value. The efficacy of any others on offer should be studied carefully in different applications.

Postprocessing

To produce a visible image, the computer converts the numeric value of each pixel into an analogue voltage pulse that is used to produce a bright spot at the appropriate point on a display screen. This is sometimes described as writing the image out from the digital map to the display. In the above example of a storage matrix of size 640×512, the pixel values in the array are written out, line by line, on a television display. The raster scan of the television spot is in synchrony with the line-by-line writing out of the matrix memory. To achieve a grey-tone display, the computer relates the brightness of the spot to the numeric value in each pixel. The whole process is repeated about 25 times per second to give a flicker-free image.

It is usual to do some processing on the numeric echo data during the reading-out process. This is called 'postprocessing'. The object of postprocessing is to allow flexibility in the allocation of stored echo-signal values to shades of grey; in other words, to allow the image data to be presented with different contrasts in the image. The operator can then select the preferred option.

One way to undertake postprocessing is to put each pixel value, as it is read out, into an intermediate storage location, called a register, prior to conversion to a voltage signal (Fig.10.8). For instance, a register which accommodates numbers in the range 0–255 (an eight-bit register). When the postprocessing is altered, pixel values are allocated to different values in the 0–255 range and, hence, each pixel appears with a different shade of grey.

Typical postprocessing options are as shown in Figure 10.9.

1. Option A — linear transfer involving no processing
2. Option B — which compresses high-level signals
3. Option C — which compresses low-level signals

There are usually about four such postprocessing options available. They may be set up to suit the user's requirements. They are often called 'gamma' options because they are analogous to changing the gamma characteristic of a film or display screen. Not all manufacturers offer as many

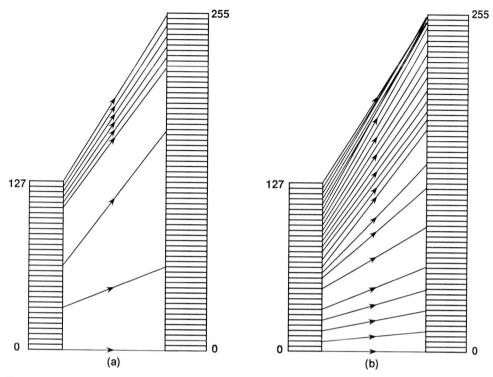

Fig. 10.8 Postprocessing of the echo signals by sending them to different storage locations in an output register: (**a**) no change in relative output values from those stored in memory, (**b**) large amplitudes compressed into a few output levels and, hence, a few shades of grey.

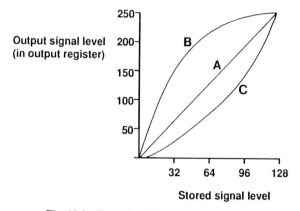

Fig. 10.9 Examples of postprocessing options.

as four postprocessing options, some preferring to offer types of known value.

The stages in a digital scan converter can be summarized as follows:

1. Sampling and digitization — to convert analogue echo signals into digital numbers (A-to-D conversion).

2. Preprocessing — to preserve weak echo information. This takes place during the writing in of the echoes signals to the computer memory.

3. Storage, updating, and image processing — to construct the image.

4. Postprocessing — to allocate data values to grey-tone levels, prior to reconstituting voltage signals by digital-to-analogue conversion (D-to-A conversion). This takes place during the reading out of the stored values from the computer to the display.

COMPUTATIONS ON STORED ECHO DATA

While echo signals are stored in numeric form, they are very amenable to computer processing techniques, which can be either simple or complex. The first priority of machine operators is to get answers to the following questions regarding a processing technique.

1. What does the processing aim to achieve?
2. How well does it achieve this goal?
3. In which applications could the processing be useful?

Having clearly established answers to these questions, the operator may or may not choose to be further involved with the details of the technique. Computer processing methods as applied to diagnostic ultrasound are at an early stage of development and have still to establish their worth. It should be borne in mind, however, that computer and digital techniques link ultrasound with one of the largest and most rapidly growing technologies. Some examples of processing will be described now to illustrate the method.

One simple technique is to select a part of an image or an echo train and to plot a bar diagram (histogram) of the number of echoes in each specified amplitude range (Fig. 10.10). The histogram distribution may depend on the type of tissue examined. Echoes from cirrhotic livers have been shown to occupy higher amplitude ranges than those of normal tissue. An associated computer process is to examine a histogram related to a region of interest to find out the range of echo amplitudes received. All of the grey tones of the display screen are then allocated to this range of

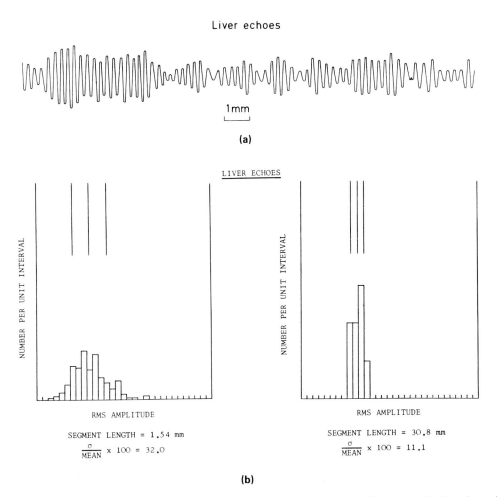

Fig. 10.10 Amplitudes measured over two different lengths of echo train (1.54 and 30.8 mm). Mean amplitude is determined more accurately using the longer train. σ/mean × 100 = coefficient of variation, σ = standard deviation. (**a**) Train of echo signals from liver, (**b**) histograms of echo amplitudes in the echo train (courtesy of Morrison D C).

amplitudes. This may allow smaller variations in tissue reflectivity to be visualized.

Techniques similar to the above are often labelled 'windowing' or 'enhancement'. In windowing, a range of echo amplitudes is selected by the operator and spread over the whole grey-shade range of the display. In CT scanning with X-rays, windowing is applied successfully to show small changes in tissue density. Enhancement selects a specific echo range and increases its brightness on the display. Care is necessary in interpreting these processed images, as some enhanced signals may have the same brightness as genuinely stronger echoes.

Smoothing techniques can be applied to the stored information, for example, by adjusting each pixel value by relating it to those of surrounding pixels. This processing option reduces noise in the image; however, in its simple form it also blurs the edges of structures. More sophisticated smoothing techniques are being developed in order to reduce speckle noise while retaining genuinely sharp boundaries (Ch. 28). Another common smoothing approach is to average echoes from several consecutive image frames. When more than about five frames are averaged, the resultant blurring of the image caused by the persistence of echoes is usually considered unacceptable.

This discussion has indicated some of the simpler computer processing techniques. If a system is purchased with the capability of performing some processing, it is possible to reprogram it to do other processing of similar or perhaps greater complexity. This provides for some adaptability in the system to take into account new developments.

The storage of an image as a matrix of pixels allows the calculation of lengths, areas, and volumes to be readily undertaken.

PERFORMANCE OF SCAN CONVERTERS

Since the ultrasonic information from real-time transducer assemblies can be passed directly to the display screen, the reader may wonder why storage memories are used. They are not essential in real-time imaging, but they add considerably to the performance of the scanners. The attractions of scan converters may be listed as follows:

1. The rapid storage, processing, and read-out of images. This rapid handling of images at around 30 per second is quite remarkable.

2. Conversion of the real-time image scan format to standard television format, making video-tape recording simple.

3. An instantaneous frame-freeze facility which makes measurements much easier.

4. Extra frame insertion to reduce flicker at low scan frame rates.

5. Extra line insertion to improve image presentation.

6. Some processing of echo data; preprocessing and postprocessing as described in the previous sections.

Digital scan converters have other features that make them very attractive from a practical point of view. These features include:

1. *Stability*. They are not affected by small voltage drifts or noise, because the echoes are stored as numbers represented by voltage levels such as 0 and +5 volts.

2. *Uniformity*. The properties of the storage technique are identical over the matrix area.

3. *Long life*. Solid-state, transistor-type technology is more likely to become obsolete than to wear out.

4. *Fast response*. Echo information is quickly and accurately stored.

5. *Accuracy* (in storing signal-amplitude values).

A few flaws in poorly designed digital scan converters may be observed. One example of this is pixels that contain zero-level echo amplitudes in regions of an image where many echoes are being produced. These pixels appear as small, dark holes in the image and look distinctly like artefacts. This situation can be produced if the updating algorithm does not store a data value when the beam direction passes through the corner of a pixel. Unfilled pixels are particularly obvious in images of high magnification.

If an echo pattern appears as single, distinct pixels rather than as groups of neighbouring pixels, it will appear to flicker slightly on the display. This arises from the way the image is generated on the display by a television-raster action. Recall that the television raster is performed in two halves. First, it proceeds down the screen, doing every alternate line; then it repeats the process, filling in the omitted lines. If the picture information is strongly dependent on single, isolated pixels rather than on groups that straddle more than one line, part of it will be absent during only half of the raster presentation.

A convenient feature of digital machines is that, to some extent, they can check their own performance. The controlling computer can generate patterns of grey tones which enable the operator to check both that the scan converter is functioning properly and that the settings of the display monitors are correct.

USE OF CONTROLS ON DIGITAL SCAN CONVERTER

We noted in Chapter 7 that a group of controls that influence the performance of a scanning machine are those of the scan converter. These controls can be classed as display and processing controls.

Display controls

Display controls consist of the following:

1. Zoom — to magnify areas of interest in the image. A region of the image is selected, and then magnified when echo information is read out from that region to fill the whole display. More scan lines may be used in the zoomed mode of operation, with a corresponding improvement in image quality (acoustic zoom). Figure 10.11 illustrates the zoom control in clinical imaging.

2. Test pattern — for setting up the display focus, brilliance, and contrast. A standard pattern can also be used to check the allocation of echo magnitudes to grey-shade levels.

3. Display subdivision — to permit a number of images to be stored and presented simultaneously.

4. Polarity switch — to present echoes as white spots on a black background, or vice versa.

Processing controls

The number of permutations of processing options may be large or small, depending on the manufacturer's design decisions. As always, it is a good policy to establish baseline settings and to change to alternative processing only once it has been established as useful in specific applications.

If options are offered in selecting which samples to use after digitization, the option of taking the peak value in each pixel is of proven worth. Using the average of the samples in each pixel also produces high-quality images.

In the case of preprocessing options, it is best to select one in which the weak echoes are allocated to most of the available levels, yet the strong echoes are not too compressed into the remaining top few. For specific studies, such as examination of liver parenchyma, an option giving high priority to the weak echoes should be considered.

A most useful updating mode for initial studies is the survey or search mode, in which the old pixel value is replaced by the new. Averaging over several frames is also common, the degree of averaging being usually a matter of personal preference.

Postprocessing options enable the stored signals to be assigned to shades of grey in a number of ways. With stored levels that already preserve the differences in weak echo amplitudes, a useful output option is a linear transfer (Option A, Fig. 10.9). Alternative postprocessing that decompresses the strong echo levels, that is, spreads them over more grey-shade values, may be worthwhile in some applications where there is interest in high-level echoes. The postprocessing options essentially alter the contrast of the grey-tone image, and their effects can be observed directly.

IMAGE QUALITY

Image quality is of paramount importance. For a given patient, it depends on the design of the machine and the expertise of the operator. The question therefore arises, 'What constitutes good image quality?' The following points contribute to the answer:

1. Good allocation of echo levels to grey shades, i.e. good contrast.

2. Low level of spurious noise signals, either electronic or ultrasonic. Liquid-filled structures should appear free of echoes.

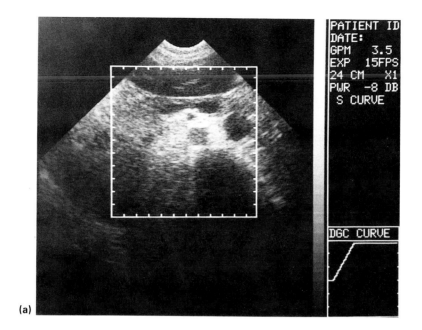

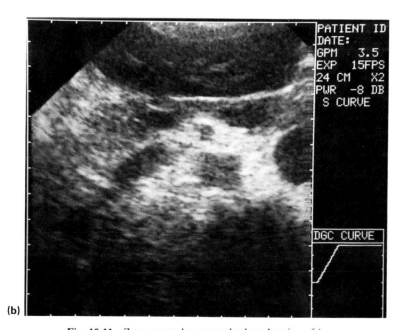

Fig. 10.11   Zoom control to expand selected region of image.

3. Sharp depiction of tissue boundaries.

4. Effective smoothing of noise without blurring of genuine edges.

5. Few artefact echoes, particularly near the transducer.

6. Good resolution, constant over all of the image.

7. Display scale appropriate to structures.

8. Individual pixels or scan lines should not be visible in the displayed image.

9. Absence of image flicker.

SUMMARY

The power of digital electronics to store and process images continues to grow rapidly. The scan converter is the heart of an ultrasonic scanner.

1. Scan converters are devices for storing echo information. They are essentially computers with sufficient memory to hold the echo information of an image. An auxiliary computer looks after the rest of the housekeeping in the machine; for example, display characteristics, measurement procedures, and, perhaps, sensitivity control.

2. Scan converters normally convert the scan-line pattern of the beam directions in the body to a TV raster-line pattern.

3. Grey-shade imaging is of crucial importance. It is achieved by matching the large range of echo amplitudes to the range of available grey shades.

4. Digital storage of echo signals was described. The power to process image data was discussed in some detail. This came under the headings of preprocessing, storage and updating, postprocessing, and computations. It was noted that since many variations in digital processing are feasible, those of particular value should be identified clearly.

5. The advantages of scan converters and digital techniques were listed.

6. Aspects of the way in which scan converters can be used were discussed.

11. Real-time B-scan instruments

In Chapter 2, we saw that ultrasonic images may be produced using pulsed ultrasound to localize tissue interfaces. A real-time pulse-echo image portrays interfaces that reflect or scatter ultrasound and that lie in a plane section through the body. Often a large number of these two-dimensional images are observed and the operator builds up a mental picture of the anatomy. Although, on first sight, an ultrasonic imager may present a confusing array of controls, a degree of proficiency is achieved quickly and this stimulates the user to try more complex procedures. On-the-spot diagnoses resulting from the combination of good-quality scanning and clinical knowledge appear to provide a satisfying area of work, well worth the effort of mastering a new technology.

Real-time B-scanning is the ultrasonic technique analogous to cine-filming in photography. Images are usually produced at a high rate, for instance, 25/s, allowing movement of the objects to be observed. Instruments designed to generate images at low frame rates, for example, 5/s, are suitable for studying stationary or slowly moving tissues. In this text, the term 'real-time B-scanner' is applied to units with the capacity to generate images at frame rates greater than about 5/s.

It is the high velocity of ultrasound in tissue that makes real-time scanning possible. The process of transmitting a pulse and collecting the resultant echoes is completed in about 0.25 ms. In one second, therefore, 4000 lines of echo information can be collected. If 100 lines are required for each image, then 40 images can be generated per second.

Portability in a real-time B-scanner may be desirable and may extend the applications to unusual areas. Variations in the degree of portability range from completely hand-held units, that is, transducer plus electronics and display in one compact structure, to large systems suitable for transport on a trolley. Compromises are involved in the reduction of the instrument size and need to be considered in light of the advantages of portability. On small instruments, the display screens may be small, and features such as image storage or control flexibility limited. The facilities available are worth noting, however, since more and more processing power can be included in small volumes as electronics becomes increasingly miniaturized.

The value of real-time B-scanning in clinical diagnosis and experimental work derives from the following features:

1. Motion of tissue is observed.
2. Searching is facilitated by rapidly altering the plane of scan.
3. The best section for making measurements is quickly determined, as for example, for crown rump length, BPD, or blood flow.
4. Image degradation caused by patient movement is eliminated.
5. Effect of patient manoeuvres can be observed (e.g. deep respiration).
6. Motion of contrast agents can be observed (e.g. microbubbles in heart or stomach).
7. The plane of scan is easily selected with little patient manipulation.
8. Biopsy needles and catheters can be observed moving through the tissues.

The label 'real-time' employed to describe this technique is, in some ways, rather unfortunate because this label is used in related fields with a different meaning. The term 'real-time' applied to a technique often indicates that the results are obtained immediately. It could, therefore, describe almost all diagnostic ultrasonic techniques. High-speed frequency analysers that are used to produce frequency spectra during ultrasonic Doppler blood-flow studies are often called real-time analysers.

PRINCIPLES OF REAL-TIME B-SCANNING

Let us briefly recall the principle of real-time B-scanning as it was described in Chapter 2. Echo information is generated when a short ultrasonic pulse is transmitted into tissue and interacts with discontinuities in acoustic impedance. The narrow beam is made to sweep rapidly and repetitively through a section of tissue (Fig. 11.1). At all times, the position of the beam is related to the direction of the line of displayed echo spots on the screen. All of the phenomena related to the propagation of ultrasound in tissue that produce both information and artefacts are relevant to this technique (Ch. 4). The ideas underlying the setting up of sensitivity controls are outlined in Chapter 7. The technology associated with grey-shade imaging is directly applicable (Ch. 10).

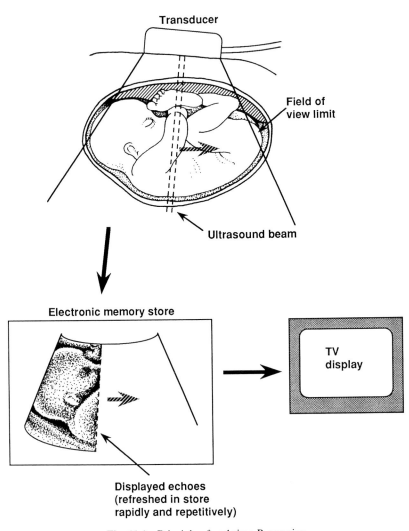

Fig. 11.1   Principle of real-time B-scanning.

Electronic system

The electronic system for the generation and detection of echoes is similar to that described for A-scanning; the basic methods of generating and processing the echo signals are the same. The main difference is that the echo signals are ultimately used to produce bright spots on the screen. Diagrams of the functional blocks of real-time B-scan and A-scan instruments emphasize their similarity as far as echo signal production is concerned (Fig. 11.2 and 9.2). With real-time array transducers, the electronic system is much more complex, but the basic aims remain the generation of a narrow pulsed beam and the processing of the resultant echo signals. Focusing of arrays on transmission and reception is described in Chapter 5, and will be further discussed when we consider specific scanners later in this section.

Figure 11.3 illustrates the component parts of an electronic system that govern sensitivity and re- lates them to the controls presented to the operator. Note that amplifier gain and TGC both influence the RF receiver. The output after the detector is the echo train in a suitable form for passing to a display or scan converter. Some instruments digitize and store the RF echo signals before they are smoothed in the detector circuitry. The echo signals typically have a dynamic range of 40 dB (100–1) and may be further processed by the computer of the scan converter.

Classification of real-time B-scanners

Real-time scanners may be classified as follows:

1. Mechanical sector oscillator
2. Mechanical linear oscillator
3. Mechanical rotator
4. Electronic linear array
5. Electronic curved array
6. Electronic sector scanner (phased array)

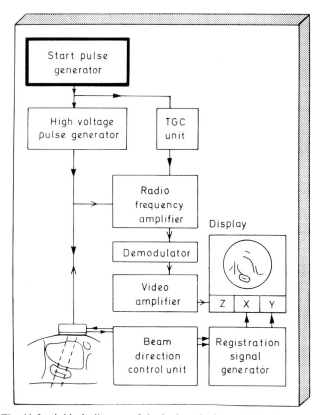

Fig. 11.2 A block diagram of the basic units in a real-time B-scanner.

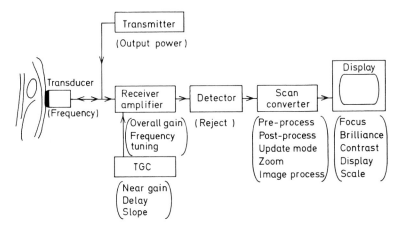

Fig. 11.3 Component parts of the echo-signal processing system and their associated controls.

7. Water-bath scanner
8. Small-parts scanner
9. Invasive scanner
10. Compound scanner

A few instances exist of scanners that combine the features of two or more of these classes.

FEATURES OF REAL-TIME B-SCANNERS

Transducers

Manufacturers offer an increasing range of transducers with their scanners. As many as 50 different transducers may be offered. Some of this range is to cover ultrasonic frequencies from 2 to 10 MHz, and to permit scanning with different fields of view. Many specialized transducers are available, such as those for internal imaging and biopsy guidance. A purchaser normally buys around four probes, but the number is increasing as the diversity of ultrasonic techniques expands. The total cost of transducers can be high; indeed, they could, in theory, cost more than all the rest of the instrumentation. One of the joys of working in diagnostic ultrasonics is the way in which the diverse transducers permit a wide range of problems to be tackled.

Frame rate

The frame rate is the number of images produced per second by the repetitive scan action. Typically,

it is in the range 5–40/s. The term 'frame' is often used to mean the image created by one scan sweep. If the frame rate is below 20/s, the real-time image flickers, as the eye fails to integrate the images. Above 40/s, the time available to perform each sweep is low, limiting the number of lines of echo information in each image. At low frame rates, the effect of flicker can be partially overcome by reading out each frame several times from the scan converter while the next new frame is being stored.

Line density

The total number of lines in a real-time image may be rather low, for example, 100. If the field is 15 cm wide and rectangular, the line density is 6.7 lines/cm. If the field is a 90° sector, the line density is 1.1 lines/degree.

Some electronic techniques may be employed to reduce the image degradation caused by low line density. For example, each line of information may be written more than once on the display so that lines with the same acoustic information are located adjacent to one another. Alternatively, new lines of information may be derived by averaging the echo information from neighbouring lines. Electronic circuitry performs these cosmetic operations very rapidly, so the new lines can be inserted among the genuine acoustic lines. Artificially increasing the number of lines in the image does improve the appearance of the real-time presentation.

Field of view

Two factors determine the size of the field of view of real-time B-scanners. The first is the limit on the number of echo lines which there is time to generate per frame. To maintain a reasonable line density in the image, one must, therefore, restrict its width. The second is the physical difficulty of making a large device that will couple conveniently to the contours of the body.

The shape of the field of view is determined by the electronic or mechanical technique used to sweep the beam. Selection of the most suitable shape for a clinical application is important, and it is done after consideration of the coupling of the transducer to the body and of the access limitations caused by bone and gas.

The three features (frame rate, line density, and field of view) just discussed are interrelated. In practice, to increase one of them requires one or both of the others to be reduced. For example, an increased frame rate can be obtained by reducing the depth or width of the field of view. Similarly, an increased line density can be achieved at the expense of a reduced frame rate or a smaller field of view. Finally, an increased field of view requires a decrease in line density or frame rate. This interrelation can be expressed as a simple equation:

$$\text{Frame rate} \times \text{Line density} \times \text{Field of view} = \text{Constant}$$

Table 11.1 presents some typical sets of values of more exact data.

Table 11.1 Relationship among number of lines in image, frame rate, and depth of field of view
Number of lines × Frame rate × Depth of field = 154 000/2

	Number of lines	Frame rate
For depth of 20 cm		
	3850	1
	770	5
	385	10
	192	20
	96	40
For depth of 10 cm		
	7700	1
	1540	5
	770	10
	385	20
	192	40

Simple scan action

The scan patterns of most real-time instruments fall into the simple scan classes as defined in Chapter 14; that is, the beam sweeps only once through each tissue region for each frame. These scanners therefore are required to make the best use of both scattered and specularly reflected ultrasound.

Display and recording units

Real-time B-scanners may have several display and recording units. In general, it is best to have one display screen for each individual task, for example, direct viewing and photography. Video-recorders and fibre-optic chart recorders are also useful. These units can represent a substantial portion of overall costs. The ease with which systems that are compatible with television can be interlinked makes expansion simple. Details of these important aspects of scanning systems are to be found in Chapter 26.

MECHANICAL ROTATING TRANSDUCER SCANNER

A transducer mounted on a wheel, such that the ultrasonic beam points radially outwards, can easily be rotated so that a sector scan is performed. Since the development of single-element transducers with small amounts of backing material, several can be mounted on a wheel of small diameter. As the wheel rotates, one element is activated on passing through the defined sector, which is the field of view. For example, each of four elements could function as it sweeps through a 90° sector, resulting in four frames for one revolution of the wheel (Fig. 11.4). If two of the elements are completely inactivated the field of view can be a 180° sector. Likewise, for internal real-time scanning, one element can be operated through 360° (Chapter 25).

Figure 2.7 shows a commercial instrument based on the principle of rotating transducers. As a means of avoiding friction between the wheel and the skin, the rotating assembly is contained in a sealed, oil-filled cylinder. The ultrasonic beam propagates through a thin oil layer and plastic window into the patient. Additional attractions of this

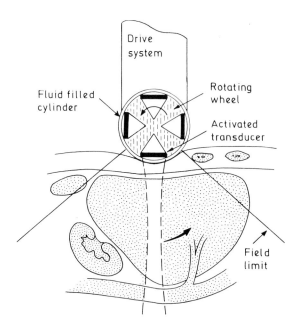

Fig. 11.4 A schematic diagram of a rotating transducer, real-time B-scanner.

arrangement are that high rotation speed is possible, the device can be pressed against the skin without loading the mechanical drive, and the coupling gel is not wiped off the skin. The excitation pulse and the echo signals pass between the transducers and the electronic system through small, gold slip rings or rotating transformers. These devices provide low-noise electronic links while allowing the transducers to rotate continuously in the one direction.

The angular position of the beam can be determined by several different types of device. A number of friction-free magnetic devices exist that can measure angle without physical contact between the moving parts. In one such device, a sensing crystal, mounted in a shaft, rotates in the magnetic field of a fixed magnet. A voltage, induced in the crystal by a phenomenon known as the Hall effect, varies with the angle between the crystal and the magnetic field.

Rotation of the wheel can be achieved directly with a mechanical link to a small electric motor. Another arrangement makes use of a magnetic link between the wheel and the driving mechanism. In this version, the transducer assembly can be completely sealed in the oil-filled cylinder.

If some compromise is made regarding the size of the wheel, several transducers of different frequency or focal lengths may be housed in it; then, at the throw of a switch, different transducers can be selected. Otherwise, like most other real-time units, changing frequencies involves replacing part or all of the transducer head.

In theory, annular-array transducers can be employed in a rotating scanner. Such devices have not been developed so far owing to the complexity of operating several arrays in one scanning head.

Because of their single-point entry (small footprint) and large field of view, mechanical rotating scanners are applied in all fields in which real-time B-scanning is relevant.

MECHANICAL OSCILLATING TRANSDUCER SCANNER

One of the simplest ways of achieving a real-time sector scanning action is to make a single-element transducer oscillate around a pivot point as shown in Figure 11.5. If the pivot point is the front face of the transducer, mechanical disturbance near the skin of the patient is minimized. The mechanical drive can again be direct or indirect via magnetic

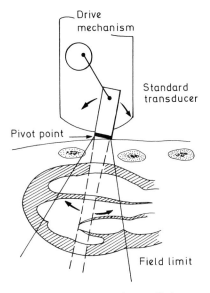

Fig. 11.5 A schematic diagram of an oscillating transducer, real-time B-scanner. The oscillations produce a sector scan.

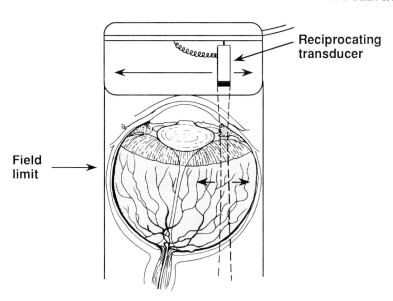

Fig. 11.6   A schematic diagram of an oscillating transducer, real-time B-scanner. The oscillations produce a linear scan.

coupling. Friction between the transducer and the skin is reduced or removed by ensuring that a layer of gel or oil is always present or by inserting a thin membrane. The electronic features of these devices for contact with the transducer and angular measurement are similar to those found in rotating transducer units.

Figure 11.6 presents an effectively linear type of oscillatory scanner. In practice, the field of view is restricted with this type of linear oscillating mechanism. Scanners based on this principle are used to image small tissue areas; for example, in eye scanning or visualization of blood vessels.

In one ophthalmic version of a linear oscillator, an 8 MHz transducer moves behind a thin methylcellulose membrane that acts as a window in a fluid filled chamber. The chamber is filled with water before use. The frame rate is 11/s, which is sufficient to allow eye motions to be observed. Direct contact with the closed eyelid is the most convenient method of use. For viewing the anterior regions of the eyeball, however, a waterbath is placed between the eye and the scanning head.

Oscillating transducer scanners are very simple in structure, containing only one element and a simple drive mechanism. They tend to be limited in their field of view (e.g. a 70° sector or a 3 cm

linear sweep), and have some intrinsic vibration caused by the mode of moving the transducer.

Annular array transducers are incorporated into oscillator scanners to obtain the benefits of electronic focusing on transmission and reception. In present designs the number of annular elements varies from 3 to 8. This number may well increase as greater flexibility of operation is sought; for example, to minimize the contributions from side-lobes or to achieve focusing over a greater range by variable aperture techniques.

ELECTRONIC LINEAR ARRAY

Modern linear arrays are constructed as shown in Figure 11.7. A commercial instrument is presented in Figure 2.4. The transducer head is made from a large number of strips of piezoelectric material laid side by side, but acoustically isolated from one another. The number of piezoelectric elements found in arrays varies from 20 to 400, with most containing around 100. The element strips have dimensions determined by the frequency of ultrasound, for instance, length 10 mm and width 1 mm in a 3.5 MHz array. An array of isolated elements is made either by using completely independent strips or by cutting parallel grooves in a piece of piezoelectric material whose dimen-

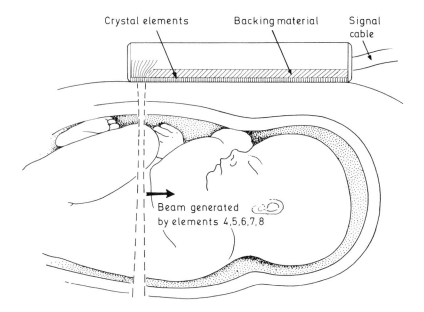

Crystal elements   Backing material   Signal cable

Beam generated by elements 4,5,6,7,8

Fig. 11.7 A schematic diagram of an electronic linear-array, real-time B-scanner.

sions equal those required for the whole linear array. Damping of the transducer by suitable backing material is similar to that for a single-element transducer.

To generate a pulsed beam of ultrasound, the device activates the small elements in groups that constitute a source equivalent to a single-element transducer. If an element was activated on its own, as a result of its small width, a divergent beam would be produced. As was noted in Chapter 5, the contributions from several strips combine to form a directional beam. The lateral resolution of a linear-array scanner depends on the success achieved in generating a well-defined beam from a number of element strips.

Stepping the beam rapidly through a succession of parallel directions is accomplished by altering the particular group of elements fired; for example, numbers 1 to 13 may be excited, followed by 2 to 14, and so on along the array. This will produce a number of lines of echo information approximately equal to the number of elements in the array, for instance, 100.

Another technique aimed at collecting slightly different acoustic information using the same group of elements is to direct the beams at slightly different angles. Small angle deflection of the beam results from introducing small differences in the time of excitation of the elements; that is, a phase difference is introduced between the contributions from adjacent elements. Since the beam deflection is, for example, 0.5°, the electronics of the display ignores it and presents the lines of echoes parallel to each other. This discussion has been concerned with methods of excitation; similar techniques and results are found in the echo-reception circuitry.

Linear-array scanners also utilize electronic focusing (see Ch. 5). This focusing results from appropriate time delays in the transmission and reception electronics. Electronic focusing may either be fixed at a particular selected range or moved along the beam so that it corresponds to the depth from which echoes are being received. We noted in Chapter 5 that to optimize the focus at different depths, the number of elements employed may be varied quite markedly. In some instruments, optimum focusing at depth results from the use of 128 elements, while, closer to the skin, 16 are functioning.

Electronic focusing by arrays consisting of parallel elements concentrates the beam in the direction parallel to the plane of scan. To assist in making the beam narrower in the direction at right

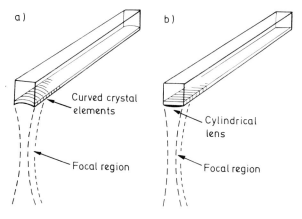

Fig. 11.8 Fixed focusing of an array to reduce the thickness of the slice of tissue examined.

The physical length of the hand-held probe varies from manufacturer to manufacturer and with the ultrasonic frequency, covering a range of 5 to 20 cm. In some devices, the electronic switching is performed in the head, an arrangement which means that the linking cable requires fewer wires and is therefore lighter. Conversely, if the switching is done in the electronic system, the transducer head is lighter, but the connecting cable requires more wires and is heavier. In general, the higher the frequency, the shorter the arrays tend to be made, since the elements become smaller. For example, the dimensions of the front face of a 3.5 MHz probe are typically 14×1 cm whereas those of a 5 MHz probe are 7×0.5 cm.

angles to the plane of scan, that is, to reduce the thickness of the slice of tissue examined, we employ curved elements (Fig. 11.8a). Alternatively, a cylindrical lens may be placed along the array (Fig. 11.8b).

The field format of an electronic linear scanner is rectangular; the width corresponds to the length of the array, the length, to the range of penetration displayed. Frame rates of up to 75/s are encountered in practice. Moving the beam by wholly electronic means allows very high frame rates to be achieved; however, the related reduction in line density puts a practical limit on frame rate. Images are presented on either a standard CRT or a television monitor. The latter is very compatible with a linear array, since the parallel lines of the television raster can be related to the parallel lines of echo signals.

ELECTRONIC CURVED ARRAY

A weakness of a linear array with a flat face is that the width of the field of view is limited to the length of the array. Making the array longer to increase the field creates difficulty in maintaining contact between the transducer and the patient. The field of view may be increased, however, by introducing curvature to the array (Fig. 11.9a). Typically, an increase of 50% is achieved, which may be sufficient to encompass the whole head or trunk of a mature fetus. If even greater curvature is introduced, the array effectively becomes a sector scanner (Fig. 11.9b), and it is then suitable for application in the upper abdomen, and may be used in paediatrics as well as obstetrics. Electronic focusing is essential in curved arrays to counteract the natural tendency of the beam to diverge. Curved arrays have proven to be popular from the

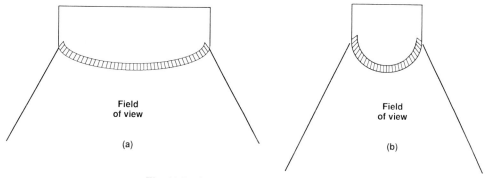

Fig. 11.9 Gently and tightly curved arrays.

point of view of both image quality and ease of use.

The principle of operation of a curved array is the same as that of the linear array described in the previous section. In its typical implementation, a strongly curved array has a radius of curvature of 25 mm and provides a sector field of around 90°. Such an array containing 50 elements may generate a directional beam with grating-lobes 40 dB down on the main beam. A weakly curved array might have a radius of curvature of 100 mm and slightly better beam characteristics.

ELECTRONIC SECTOR SCANNER (PHASED ARRAY)

The electronic sector scanner is another example of an instrument that can alter the path of an ultrasonic beam from a transducer by purely electronic means. In this case, rapid sector scanning is achieved by applying electronic delays to both the excitation pulses and subsequent echo signals at each transducer element in a small array. The principles of steering and focusing an ultrasonic beam by electronic delay of the signals have been discussed in detail in Chapter 5. A phased array scanner is schematically illustrated in Figure 11.10. Light weight and ease of manoeuvre

are two of the attractions of this type of transducer assembly. The small footprint of the transducer face (10–30 mm) is a third attraction since it permits access to the heart. At present, the number of piezoelectric strip elements in a phased array ranges from 16 to 128.

In an example of a 3 MHz array, the beam, during transmission, may be directed at an angle of 20° to the central axis, by delaying the excitation of the elements by equal time intervals of 0.23 μs (Fig. 11.11a). The delay between firing of the two outside elements is then 4.7 μs.

To provide focusing, the device ensures that the time delays between elements are no longer equal, but are arranged such that the emitted wave front is curved (Fig. 11.11b). In this instance, for focusing at a range of 8 cm, the time of excitation of the central and outside elements would differ by 0.4 μs. Note that, for transmission, the focal region is determined by the delay pattern when the elements are being activated and is fixed in that region.

During reception, the directional sensitivity of

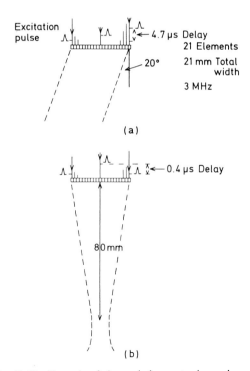

(a)

(b)

Fig. 11.11 Example of electronic beam-steering and focusing with a phased array.

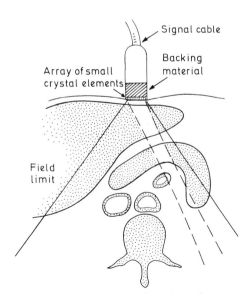

Fig. 11.10 A schematic diagram of an electronic sector, real-time B-scanner (phased array).

the array is made the same as that of the transmitted field by delaying the echo signals detected by the element strips, by the same time intervals as were used during transmission. The final echo signal is produced by adding the contributions from all elements after they have passed through the requisite electronic delay lines. As for the transmission situation, the directivity of the reception zone can be focused on a particular region by modifying the delays applied to the signals from the elements.

Greater flexibility of focusing is possible during reception than during transmission. During reception, the electronic delays can be manipulated as the echoes are being received such that the focus is quickly moved along the axis to coincide at each instant with the depth from which echoes are being detected. For example, during the echo-reception time, the focal region may move from 3 cm in front of the transducer to 15 cm from it.

The alteration of the pattern of delays, both for transmission and reception, is carried out rapidly and precisely for each scan line. Control of such a complex procedure is usually achieved by a microprocessor or minicomputer.

As for linear arrays, focusing achieved by such electronic methods is in the direction perpendicular to the lengths of the strip elements, that is, parallel to the plane of scan, and it improves the lateral resolution in only that direction. Quoted

results are often misleading if they refer to the beam being halved in its width. To produce some focusing perpendicular to the plane of scan, one can attach a cylindrical lens to the front of the array.

It has been found to be difficult to produce highly defined ultrasonic beams at all angles in the sector sweep. In some instances, grating-lobes have created problems. Several techniques are used to improve beam shapes. One technique is to apply logarithmic compression to the echo signals from the crystal elements prior to summation. The image quality associated with phased arrays has improved in recent years, but they still require to be assessed carefully from the aspects of resolution, noise, and artefact echoes.

Commercially marketed phased arrays have fields of view with sector angles up to 90°. Steering the beam to larger angles is difficult. To increase the frame rate or the line density, one can reduce the sector angle to a smaller value (e.g. 30°).

Electronic and mechanical sector scanners are in direct competition. Their strengths and weaknesses are summarized in Table 11.2.

WATER-BATH REAL-TIME SCANNERS

The combination of a water-bath and a real-time scanning mechanism offers advantages in some situations. Increased bulk of the scanning assemb-

Table 11.2 Strengths and weaknesses of sector scanners

Feature		Mechanical	Electronic
Size		★★★★	★★★★★
Focusing	(fixed)	★★★	Not applicable
	(dynamic)	★★★★★	★★★
M-mode		★★	★★★★★
High-frequency transducers		★★★★★	★★
Doppler	(CW)	★★	★★★★
	(PW)	★★★★	★★★★
	(Colour flow)	★★★	★★★★
Invasive transducers		★★★★★	★★★★
Biopsy		★★★★★	★★★★★
Cost		★★★★★	★★★★
Reliability		★★★	★★★★★

ly in contact with the patient is the price paid. The reasons for including a water bath in the design of a system include:

1. The transducer may be more easily coupled to the patient.

2. Large-diameter transducers can be used to give sharper focusing and greater sensitivity. Large transducers constructed from annular elements can incorporate electronic swept focusing that is effective over a large range.

3. With a sector-scanning mechanism, the resultant field shape in the tissue is virtually rectangular, giving good visualization of superficial tissues.

4. The scanning procedure can be fully motorized.

Examples of the principles of real-time, water-bath machines are presented schematically in Figure 11.12.

Two problems arise with water-baths in real-time scanning. Because of the depth of water, the echo signals take at least twice as long to return to the transducer as in contact real-time scanning. The pulse repetition frequency and, hence, the line density in the image is therefore reduced. An alternative to reducing the PRF is to reduce the range of penetration into the body (e.g. to 15 cm). This is rarely satisfactory in an instrument for abdominal examinations. The second problem relates to reverberations in the water-bath. To prevent the reverberations from one transmission still being present when the following one is made, one may have to lower the PRF even further. A water-bath constructed with highly absorbing walls can help to alleviate this problem. Nonetheless, it is advisable to check water-bath scanners for the presence of reverberation echoes. To counteract the low line density resulting from the lower-than-optimum PRF and to ease the problems of moving a large transducer assembly in water, several water-bath machines operate at frame rates below 15/s. Such machines cannot depict fast-moving structures, but they can present high-line-density images at frame rates around 10/s. With a scan converter, frame insertion reduces distracting flicker.

Oscillating and rotating transducer mechanisms can be incorporated into a water-bath (Fig. 11.12a, b, c). The transducer and bath structure is placed on top of the patient, and the ultrasound is transmitted via a thin flexible membrane to the tissues. In one commercial version of a rotating transducer plus water-bath, the main use is to visualize superficial blood vessels. This instrument has three equally spaced, 5 MHz transducers mounted on a wheel. The frame rate is 0–25/s and the field of view shape is approximately 6 × 4 cm.

Figure 11.12d shows a multi-element, annular array transducer that oscillates in a water-bath. The reduction in effective beam width with these more complex transducers is, at least, a factor of 2.

One of the earliest real-time scanners was produced by Siemens (Fig. 11.12e). A rotating transducer, situated at the focus of a parabolic acoustic mirror, transmitted an ultrasonic pulse toward the mirror at successive positions in its rotation. At each position, a pulse travelled from the transducer to the mirror and was reflected into the patient. The transducer transmitted only when

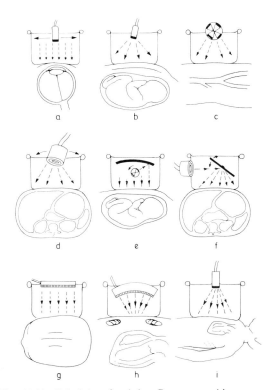

Fig. 11.12 Principles of real-time B-scanners with water-baths.

it was facing the mirror. Because the transducer was at the focus of the mirror, the successive ultrasonic beams entered the patient along neighbouring parallel paths. Echoes returned to the transducer by the same path as the related transmitted pulse. Two transducers of 2.2 MHz each were fitted to the commercial version of this instrument. They pointed in opposite directions, each being activated at the appropriate time. A variable frame rate of 15–30/s and a field of view of 22 × 16 cm were features of this instrument.

Another instrument utilizing an acoustic mirror is illustrated in Figure 11.12f. Rapid sweeps of the beam are implemented by reflecting it from an oscillating acoustic mirror that is contained in a water-bath. A large-diameter, annular array transducer is the source of ultrasound. With this type of device, it should be easy, in theory, to interchange transducers of different frequency since they are not part of the moving mechanism. A commercial unit of this type has a frame rate of 12/s and a trapezoidal field of view measuring 7.4 cm along the top, 17.7 cm along the bottom, and 20 cm in depth.

Other examples of combining a real-time scanner and a water-bath are outlined in Figure 11.12g, h, i, in which electronic array scanners are inserted at the top of the bath. The electronic array could be either a sector scanner or a linear scanner.

SMALL-PARTS SCANNERS

When water-bath scanners are designed for the examination of superficial structures, they are often called 'small-parts scanners'. This is a commonly mentioned category, but it is not defined by any new design features. All of the above water-bath scanners can be made to operate at high ultrasonic frequencies and are therefore suitable for imaging structures close to the skin surface. Some types of small-parts scanner do not involve a water-bath. Linear arrays are convenient for small-parts scanning if the dead space in front of the transducer is less than 2 or 3 mm.

INVASIVE SCANNERS

The versatility of ultrasonic technology is evident from the number of small transducers which have been made for invasive scanning. Since invasive procedures are often specialized, the discussion of invasive real-time B-scanners is deferred until Chapter 25. To date, all invasive scanners operate on the principles described in the preceding sections.

REAL-TIME COMPOUND B-SCANNING

Real-time compound scanning is a technique which is technically feasible, but has not yet been shown to be clinically advantageous. The main attraction of compound scanning is that tissues are interrogated by the ultrasonic beam from more than one direction, resulting in more information being collected. Some degradation of a compound image may be caused by echo-registration errors on the display; these errors are due to different average velocities of ultrasound along the different tissue paths. Further degradation is due to poor lateral resolution which results in point targets writing as asterisks or crosses on the display.

Figure 11.13 illustrates a mechanical and an electronic approach to real-time compound B-scanning. The scanning heads contain several spatially separated transducers that are fired in sequence to send ultrasonic beams in different directions into the body. The unit in Figure 11.13a achieves this end by enlarging on the rotating transducer principle; that in Figure 11.13b, by using more than one phased array.

Ultrasonic imaging technology has matured to the stage where it is very compatible with routine use in the clinical situation (Fig. 11.14).

SUMMARY

In this chapter, the principles of real-time B-scanning were studied. The pulse-echo mode of data collection was seen to be common to all types. Real-time B-scanners differ primarily in the methods used to sweep the beam rapidly and repetitively through the scan plane.

1. The value of real-time B-scanning was presented by noting six attractive features.
2. Ten types of scanner were listed in their classification. Each was described in detail. It is

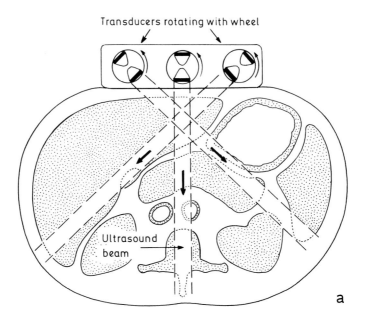

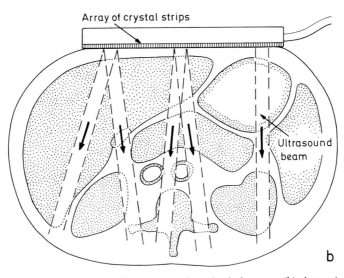

Fig. 11.13   Real-time compound B-scanning: (**a**) mechanical system, (**b**) electronic system.

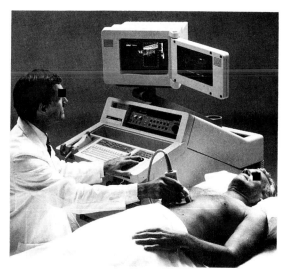

Fig. 11.14 The compatibility of real-time B-scanners with routine clinical use (courtesy of Philips).

important to build up a knowledge of the most appropriate type of transducer for each clinical application.

3. Features of real-time transducers and displays were considered. The large number of hand-held transducers was seen to be a major attraction of real-time B-scanning.

4. Since transducer selection is so central to work in diagnostic ultrasound, knowledge should be accumulated of the strengths and weaknesses of each type.

REFERENCES

Barber F E, Baker D W, Strandness, Jr, D E et al 1974 Duplex scanner 11: For simultaneous imaging of artery tissues and flow. IEEE Ultrasonics Symp Proc 744–748

Bom N, Lancee C T, Honkoop J et al 1971 Ultrasonic viewer for cross-sectional analysis of moving cardiac structures. Biomed Eng 6: 500–508

Bow C R, McDicken W N, Anderson T et al 1979 A rotating transducer real-time scanner for ultrasonic examination of the heart and abdomen. Br J Radiol 52: 29–33

Davidorf F H 1975 A simplified B-scan ultrasonoscope for ocular diagnosis. Ann Ophthalmol 7: 927–933

Griffith J M, Henry W L 1974 A sector scanner for real-time two-dimensional echocardiography. Circulation 49: 1147–1152

Holm H H, Kristensen J K, Pedersen J F et al 1975 A new mechanical real-time ultrasonic contact scanner. Ultrasound Med Biol 2: 19–23

Iinuma K, Kidokoro T, Ogura I et al 1979 High-resolution, electronic-linear-scanning ultrasonic diagnostic equipment. Ultrasound Med Biol 5: 51–59

Ligtvoet C, Rijsterborgh H, Kappen L et al 1978 Real-time ultrasonic imaging with a hand-held scanner. Part I — technical description. Ultrasound Med Biol 4: 91–92

McDicken W N, Bruff K, Paton J 1974 An ultrasonic instrument for rapid B-scanning of the heart. Ultrasonics 12: 269–272

McDicken W N, Anderson T, McHugh R et al 1979 An ultrasonic real-time scanner with pulsed Doppler and T-M facilities for foetal breathing and other obstetrical studies. Ultrasound Med Biol 4: 333–339

Somer J C 1968 Electronic sector scanning for ultrasonic diagnosis. Ultrasonics 6: 153–159

von Ramm O T, Thurstone F L 1976 Cardiac imaging using a phased array ultrasound system. I. System design. Circulation 53: 258–262

Winsberg F 1979 Real-time scanners: A review. Med Ultrasound 3: 99–106

12. Performance of real-time B-scan instruments

The factors that determine the performance of real-time B-scan machines will now be considered. Not all aspects of the performance of real-time B-scanners have been fully investigated. For example, real-time images on a display usually look superior to any static recording of that image. It is probable that small motions of structures such as the liver help the eye to differentiate between true echoes from structures and spurious echoes formed by multiple reflections. Likewise, the effect of a limited frame rate (e.g. 30 frames/s) on imaging fast-moving structures has not been evaluated in detail.

LIMITATIONS OF REAL-TIME B-SCANNING

The limitations of ultrasonic imaging techniques are not always easy to quantify. Accurate knowledge does not always exist of the physical quantities and effects associated with the propagation of ultrasound in tissue. The 'suck it and see' approach is often a good way of finding out if a particular application is feasible. Though future developments may well reduce the various limitations, the demands on the subject are also growing. The limitations are now briefly reviewed before we consider them further in this and the next chapter.

Resolution

The spatial and contrast resolutions in images are lower than might be desired. They are improving slowly as focused transducers, image processing, etc; find application. Resolution is discussed later in this chapter.

Line density

The interdependence of line density, frame rate, and field of view has been noted in the previous chapter. If any one of these parameters is made large, one or both of the others must be reduced. Line density in real-time B-scanning is restricted, in practice, to the order of 150 lines per image. This may be compared to slower scanning methods where there is time to put several hundred lines in the image. The limited line density of a real-time image degrades the resolution, but, since beams have a finite width, this is not too serious and may hardly be noticeable.

Uniformity of line density in a linear-array or water-bath instrument is constant, or nearly so, throughout the image. A sector field of view has increasing line density towards its apex. Sector images can be significantly degraded at greater ranges because the line density decreases continuously with depth as the scan lines fan out.

Field of view

The image from the majority of real-time instruments is often only part of the section of interest; for instance, it may not be possible to image a whole fetus. Some instruments, by their inherent design, suffer more from this limitation than do others. The problem is basic to this mode of scan. Suppose that it is possible to generate echo lines at a rate of 3000/s before the tail of one echo train overlaps the start of the next. If 30 frames per second are presented, each frame will contain 100 lines of acoustic information. To maintain a reasonable line density (e.g. 1 line/mm or 1 line/degree), one must restrict the area swept out by the beam.

Practical factors may affect the size of the field of view. When scanning a curved abdomen, linear-array and water-bath scanners may have difficulty in making contact with the skin surface for the full width of their theoretical field shape. In cardiac examinations, access to the heart can be limited by the lung gas, and bone.

The field shape, as distinct from the size, may also be a limitation. The narrow region at the top of a sector presents limited information on superficial structures. In general, water-bath scanners are best for viewing superficial regions, followed closely by some linear-array instruments.

Simple scan action

Simple scan actions are satisfactory for many applications and may, indeed, be the action of choice. The option to try compound scanning is not usually open to the operator.

Noise

There are three sources of noise in ultrasonic images — electronic noise, spurious reflections, and image speckle.

Interpretation of images

Difficulties arise from uncertainties in the sources of some echoes. The image of a plane section through an object can often be intrinsically difficult to interpret.

Unknown distortions of the ultrasonic beam

In any ultrasonic technique, the ultrasonic beam can be deformed in tissue in an unknown way by phenomena such as refraction, absorption, and reflection.

Assumption of average properties for tissue

Calibration of picture scale and accurate registration of echo spots in the image depend on an assumption of an average value for the velocity of sound in tissue. We noted earlier that this assumption can produce range measurement errors of 2 or 3 mm. This results in a slight misregistration of echoes that may degrade the definition of interfaces in an image, though it is not usually a serious problem with the simple scan actions used in most real-time scanners.

The assumption of an average rate of attenuation in different tissues when setting up the TGC will be inaccurate in many situations, for example, the attenuation of ultrasound in a fetal head is much greater than that in amniotic fluid.

Display limitation

In ultrasonic scanning, the significant range of ultrasonic echo size may be 100:1 (40 dB). The limited dynamic range of displays and of our ability to appreciate grey shades require the echo-signal dynamic range to be compressed to around 25 dB (approximately 16:1).

Operator bias

Preconceived ideas may influence the way in which results are interpreted or the sensitivity controls manipulated.

Image variability

An ultrasonic image is dependent on the machine, the operator, and the patient. Machine and operator variability are being reduced as equipment design develops and expertise spreads. Variability owing to the patient is also being reduced, to some extent, by improvements in instrumentation. However, it is likely the variability in ultrasonic images will remain higher than that in other imaging modalities for the foreseeable future.

Image flicker

For the eye to combine a series of rapidly presented images into a moving picture, a frame rate greater than 15/s is desirable. It is necessary to have a frame rate of at least 20/s to remove image flicker. For instance, a domestic television presents complete images at a rate of 25 or 30/s, that is, 50 or 60 interlaced rasters (see Ch. 1). Cine-film projectors commonly operate at 24 frames/s.

With a digital scan converter, an image from one beam sweep can be stored and presented several times before the next sweep is complete. Thus, the scan frame rate could be 8/s, but the display frame rate, 24/s. In this situation, the true image content changes at a rate of 8/s but the flicker is acceptable. A low true frame rate may be employed to give a high line density, or because it is difficult to move a large transducer quickly.

EFFECTIVE ULTRASONIC BEAM SHAPE

We must now consider beam shape in more detail before studying resolution in ultrasonic images.

For a particular frequency bandwidth in the transmitted pulse, the shape of the transmitted intensity field is determined primarily by the dimensions and shape of the transducer elements (Fig. 1.2a). The degree of blackness in the figure is related to the intensity of ultrasound at each point. After rising to a maximum at the focus, the intensity can be considered to fall off slowly with distance along the axis from the transducer. It decreases rapidly in the direction at right angles to the central axis.

As well as considering the transmitted intensity field, we must consider the sensitivity reception zone. For a single-element transducer, reception is the converse of transmission; therefore, the reception zone sensitivity pattern is the same as that for the transmitted intensity field (Fig. 5.7a). Where electronic focusing is employed, the transmission field and reception zone may be very different in shape (Fig. 5.7b).

The combined effect of the field and zone determines the ultrasound beam shape (Fig. 5.9) and, hence, plays a large part in determining the echo magnitudes received from targets in front of the transducer. For pulsed-echo use, the beam of a transducer may be described as that region within which echoes can be detected from a standard target. The beam is usually plotted by moving a standard ball bearing systematically in front of the transducer and noting the echo amplitude at each point (see Ch. 27).

From the standpoint of diagnostic ultrasound, we are interested in the size of echoes that can be detected from targets at points throughout the beam. Therefore, with the sensitivity controls of

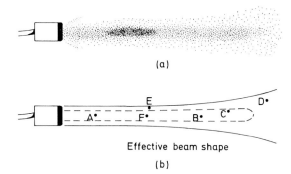

Fig. 12.1 (a) Pictorial representation of an ultrasonic beam, (b) effective beam width for particular target and sensitivity settings.

the instrument fixed, let us consider the echoes detected by the transducer from a tissue target positioned at different locations in the beam. Because the target is close to the transducer and on the central axis of the beam at point A (Fig. 12.1), a strong echo is detected. It is still on axis at B, but the incident intensity is less, and it is further from the transducer; hence, a weaker echo is detected. The echo is weak at C because the target is off axis. The echo is probably not recorded at D as the target is far off axis and distant from the crystal. The target may escape detection at E since, although it is fairly close to the transducer, it is very far off axis. The echo strength from E may be more than −40 dB below that from F.

It is thus evident that only part of the ultrasonic beam may be effective in producing detectable echoes. In ultrasonic imaging, it is very relevant to think in terms of 'effective' beam shape. The broken line in Figure 12.1b represents the effective beam shape for the above target and instrument settings.

During the previous discussion, the sensitivity of the instrument was held fixed. If the sensitivity is increased, for example, by putting up the gain or intensity, or decreasing the suppression level, the previously undetected echo from E can be recorded. When the sensitivity is increased still more, an echo may be picked up from position D. Similarly, decreasing the sensitivity could mean that the originally weak echoes from B and C are no longer displayed. Thus, the effective beam shape varies with the sensitivity settings.

The effective beam width also varies with the

reflectivity of the target, and this is relevant to considerations of detail in clinical images. Consider an electronic detection system that can process echoes with a 40 dB dynamic range without distortion. Consider also a strong reflector on the central axis, and let its echo size be the maximum the system can handle. Now let it move towards the side of the beam. The echo magnitude drops, and when it is 40 dB below its on-axis value, it is no longer detected. This may occur at a distance of as little as 5 mm from the central axis. If the procedure is repeated with a weak reflector of −20 dB reflectivity compared to the strong reflector, then its echo may be lost after it has moved 2 mm from the axis.

Two points can be made from this experiment. First, when the controls are set for a scan, the weaker the reflector, the narrower the effective beam width. This explains why within an organ such as the liver, structures formed by weak reflectors are often depicted with high resolution, while the surrounding major interfaces look fairly coarse. Second, if the dynamic range had been 50 dB, the effective beam width would have been wider for each target. Systems are therefore designed with a dynamic range large enough to detect weak reflectors near the central axis, but not so large as to allow strong reflectors to be detected when they have passed well to the side of the beam.

From these considerations, we can see that the effective beam width is variable and highly dependent on how the operator drives the machine. In other words, the image quality is highly dependent on the operator. Note the distinction made between transmitted ultrasonic field and ultrasonic beam which depends on both the transmitted field and reception zone. The ultrasonic beam is of more direct relevance to diagnostic techniques than the ultrasonic field on its own.

RESOLUTION IN REAL-TIME B-SCANNING

The detail in a real-time image depends on the resolution achieved by the scanning instrument. The minimum size of structure and the minimum detectable difference in tissue reflectivity, or contrast, are of major interest in determining possible applications. It is essential to have an appreciation of these limits so that echo patterns are not interpreted wrongly.

Axial resolution (range or linear resolution)

Axial resolution is the minimum separation of two objects along the beam axis for which two separate echoes can be identified. It is determined by the ultrasonic pulse length, which can be made shorter at high frequencies. In theory, the axial resolution is equal to half the pulse length, as has been noted already for A-scanning.

The axial resolution of all types of single-element and array scanners is fairly similar at a particular ultrasonic frequency. Occasionally designers appear to sacrifice axial resolution slightly by making the pulse length longer with a view to producing a better beam shape.

Lateral resolution (azimuthal or beam-width resolution)

Lateral resolution is the minimum separation of two objects placed at the same range for which two separate echoes can be identified. The way in which lateral resolution contributes to the final image and depends on effective beam width is most clearly shown by considering a simple scan of two point targets, equidistant from the transducer.

First the scan is performed with the targets separated by several beam widths (Fig. 12.2), and echoes are received at the transducer as the beam sweeps across each target. For the whole time that a target is within the beam, it is reflecting echoes back to the transducer. Because the line of presentation of echoes on the screen continuously follows the motion of the beam, the echoes write a short line on the screen as the beam sweeps across a target. The length of the line is equal to the effective width of the beam at the position of the target. Thus, because of beam width, point targets are registered as short lines.

Now move the targets closer together and perform another scan. The recorded short lines on the screen also move closer together. When separation of the targets is almost reduced to the beam width, the lines on the screen virtually form one line (Fig.

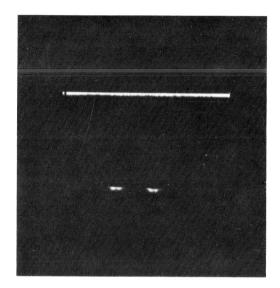

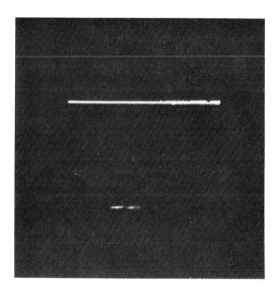

Fig. 12.2 Lateral resolution in B-scan imaging. Top, well separated targets: bottom, neighbouring targets.

12.2). Targets in this position are separated by the minimum distance for registration as two separate objects on the display. This minimum separation is the lateral resolution.

We noted above that effective beam width, and hence, lateral resolution are variable quantities depending on the instrument sensitivity, the nature of the target, and its position in the beam. Lateral resolution is the main factor in determin-

ing detail in an ultrasonic scan. It degrades the image more than axial resolution; for example, at 3 MHz, a typical value for lateral resolution may be 3 mm while that for axial resolution is 1 mm.

The lateral resolution is highly dependent on the focusing of the beam. Single-element transducers have a narrow beam close to their focus, but the resolution may be quite poor away from the focus. Electronic focusing in all types of array scanners greatly improves resolution over an extended range (Fig. 12.3).

If a beam is symmetrical in shape about its axis, the lateral resolution is the same in the directions parallel to the scan plane and perpendicular to it (Fig. 5.15). Beams from linear and phased arrays are, however, electronically focused only in the direction parallel to the scan plane. For these types of transducer, the 'in-plane' is superior to the 'out-of-plane' lateral resolution. Although the effect of the latter is not easily recognized in the image, it does, in fact, determine the thickness of the slice of tissue examined during a scan.

Electronic insertion of lines of echoes among the genuine acoustic lines helps to improve the acceptability of the image for viewing. However, it is unlikely to do much for the lateral resolution, even if averaging and smoothing techniques are used in the electronic generation of the echo information for the new lines.

An estimate of both axial and lateral resolution may be obtained from the image of a small target in a tissue-mimicking test-object. The thickness of the image line provides the axial resolution and the width the lateral resolution (Fig. 12.3).

Contrast resolution (reflectivity resolution)

Contrast resolution is the minimum change in reflectivity of tissue which can be depicted in an image. The detail in an image depends strongly on the power of the system to depict differences in the reflectivity of targets. In theory, this can be achieved for distinct interfaces to a high accuracy; for example, interfaces may be resolved for which the echo amplitudes differ by 1%. In practice, angulation of the interface to the beam and the shape of the interface create uncertainties that reduce contrast resolution to worse than 10%.

Contrast resolution for neighbouring tissue areas

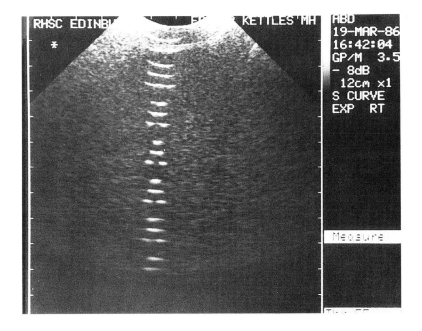

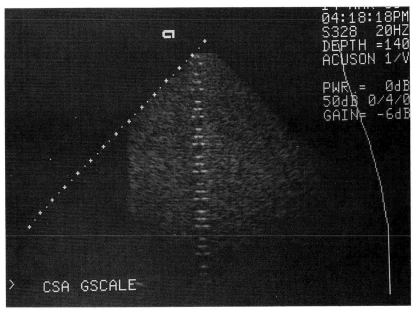

Fig. 12.3   Images of wire targets in a tissue-mimicking test-object. Top, image using a single-element, fixed-focus scanner — note degradation of image away from focus. Bottom, image using phased-array transducer with electronic focusing — note extended focal region.

in which signals are generated by closely spaced targets is more difficult to determine. The reflected and scattered echoes from each target overlap and interfere to produce the resultant signal for that area. The size and shape of the resultant signal depends not only on the amplitudes of the individual echoes but also on the relative positions of the targets (Fig. 12.4).

These interference effects produce statistical fluctuations in the resultant signals and, hence, a speckle-pattern appearance in neighbouring areas of the image. This speckle is, in effect, noise in

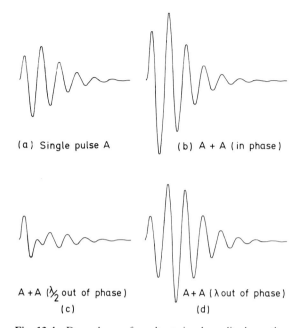

(a) Single pulse A (b) A + A (in phase)

A + A (λ/2 out of phase) A + A (λ out of phase)
(c) (d)

Fig. 12.4 Dependence of resultant signal amplitude on the relative positions of closely spaced targets. (a) Echo from one target (b) echo from two adjacent targets (c) echo from two targets separated by $\lambda/2$ (d) echo from two targets separated by λ.

Minimum resolvable structure size

Having studied axial, lateral, and contrast resolution, we can now attempt to define the minimum size of structure that can be imaged with present-day techniques. There is no easy answer to the question of minimum detectable detail; it can be answered with reasonable accuracy only when the particular examination is specified for a particular type of patient. When scanning the abdomen with 3 MHz ultrasound, one can image structures of dimensions around 2 mm in some situations, but more typically the minimum size is 5 mm. Similarly, in eye scanning at 10 MHz, structures of 0.5 or 1 mm can be outlined. This ties in reasonably with our notion of effective beam width.

Note that the smallest resolvable structure is not necessarily the smallest structure that can provide useful information. In many situations, the mere presence of echo-producing interfaces is valuable information. Also note that when working with images on a reduced scale (e.g. one-third life-size), it is easy to develop a false sense of high resolution. If echoes are displayed on a life-size scale, then most reflectors, in fact, register as short lines.

In obtaining the best possible resolution, two points are of importance. First, the operator must use the highest frequency that will give the necessary penetration, because high-frequency transducers can be designed to generate short pulses and narrow beams of ultrasound. As noted earlier, in most applications the best frequency for the task has been established by workers in the field. Second, unnecessarily high sensitivity is not recommended because this produces a large effective beam width and, hence, degrades the resolution. This latter point of technique has to be treated with some caution in case some valuable echoes are lost. It is probably best to start with a slightly high level of overall gain or ultrasonic intensity to detect the required echoes, and then to reduce the gain or intensity to optimize image detail. If the operator has the sensitivity controls well set up, then the effective beam width can be made narrow, and a surprisingly good resolution obtained.

A few test objects and phantoms for the measurement of resolution have been developed and are

the image which reduces the power of the system to depict small contrast changes; that is, it reduces the contrast resolution. The patterns from the parenchyma of the liver, spleen, and kidneys are common examples of such speckle patterns. Since the fluctuations in the speckle are of a statistical noise nature, the larger the area of tissue examined, the more accurately can its reflectivity be determined. The contrast resolution for a 5 mm tissue mass surrounded by other tissue might be 30%, as compared to 10% for a 3 cm mass of the same tissue. Contrast resolution can be improved by image smoothing techniques.

Contrast resolution is dependent on the transducer type only in a limited way; a narrow beam reduces the echoes from structures outside the tissue of interest. Contrast resolution is influenced more by the way echo-signal size is translated into grey shades and image processing in the scan converter. This is one of the reasons why single-element scanners often provide images which are comparable to those of array scanners. Another reason is that good design of array scanners is difficult.

commercially available. These permit resolution to be checked at regular intervals. The most useful test pieces are designed to generate echoes of magnitude similar to those encountered in clinical applications. Information on test objects is supplied in Appendix 1.

Temporal resolution

Since real-time B-scanners often present the changing of structures with time, we will briefly consider temporal resolution. Temporal resolution is the minimum separation in time for which two events can be observed. With a frame rate of 25/s the images recorded are separated in time by 40 ms. Detailed study of motion is obviously not possible if significant changes occur in less than this time interval. This image production rate is adequate for many movements in the body, such as movements of a fetus or the pulsations of the abdominal aorta. Most heart movements can be observed well with frame rates in the 20–30/s range. The more rapid excursions present in the heart, however, cannot be depicted satisfactorily at a frame rate of 25/s.

Some instruments can operate at 50/s or more, with a corresponding reduction in the line density or field of view. The time interval between images is then 20 ms or less. When even faster actions are of interest, for example, the flutter of a heart valve, M-mode recording is required.

A final point to bear in mind is that the tissue structure positions depicted in a single frame do not all correspond to the same moment in time. The ultrasonic beam takes a finite time to sweep across the field of view; for example, 40 ms for a frame rate of 25/s, and 20 ms at 50/s.

With a mechanical oscillating real-time scanner, in which the beam sweeps back and forth, the time interval between renewal of any line of echo data in the image depends on the position of that line in the field of view. This is a result of the non-uniform sweep speed of the beam.

Display size

The advent of the presentation of ultrasonic images on large grey-tone displays was of considerable importance in the development of diagnostic ultrasonics. There has been a tendency to retreat from this position in the development of real-time scanners. The reasons for this are the desire for portability and lower line density in the images. It is not desirable to take this trend too far. Apart from the inconvenience in viewing small screens, the display spot size does not usually decrease in direct proportion to screen size. Unless portability is of paramount importance, a reasonable size of grey-tone screen (e.g. 15 × 15 cm) is indicated. Some instruments do manage to combine compactness and good screen size.

A zoom control permits magnification of a portion of an image and may enable small movements, of perhaps a few millimetres, to be appreciated on a small screen. Such small movements may be encountered in pulsating blood vessels or fetal breathing actions.

From this discussion, it may be seen that a number of factors influence resolution. Table 12.1 summarizes these factors and attempts to assess their significance. The operator is cited as a factor because of the large influence of the settings of the sensitivity controls.

MEASUREMENT FROM IMAGES

Dimensions of the tissue structures are measured from an image and presented to the operator as numeric values of their true physical size. Linear dimensions, such as the diameter of a fetal head, the axial length of an eye chamber, or the diameter of a blood vessel, are measured using an electronic calliper or a calibration scale. Calliper systems are also used to evaluate area or circumference, and to calculate volume. These callipers are normally an integral feature of the scanner and measurements are made from the display screen; measurements may also be made from recorded images or charts, using separate instruments.

Considerable care is required to make accurate absolute measurements. When making measurements of biological structures, it is often much easier to record changes in dimensions and to follow these changes in serial studies. Changes can often be interpreted more reliably in this way, since some of the errors will affect all the measurements in the same way.

Table 12.1 Factors which influence the resolution in a pulse echo image

Factor	(Related parameter)	Importance
Pulse length	(Transducer, Frequency)	7
Beam width	(Transducer, Frequency, Focusing, Dynamic range)	10
Contrast	(Grey shade, Noise)	8
Propagation	(Attenuation)	8
	(Refraction)	2
	(Diffraction)	2
	(Non-linear propagation)	2
Signal processing	(Edge enhancement, Compression)	7
Image processing	(Filtering, Adaptive TGC)	6
Recording systems		8
Operator	(Sensitivity)	10
Frame rate	(Line density)	3

Measurement on a straight line

To make a measurement of a linear dimension such as the biparietal diameter of a fetal head, we use a feature of the scanner known as an 'electronic calliper'. Superimposed on a frozen image, two marker spots are adjusted to lie on the boundaries of the structure of interest (see Fig. 2.11). It is usually recommended that the calliper markers be placed on the leading edges of the displayed echoes; however, some compromise is necessary if the leading edges are not clearly depicted. For example, in the measurement of a liquid-filled structure such as a cyst or heart chamber, the trailing of the first echo and the leading edge of the second are commonly used. The numeric value for the distance between the spots is displayed on the instrument. Several dimensions may be measured on the same image with additional markers.

An alternative calibration approach is to include in the image a line of regularly spaced marker spots to provide a scale for measurement.

An error of ±1 mm is typical of measurement along a line on a 9 inch (23 cm) display screen. The greatest accuracy is achieved by displaying the image on the largest convenient scale.

When measurements are made from recorded images, a check should be made to see whether the recording device has altered the scale of presentation. It is not uncommon for a camera to alter the scale of an image recorded from a display screen.

Measurement in a plane (length, area, circumference, 'volume')

For measurements on a curved line in an image, a bright indicator spot on the display is moved along the line, and at small regular intervals a mark is superimposed on the line. The length is automatically computed and displayed on the screen. If the line is a closed loop, the circumference value is obtained when the indicator spot returns to its starting point (Fig. 12.5). The area of the loop is usually automatically calculated and displayed at this time. Reasonably smooth movement of the indicator spot is possible with a variety of measurement devices. Areas in images from parallel planes of scan of known separation enable the volume of an organ to be calculated.

When the indicator is placed at a point on the image, two coordinates are recorded that define the position of that point in the plane. These coordinates are usually the X and Y Cartesian coordinates that, respectively, define the horizontal and vertical distances of the point from the origin (Fig. 12.6). When the operator positions the indicator at an appropriate point, the coordinates

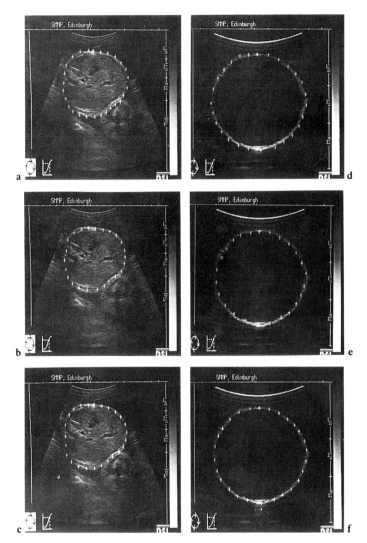

Fig. 12.5 Effect of measurement decisions on value obtained; (**a**) and (**d**) markers on outside of boundary; (**b**) and (**e**) on inside of boundary; (**c**) and (**f**) in centre of boundary. Value obtained for (**a**), 304 mm; (**b**) 283 mm; (**c**), 292 mm; (**d**), 218 mm; (**e**), 205 mm; (**f**), 211 mm. The images (**a**), (**b**), and (**c**) are of the cross section of a fetal abdomen; images (**d**), (**e**), and (**f**) are of a circular test-object.

are recorded and stored in the computer memory. The indicator may then be moved to a second point and the process repeated. Usually the indicator is moved continuously, and coordinates of neighbouring points are recorded automatically.

Measurement devices

A long-established method for making measurements directly on a display screen utilizes a television-raster display and a light pen. The light pen has a light detector at its tip that is placed on the point to be recorded. The position of the tip on the screen is recorded by noting the time delay between the start of the television raster at the top corner of the screen and the scanning spot sweeping past the pen tip. This time delay is converted into X and Y coordinates. Points at which coordinates have been recorded and stored in memory are marked on the displayed image to show where

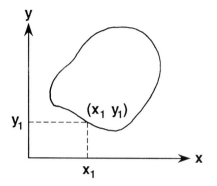

Fig. 12.6 Coordinate systems employed in measuring devices (Cartesian coordinates)

measurements have been made. Coordinates can be measured with an error of 1 mm on a 9-inch television screen.

The joy stick and the roller ball are two common devices for measurement from frozen images on a display screen. They generate voltages corresponding to the X and Y coordinates of the bright indicator spot, which is overlayed on the display and which may be freely moved around it.

An advantage of techniques which make measurements directly on the display screen is that sources of error, such as distortion by the CRT display, affect equally the location of the indicator spots and the echoes in the image. The errors, therefore, cancel out. It has been shown that errors of around $\pm 2\%$ are incurred with this type of system in measuring the circumferences of test objects of the size of a fetal head or kidney.

When one is purchasing an ultrasonic scanner, it is very advisable to check that the measurement system is, in fact, easy to use, since it may be employed to make a large number of time-consuming measurements. Check to see that the markers can be moved rapidly, smoothly, and accurately to the desired location. A major defect in some systems is that an indicator-spot-positioning error can be corrected only by restarting the whole procedure, and not by erasing the last few points.

A variety of principles are applied in coordinate-measurement devices which are suitable for use with recorded images or charts and which are independent of the scanner. Electric potentiometers, whose variable electrical resistance is governed by the position of an indicator or pointer, may be at-tached to the side of a board on which the image or chart is laid. Other devices have an indicator that transmits low-frequency ultrasound toward detectors at the side of the measuring frame. The transit times from the indicator to the detectors are converted into XY coordinates. Other electric position-sensing methods are also used. These devices are usually accurate to better than 1%. They have been developed for fields such as engineering drawing and cartography.

Accuracy of dimension measurements from images

The accuracy of a measurement using an image depends on a number of factors:

1. The selection of the correct section through the tissues
2. The clear and complete depiction of the structure of interest
3. The decision as to the correct place to put the calliper markers
4. The use of the correct value for the velocity of ultrasound in tissue to calculate the image scale
5. The accuracy of the electronic measuring device

From the first three points in this list, it can be deduced that the operator has a bigger influence on the accuracy of the measurement than any technical factor associated with the instrument. Deciding where to place the calliper markers is particularly difficult. Figure 12.5 illustrates the measurement of a circumference using three different criteria. Placing the markers on the outside rim of the echo pattern (Fig. 12.5a) is a common approach, which is practical, but which is subject to obvious error, since the outside does not represent the true circumference. The same criticism can be levelled at placing the markers on the inside (Fig. 12.5b). Alteration of the sensitivity of the scanner changes the results obtained with these two approaches. The most logical technique, but still not perfect, is to put the marker spots in the centre of the echoes (Fig. 12.5c). At the top and bottom of the image, the centre of the echoes does not necessarily represent the circumference. It is worth noting the significant difference in the cir-

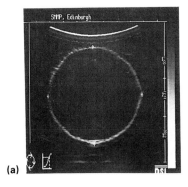

(a)

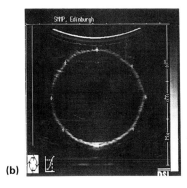

(b)

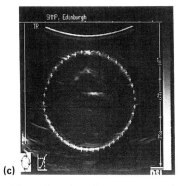

(c)

Fig. 12.7 Effect of number of measurement points on the result obtained for the circumference; (**a**), 197 mm; (**b**), 212 mm; (**c**), 213 mm.

cumference and area provided by the three measurement methods.

A few calliper systems have been designed for quick, convenient use. Typically, they estimate circumference and area by using a limited number of measurement points, or, equivalently, by matching an elliptical shape with the cross section to be measured. Figure 12.7 shows that reducing the number of measurement points reduces the ac-

curacy, but this method may be adequate for rough estimations.

Most callipers now assume a value for the average velocity of sound in tissue of 1540 m/s for all measurements, including that of the biparietal diameter of the fetal head. The older practice in some quarters of using 1600 m/s for the fetal head has been abandoned in the interests of simplicity. The assumption of one value for the average velocity is not a serious source of error since abnormal growth can still be detected, and the other sources of error are often larger than the typical error of 4% resulting from this assumption. Tissue dimensions quoted in the literature are only comparable with those from a machine if the literature dimensions were produced using the same velocity of sound as that of the machine. Care should therefore be exercised before using a growth curve from the literature.

Electronic callipers can be made very accurate; they contribute little to the total error. However, it is worth checking callipers, since it is not uncommon to find them badly set up. For instance, measurement in the vertical direction may be accurate while that in the horizontal has a substantial error.

On a large-scale image, linear dimensions can be measured with an error of only ±1%, for example, ±1 mm on a life-size image of a fetal head at term. The instrumentation is also capable of measuring cross-sectional areas with an error of about ±3% if the tissue boundaries are clearly defined. Two points should be made to qualify this statement of attainable accuracy. First, if the image is stored on a small scale (e.g. one-fifth life-size), the measurement of an area of 100 cm^2 could have an error as high as ±10%. On such a small scale, a line thickness in the image of 1 mm corresponds to a 5 mm tissue thickness. Second, absolute measurement of area is affected by any error in the assumed velocity of sound. For an assumed velocity of 1540 m/s, instead of the correct value of, say, 1500 m/s, a 5%-error arises in the measurement of 100 cm^2.

The accuracy achieved in the measurement of organ volumes appears to be at best about ±10%.

When using or devising a measurement procedure, we should ask some technical questions:

1. Is the scale of presentation of the image as large as possible?

2. Would alteration of the sensitivity or frequency make the image sharper?

3. What accuracy can be achieved by the procedure, and is it able to give a clinically significant result?

4. Is the measurement reproducible by the same operator or by another operator?

5. Would serial measurements improve the value of the technique?

6. Can the measurement be directly compared with those of other workers in the field? Comparison with the results of other workers requires checks on factors such as calliper velocity and similarity of population. The type of scanner, for example, sector or linear, should not affect the results, but the quality of the images will.

7. How many parallel sections are needed for accurate calculation of organ volume? A large number of sections increases the accuracy. In practice, the parallel sections are usually separated by a distance similar to that of the diameter or array width of the transducer.

8. Could a useful ratio of measured quantities be devised, for example, the head cross section to trunk cross section of a fetus? Some errors common to both measurements may cancel out when a ratio is taken. The use of ratios has proven successful in several applications of diagnostic ultrasound.

9. How could the measurement be improved?

10. Is this the best quantity to measure?

Accurate measurement from ultrasonic images is never easy. If a complex quantity is to be calculated from a few simple measurements, the error is liable to be large. For example, various formulae advocated for the estimation of fetal weight can give errors of 30%.

Accuracy of echo amplitude measurement from images

By the time echoes are presented on an image, much of the echo-amplitude information has been sacrificed. The grey tones in an image, however, do provide a measure of echo amplitude and, in particular, allow the reflectivity of areas of tissue to be assessed. Reflectivity can be measured with an error of ±20% from a grey-shade image. For more accurate values of reflectivity, A-scans or stored echo signals should be studied. Storage in digital scan converters allows echo magnitudes to be studied, but such techniques are rarely sufficiently accurate to be of clinical value.

SUMMARY

The accurate interpretation of images depends on knowing the limitations of the technique. Twelve areas of limitation of real-time B-scanning were considered. The resolution in an image is also of central importance, so the factors which influence resolution were assessed and listed. Since the effective beam width was seen to be variable, it was concluded that the resolution achieved with a scanner was strongly dependent on the operator. Measurement of anatomical structures is often un- often undertaken from images; therefore, the methods and devices were considered in detail. The accuracy which can be attained was examined and found to be a few per cent for spatial dimensions, but at least 10% for tissue-reflectivity measurement.

REFERENCES

Alasaarela E, Koivukangas J 1990 Evaluation of image quality of ultrasound scanners in medical diagnostics. J Ultrasound Med 9: 23–34

BMUS Ultrasonic fetal measurement survey 1990. British Medical Ultrasonic Society, 36 Portland Place, London WIN 3DG

Deter R L, Harrist R B, Birnholtz J C, Hadlock F P 1986 Quantitative obstetrical ultrasonography. Wiley, New York

Feigenbaum H 1986 Echocardiography. 5th edn. Lea and Febiger, Philadelphia

13. Using real-time B-scan instruments

In clinical applications, the role of a real-time B-scan instrument may vary from that of a screening instrument to that of one used to perform and record a complex examination.

SCANNING PROCEDURE

For completeness and for guidance to beginners in the field, the scanning procedure with a real-time unit will now be described. Many of the points raised are obvious; however, it is useful to consider the process as a whole.

The patient is positioned on the couch usually in the prone, supine, or decubitus position. Some applications are helped by specific postures such as raising the feet to move an engaged fetal head or arching the back to spread the ribs for kidney scanning. The real-time aspect of the scans permits movement of tissues to be observed as the patient is manipulated, for example, in ophthalmology and infant hip studies. Great flexibility in the scanning procedure is feasible as a result of the compact dimensions of most transducer assemblies. Scanning with the patient standing or performing a stress test is possible.

The transducer head is coupled to the skin of the patient with a liberal amount of oil or gel. With any scanner in which the front surface is curved, care should be taken to ensure good contact with the skin for a large part of its surface area. Otherwise, the edge of the ultrasound beam at the transducer/air interface, may produce multiple reflection signals that are added to the genuine echoes. This is shown on the screen by a reduction in the usable angle of the sector scan. Slight pressure on the skin or the addition of more gel will exclude the air and remove the multiple reflections. The essential rule for good coupling is that all air must be excluded if it can interfere with the passage of ultrasound between the scanner and the patient.

The transducer head is placed on the skin surface to image a section that is expected to be readily understood from an anatomic point of view; for example, a longitudinal section of the pregnant uterus, a transverse section of the eye, or the four-chamber view of the heart.

A check is made to ensure that the sensitivity and scan-converter controls are set at recognized baseline positions for the particular transducer and application. Baseline settings can be established initially by using the method described in Chapter 7 and in the light of subsequent experience with each machine. Many machines allow baseline settings for particular applications or operators to be stored in the computer memory and to be simply recalled.

Observing the image on the display, one adjusts the sensitivity controls to produce the best possible grey-tone image. Weak echo signals should be checked to ascertain if they are being presented in the lowest shades of grey. Strong echoes should not appear as long white spots, indicating saturation.

Automatic gain control (AGC), in which the machine sets up the TGC by relating it to the magnitude of the received echoes, works well in several instruments. AGC may provide the best sensitivity for searching through the body.

In addition to checking the sensitivity controls, the operator should note the display controls such as image orientation, postprocessing curve, field-of-view size, and frame rate. A quick check of the recording equipment is also worthwhile. The searching process and the clinical interpretation of the images can now begin.

The key to success in ultrasonic scanning is often the identification of familiar landmarks; for example, the diaphragm in liver scanning, the mitral valve in the heart, and the network of blood vessels adjacent to the pancreas. These landmarks not only serve to identify tissue structures, but also indicate, through their appearance on the screen, the suitability of the instrument settings for that patient and that examination.

Several techniques exist for recording images. These rarely capture the full image quality or information content of a real-time examination. Photography of frozen images provides a permanent record. Television video-tape recording best retains the information (Ch. 26).

Measurement by the real-time mode is an attractive proposition because of the ease with which relevant sections can be visualized and recorded (Ch. 12).

The capacity of real-time B-scanners to perform dynamic studies and their compact size has resulted in their being combined with other procedures. Time-motion scanning, Doppler-flow detection, and tissue-puncture biopsy are examples of these procedures. Here the role of the real-time technique is primarily to identify anatomic structures.

For the operator to reproduce a result accurately, the following contributing factors need recording:

1. Sensitivity and display-control settings
2. Transducer identification
3. Real-time scan-control settings
4. Recording system parameters
5. Plane of scan (App. 5)
6. Patient posture and manipulation

Much of this scan specification information appears automatically on the display screen or can be typed on to it.

A few points are worth remembering when considering real-time B-scanning. The plane of scan can be swept smoothly and continuously through complex anatomy, a facility which greatly assists in the understanding of the relative positions of the component structures. At first, one may think that because the beam width is several millimetres,

there is little to gain by viewing planes that are more closely spaced. In practice, however, if the operator observes an image as it changes with the scan plane, then a three-dimensional mental image of the tissues can be built up. Note that if the scan plane is altered by pivoting the transducer about its face, the plane sweeps through deep tissues much faster than superficial ones. For example, a 30° tilt will move the plane of scan 3 cm at a depth of 5 cm, but 12 cm at a depth of 20 cm.

EFFECT OF SENSITIVITY CONTROLS ON IMAGE

During ultrasonic scanning, the number and size of echo signals presented on the display screen depend mainly on how the operator manipulates the sensitivity controls. Gain, TGC, ultrasonic intensity, suppression, and frequency have been linked together in this text and called the sensitivity controls. These controls must be operated in an interrelated fashion rather than as five independent variables (Ch. 7). Another reason for treating them collectively is that, in some respects, they have similar effects on the echo pattern. This is particularly true of gain, intensity (power), suppression, and frequency. In fact, in a number of machines, only two or three of these controls may be variable.

Effect of sensitivity controls

It is worthwhile to scan a complex tissue structure and carefully note the effect of changing each sensitivity control. Figure 13.1 illustrates the effect of altering the intensity control while leaving other sensitivity controls fixed. A 10 dB change can be seen to have a marked effect on the displayed image.

Figures 13.2 and 13.3 show that the effect of changing gain is similar to that of changing intensity. Indeed, Figure 13.4 shows that a -10 dB decrease in intensity can be compensated by a $+10$ dB increase in gain.

Alteration of the suppression control is usually more difficult to quantify. It can be seen from Figure 13.5, however, that, although suppression acts by rejecting weak echoes, its effect on the final

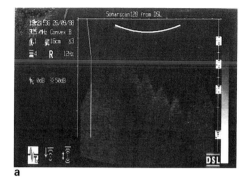

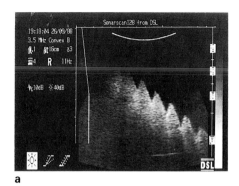

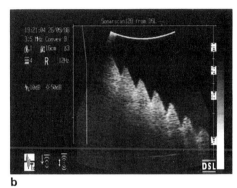

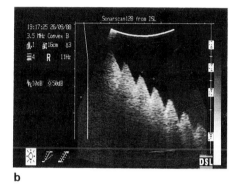

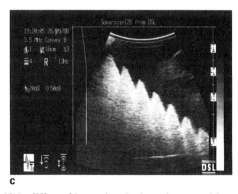

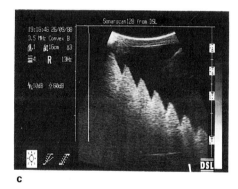

Fig. 13.1   Effect of increasing the intensity control by 10 dB steps.

Fig. 13.2   Effect of increasing the gain control by 10 dB steps.

display is similar to that of gain and intensity changes.

The sensitivity of an instrument is affected by the frequency selected. Figure 13.6 shows that 3.5 MHz ultrasound is the highest frequency, of those available on the instrument, to give adequate penetration for scanning the test-object.

TGC was discussed fully in Chapter 7 and is the most difficult of the sensitivity controls to set up correctly. Figure 13.7 demonstrates some of the

consequences of poorly adjusted TGC controls.

In the overall assessment of the ability of a system to display echo information in an image, there are other contributory factors. The first of these is the display system controls. The effect of having the brilliance control too low is that only the strong echoes are recorded. The picture scale also is of importance. Figure 13.8 shows a scan for three different display scales.

Manipulation of an ultrasound beam-focus con-

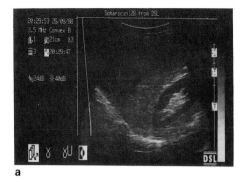

a

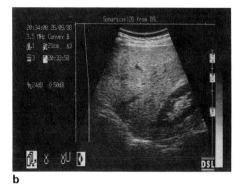

b

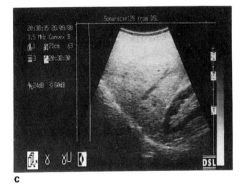

c

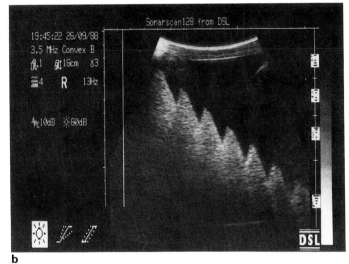

a

b

Fig. 13.3 Effect of increasing the gain control by 10 dB steps.

Fig. 13.4 (a) Intensity 20 dB, gain 50 dB; (b) intensity 10 dB, gain 60 dB. Note decrease in intensity by −10 dB is compensated for by an increase in gain by +10 dB.

trol also affects the sensitivity throughout, or in localized regions of, the image. In the focal region, the structures are presented not only more sharply than outside the focal region but also somewhat more strongly (Fig.13.9).

To include the digital scan converter controls among those that are manipulated during the scanning creates too many variables in the procedure. It is recommended, therefore, that the preprocessing option most suited to the application be fixed at the start as described in Chapter 10. Once the image has been recorded, the postprocessing options may be tried to see if they add diagnostic information.

We can conclude that a number of factors produce the final result. Assuming that display and scan converter controls are set up, the operator then concentrates on the problem of how best to use the sensitivity controls collectively.

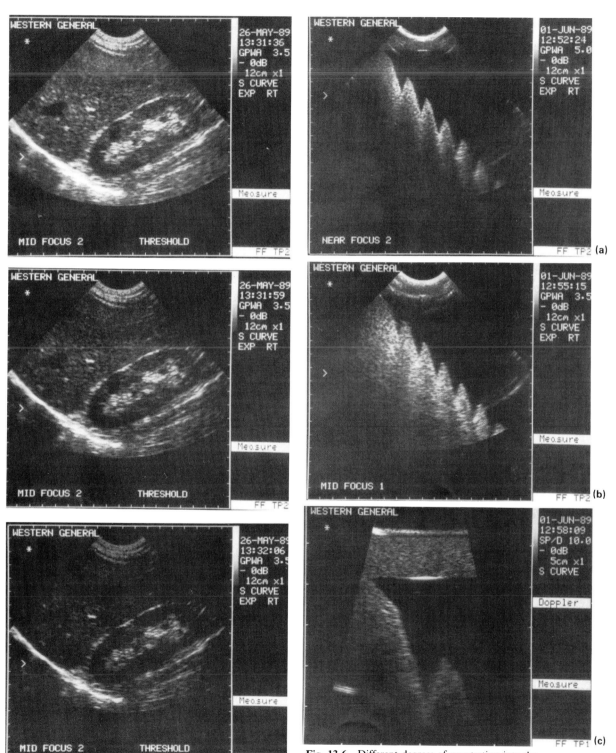

Fig. 13.5   Effect of change in the suppression level.

Fig. 13.6   Different degrees of penetration into the test-object using frequencies (**a**) 3.5 MHz, (**b**) 5.0 MHz, (**c**) 10.0 MHz.

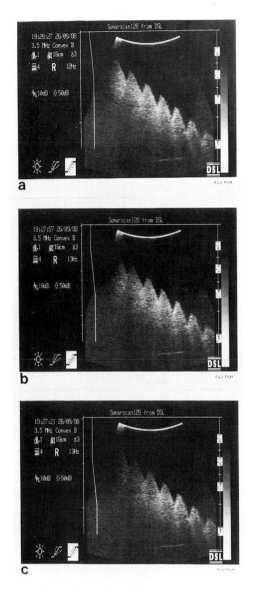

Fig. 13.7 Loss of echo signals in (**b**) and (**c**) as TGC function is made less suited to structures scanned. The TGC function can be seen next to the left-hand calibration axis. Increasing gain with depth moves the function further from the vertical axis.

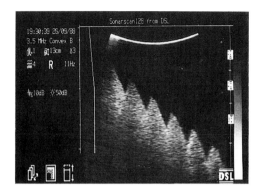

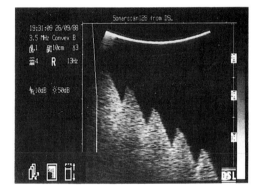

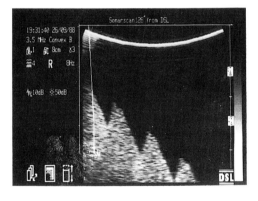

Fig. 13.8 Effect of picture scale on presented image detail.

Collective use of sensitivity

We will now briefly recall the procedure of setting up the sensitivity from the standpoint of imaging, and we will consider a few practical points. Observing the display, we perform a scan through the tissues of interest, and set up the sensitivity controls as in Chapter 7. For most practical purposes,

intensity and gain can be considered to have the same effect on sensitivity unless the echoes are very weak and have to be made larger by using an incident pulse of higher intensity. Frequency is the first sensitivity control to be set up and is normally adjusted automatically when the selected transducer is plugged into the machine. The frequency chosen by the operator is the highest that will give adequate penetration. For optimum

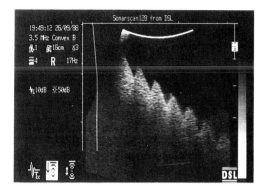

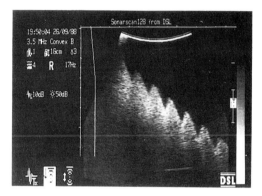

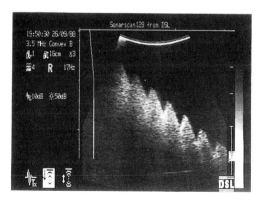

Fig. 13.9 Effect of position of focus on image; near the focus the image is sharper and sometimes the echo signals are larger. The white rectangle on the right axis shows the position of the focus.

results after a frequency change, the TGC must be reset. Changing the frequency is therefore one of the more time-consuming operations. If it seems necessary to reduce the frequency to get more penetration, the operator should check to see if the

sensitivity may be increased via the gain or intensity. So far as transducers are concerned, similarly labelled ones may not have exactly the same characterics. Discrepancies in the sensitivity of identical machines can often be attributed to the transducers.

Diagnosis by sensitivity change

In a few clinical techniques, the diagnosis is made by observing the effect produced in the image by discrete changes in the sensitivity. Masses in the eye and breast have been studied by changing the gain by steps of a few decibels (e.g. by 2 or 5). When these techniques are described in the literature, the authors usually refer specifically to a particular type of change, such as in ultrasonic intensity. It is important to note that the same value of change in intensity or gain decibels results in the same effect on the image. This equivalence of intensity and gain shifts has been illustrated in Figure 13.4. It does not matter, therefore, whether a machine has one of these controls fixed, as the other can be used to apply techniques involving diagnosis by sensitivity change.

Finally, when using techniques that rely on observing effects due to sensitivity change, it is necessary, initially, to have the sensitivity settings at some reasonably well-defined baseline, or to have first produced a standard image. A technique that is less dependent on the starting point is to observe the change in the number of echoes in an image on introducing a series of small decibel alterations; for example, steadily increasing the gain in steps of 1, 2, or 5 dB.

Diagnosis by sensitivity change is not widely used, but it has found application in the study of breast and abdominal masses.

INTERPRETATION OF IMAGES

The interpretation of an image is basically a pattern-recognition procedure. It may be linked with a manoeuvre to obtain additional information; for example, alteration of the plane of scan or of the output intensity. Manipulation of the patient, such as deep inspiration to move organs to more accessible positions, is also used. The final diagnosis may well depend on the addition of other clinical information. We can help to improve the contribution of the ultrasonic technique by asking some questions about the ultrasonic image. The answers to those questions assist the pattern-recognition process and the avoidance of errors.

When confronted with an ultrasonic image, the operator should ask the following questions. All of them need not be asked, particularly if the same person performs the scans and reports the results.

1. What were the machine settings during the scan? A basic list of sensitivity settings should be considered.

2. What is the plane of scan?

3. Has any processing been carried out by the scan converter?

4. What type of scanner was employed?

5. What degree of resolution is there in the image and have the controls been set to optimize it? The presentation of familiar landmarks, such as arteries, veins, fetal anatomy, etc., shows if the sensitivity and grey-shade settings could be improved.

6. What artefacts are in the image? With experience, many artefacts are subconsciously disregarded. The artefacts to pay particular attention to are those resulting from the limited effectiveness or poor adjustment of TGC. Spurious echo signals produced by multiple reflections and other complex influences on the ultrasound are unlikely to be explained completely.

7. Can the echo amplitudes in a region of interest be reliably interpreted? The path traversed by the ultrasound to generate the signals is worth considering here. Recall that superficial structures in the image influence the signals from deeper ones since both the transmitted pulse and the echoes cross them. Another useful point when assessing reflectivity is to compare the patterns from tissues situated at similar depths and examined along similar beam paths, for example, normal and abnormal liver patterns. The effects of inaccurate TGC are reduced by this approach. Echo amplitudes are interpreted, at present, on a gross scale. Interpretation of finer details in signals awaits developments in the field of tissue characterization.

It is worth noting the true frame rate of the scanner when moving images are being studied. The operator then knows the velocities that can be presented accurately. With a frame rate of 25/s, velocities up to 50 mm/s are accommodated, as an echo is obtained from the structure at each 2 mm interval in its range of movement; an example of this is the adult heart wall. Details of the motions of higher-velocity structures, e.g. heart valves or fetal heart walls, may be more difficult to interpret because fewer echoes are obtained per centimetre of range of motion. A velocity of 300 mm/s results in an echo at each 12 mm interval of range when the frame rate is 25/s.

Apart from simple blood vessels, the structures imaged often have a complex motion in three dimensions. It is often difficult to separate the component of change in the image resulting from true motion in the plane of scan and that resulting from movement of the structure out of the plane of scan.

When studying small movements such as fetal breathing, one should ask whether the observed action is truly characteristic of the tissues, or whether it is merely a transmitted motion from a cardiac impulse or the patient's respiration.

Structures that pulsate slightly may produce variations in the associated echo amplitudes and cause brightness variations in the displayed echo spots. When the image is enlarged, small excursions in the positions of these structures may actually be seen.

Small movements of the internal parenchyma of organs partially smooth the speckle interference pattern of echoes from closely spaced scatterers. This helps in the identification of genuine structures in a real-time image. The motion of the speckle pattern does not accurately depict the motion of the parenchyma, and in some circumstances it may be very different.

As soon as one begins to use a real-time B-scanner, it becomes obvious that tissues that were taken to be reasonably static are, in fact, quite mobile. A high degree of image clarity is a bonus arising from the capacity of real-time B-scanners to eliminate movement blur artefacts. Good examples of this are to be found in the scanning of ducts and blood vessels in the liver and of the internal anatomy of the fetus.

Pattern recognition

The process of pattern recognition is greatly assisted by an understanding of how the pattern is produced by the interaction of the sonic pulse and tissues. A few examples of this type of analysis will now be considered. It can be applied to most images and is also of value in understanding abnormal patterns.

1. *Cysts*. The wall image is smooth and bright from the smoothness of the tissue/fluid interface and the relatively large acoustic impedance change. Echo amplitudes on the far side are enhanced due to the low absorption in the fluid. At the sides of the cyst, where the ultrasonic beam is partly in the liquid and partly in the tissue, processes such as defocusing and refraction weaken the beam so a shadow is cast since weak echoes are generated beyond the cyst. Irregularly spaced spurious echoes within the cyst are probably due to multiple reflections or debris. A uniform pattern of weak echoes militates caution in the diagnosis of a cyst, and guidance may be had by comparison with a known, fluid-filled structure at a similar depth.

2. *Gallstone*. Disruption of the smooth wall shape arises from the presence of stones. A strong echo results from the large acoustic impedance difference at the liquid/stone interface. A shadow results from high reflection and absorption at or in the stone.

3. *Diaphragm*. This strong reflecting interface is a prominent landmark at the back of the liver. At the gas/tissue interface, the acoustic impedance change is very large.

4. *Detached retina*. At this weakly reflecting structure within the vitreous body, the echo strength is highly dependent on the angle of incidence of the beam at the smooth membrane.

5. *Organ parenchyma*. A speckle pattern results from interference of echoes from closely packed, weakly reflecting targets. The bright and dark regions of the image do not necessarily correspond to physical structures, but are, rather, an interference pattern (Fig. 15.5). Diagnosis is made on the basis of large changes in the speckle pattern.

6. *Abdominal aorta*. Clear, distinct echoes are detected from the wall/blood interface. Scattering from the blood cells provides weak signals that are not normally depicted. Pulsations are observed as changes both in position and echo amplitude.

7. *Fetal spine*. The properties of cartilage are not as disruptive as those of adult bone, although strong shadows may be cast across the fetal trunk. An image of the spinal canal can still be obtained despite the non-average tissue properties.

8. *Pancreas*. This organ has an echogenicity that is very close to that of the tissues overlying it. Use of good grey-tone imaging and anatomic landmarks is required.

9. *Fat*. Fat layers can be imaged. However, variations in the consistency of fat and its slightly unusual physical properties, for example, a velocity of sound of 1470 m/s, appear to degrade the ultrasonic beam and, hence, the image quality of underlying organs.

10. *Placenta*. As mentioned earlier, the vascular dimensions are less than can be resolved by the scanner, but the characteristic pattern provides means of identification.

11. *Muscle*. When muscle is scanned in a particular direction, we observe characteristic striations related to the fibre structure.

12. *Peristaltic motion*. Resolution of the complex anatomy of the abdomen may be assisted by the observation of peristaltic motion.

This list illustrates some common physical considerations relevant to pattern recognition.

MANIPULATION OF THE PATIENT

Ultrasonic techniques at present involve little manipulation of the patient. Most scans are performed with the patient lying supine. Occasionally, rotation to one side may improve access for the ultrasonic beam into particular tissues. Kidneys are often examined with the patient in the prone position. Deep inspiration helps to push the liver from behind the rib cage and reduces patient movement for long enough to perform biopsy sampling.

Versatile adjustable beds are available. Tilting the bed allows the feet of obstetric patients to be raised, and results in movement of the fetal head. Tilting half of the bed in the opposite direction lowers the feet. With the patient in the prone position and a pillow under the abdomen, the rib spacing is increased, giving access to the kidneys.

Only in ophthalmic applications is patient manipulation widely practised. Useful information can be obtained on occasion if scans are made with the bulb of the eye in different rotational positions.

A full bladder provides a 'window' to the lower pelvic regions. This window technique is particularly successful in early pregnancy, and in moving the fetal head upward later in pregnancy, thus allowing BPD measurements to be made. A liquid-filled stomach can provide a similar window to the upper abdomen, particularly with the patient in the upright position when gas gathers at the fundus of the stomach. A starch preparation is retained longer in the stomach than is water.

Clarification of structures may be achieved in orthopaedic studies by manipulation of limbs.

CONTRAST MEDIA

Virtually no contrast media are used routinely in ultrasonic scanning, at present. The most profitable application of a contrast medium has been in heart studies. Small bubbles are detected when saline, indocyanine green, or 5% dextrose in water is injected quickly through a catheter; for example, 2–3 ml at a rate of 10 ml/s. They can be observed passing into the various chambers of the heart. A negative contrast effect is seen when normal blood enters a chamber containing bubbles. The microbubble approach is being further developed to give more reproducible results by incorporating the bubbles in protein material which dissolves quickly in the bloodstream. Agents which can pass through the lungs are also being developed. Gas in the stomach, after water has been swallowed, has also been used to localize it in the abdomen. Other agents are being developed, but they have not been routinely applied (Ch. 28).

LABELLING PLANES OF SCAN

Once the operator has set up the instrument and performed and recorded the scan, it may be desirable to label the plane of scan to allow the procedure to be repeated at a later date, or scans

in different planes to be correlated. Some instruments show a diagram on the screen on which the scan plane may be marked by the operator.

Longitudinal and transverse scans

A simple method of labelling is shown in Figure 13.10. It is limited in that it applies only to exactly transverse or longitudinal scans. Distances are measured from a reference point, for example, the umbilicus, xiphisternum, symphysis pubis, middle point of the line joining iliac crests, or the centre of the eye. Transverse scans are labelled T plus the distance moved in centimetres towards the head (e.g. $T + 6$) or T minus the distance towards the feet (e.g. $T - 5$). Similarly, longitudinal scans are labelled 'L plus distance' for displacements to the right of the patient, and 'L minus distance' for those to the left. Transverse and longitudinal scans through the reference point are labelled T and L, respectively. The angle of tilt from the vertical of a plane of scan is also measured and prefixed with a plus sign if the plane slopes towards the central

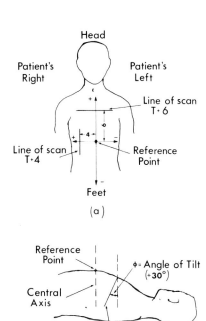

Fig. 13.10 Labelling longitudinal and transverse scans.

axis within the body, and with a minus sign for planes sloping away from the central axis. In addition to the fact that it defines only longitudinal and transverse planes, the system has the disadvantage that the angle of tilt to the vertical of longitudinal or transverse planes that pass through the reference point is not uniquely specified.

A convention for labelling all planes of scan is described in Appendix 5.

Orientation of an image on a display screen or photograph

A widely accepted convention exists for presenting ultrasonic images on a CRT display screen or photographic record. For transverse scans, the image is presented as though the patient were viewed from the feet. Longitudinal scans are orientated on the display with the feet of the patient to the right-hand side. For an oblique scan, the end of the line of scan closest to the feet is presented on the right-hand side of the image. An exception to this is in cardiac imaging, in which longitudinal sections are presented with the feet of the patient to the left.

In Chapter 25, it will be seen that there has been a rapid growth in the use of internal scanners. No convention for the orientation or labelling of the images from such scanners has been established. Considerable care has to be taken in their interpretation.

SPECIFICATION OF AN ULTRASONIC TECHNIQUE

For a published clinical article to be completely meaningful, it is helpful to specify the technique in an introductory paragraph. Specification of the following quantities helps to make results reproducible by other investigators.

1. Plane of scan
2. Make of commercial instrument
3. Particulars of transducer (i.e. frequency, type)
4. Frame rate
5. Machine settings (e.g. calibration velocity)
6. Sensitivity controls (e.g. ultrasonic intensity, TGC slope)

7. Sensitivity changes in diagnostic techniques
8. Scan converter processing
9. Display and recording systems (picture scale)
10. Reference to any data taken from the scientific literature

In practice, it is difficult to compile a complete list. As a way to overcome this difficulty, presentation of an echo pattern from a test system has been advocated, but this is rarely included.

REAL-TIME B-SCANNING PLUS M-MODE

On viewing a real-time B-scan image, the operator may wish to make M-scan traces of the motion of particular structures. This allows their motion to be recorded in detail or to be related to other physiological signals. There are two basic approaches to obtaining M-scan records from a real-time system. The first is to select electronically any line of echoes from the image and to feed it simultaneously into a fibre-optic chart recorder during the scanning procedure. Lines of echo information will be fed into the recorder at a rate equal to the frame rate of the scanner (e.g. 30/s). This is a slow rate and is effectively a low PRF, M-mode system. It is adequate for recording slow-moving tissues as in fetal breathing or heart-wall studies. It is not acceptable, however, for examining rapid actions.

The second approach is to transmit ultrasonic pulses in a selected direction at a rate much higher than the imaging frame rate; the result is a high-quality trace. The technique with a mechanical scanner is to select a scan line in the image, and then to stop a transducer with its beam pointed in that direction. The M-mode trace is then recorded at a high PRF. The image is obviously lost when the M-mode is engaged in this manner. With electronic real-time instruments, it can be arranged that an ultrasonic pulse is transmitted along the selected direction much more often than along other beam paths in the scan sweep. For example, the pulse rate in the selected direction may be 1000/s while that of other image lines is 15/s. Because the system is regularly jumping back to the selected direction during the sweep, the rest of the image suffers degradation in terms of frame rate or line density. The image is still observed when the trace is being recorded, however.

More than one trace can be recorded during a real-time B-scan, provided suitable recorders are available. Normally, beam directions are selected from the image and the appropriate echo trains are passed to a chart recorder that presents the traces side by side. Electronic scanners are best suited to this technique, a common example being the use of phased arrays in cardiology.

If a series of real-time image frames can be stored in an electronic memory, M-scan records can be made from selected lines in any direction across the image, not only in those corresponding to ultrasonic beam directions. This facility is not widely available at present and has still to be evaluated.

Real-time B-scan and M-modes are obviously complementary to each other. Equipment offering both approaches represents a powerful tool for studying internal tissue motions.

REAL-TIME B-SCANNING PLUS STOP-ACTION RECORDING

The stop-action mode is used to obtain an image at a particular phase in a cyclic motion. In real-time B-scan imaging, a particular phase of heart action can be frozen on the display screen by using the ECG as a timing signal. One should recall that the sweep time of the ultrasonic beam across the field of view is typically 40 ms. This variation in time of recording across the image is not important for calculations of quantities such as chamber size, but could be important in observation of the position of a fast-moving valve flap.

Several machines offer the facility of recording a large number of consecutive frames in computer memory, for example, 64. It is then possible to examine each image, in turn, to select that of interest. Replaying these images repetitively at a slow rate is a convenient way of studying motion in detail.

REAL-TIME B-SCANNING PLUS DOPPLER TECHNIQUES

The combination of real-time B-scan and Doppler methods to detect moving structures and blood flow offers great potential for the examination of the cardiovascular system. A blood vessel is located on the real-time B-scan display, and an associated Doppler transducer is then manipulated to make its beam intersect the blood vessel. The direction of the Doppler probe beam is indicated on the display screen.

If the Doppler unit is a simple continuous-wave device, movements of tissues in the ultrasonic beam other than blood flow in the vessel contribute to the output signal. A pulsed-Doppler unit can eliminate this problem because it detects blood flow from specific sites. The pulsed-Doppler type of instrument may, however, run into difficulties related to the maximum velocity of flow that it can measure.

It is often difficult or even impossible to run a real-time B-scanner and a Doppler unit simultaneously. Both modes must transmit and receive ultrasound for a large percentage of the available time, and, therefore, they interfere with each other. Discussion of the combined use of these two modalities will be deferred until the chapters on Doppler instruments. The combination of real-time B-scan imaging and colour-flow imaging is also discussed in these chapters.

REAL-TIME B-SCANNING PLUS BIOPSY

A biopsy needle moving through tissue is often observable on a real-time B-scan image. The location of the tissue and the best direction for inserting the needle are ascertained using the real-time imager. The needle is inserted through a guidance hole incorporated into the transducer assembly. In this way, the needle path has a fixed and known spatial relationship to the displayed image. The tissue to be sampled is therefore presented in a particular region of the image before insertion of the needle. With real-time, B-scanner puncture systems, the needle path need not be parallel to the direction of the ultrasonic beam; this fact makes easier the identification of the needle tip. Further discussion of invasive techniques is in Chapter 25.

SELECTION OF A REAL-TIME B-SCANNER

A bewildering range of instruments confronts the purchaser new to the real-time B-scan field. The most expensive instrument costs about 20 times more than the cheapest. One way to clarify the situation is to define the applications as exactly as possible and to try out some instruments in these fields. For routine, well-established tasks, simple instruments may prove adequate. Where there is doubt concerning the full range of present and future applications, and if it is hoped to implement more recent clinical developments, only instruments with the best performance are relevant.

The features of an instrument relevant for selection from a clinical viewpoint are presented in the following check list:

1. *Transducer selection* — Large (linear, sector, small parts, invasive, intra-operative, Doppler) with a range of frequencies (3–10 MHz). The performance of each transducer should be carefully checked in the intended application.

2. *Measurement system* — Accurate and easy to use. It should not be necessary to start again when a small mistake is made.

3. *Recording device* — Chosen from the range of good devices available (Table 26.2).

4. *Biopsy attachment* — A device which is proven to work well. Many devices have been purchased, only to lie in drawers. Sterilization should be borne in mind.

5. *Image quality* — Low noise in fluid structures, high resolution in focal regions, clear detail near the transducer, crisp delineation of boundaries, good contrast resolution, suitable field-of-view size.

6. *Servicing* — Good local support.

7. *Transportability* — Able to survive the rigours of being moved around hospitals (good wheels, light weight, no trailing cables, easy to move, solid electronic construction). The transporting of equipment should only be undertaken if there is no alternative.

8. *Doppler* — The Doppler mode should be thoroughly checked in the fields of intended application. The clarity of a sonogram or image should be carefully scrutinized. The feasibility of detecting subtle changes in velocity due to disease should be tested. Pulse-echo imaging is a fairly mature technology with limited pitfalls for the purchaser; much of Doppler technology is still immature.

9. *Controls* — Easy to use with a limited number of manipulations. Machines for use in a wide range of purposes should not be limited in their flexibility by having few controls. The sensitivity controls should be altered to check that the changes in the image are logical and of the desired magnitude.

10. *Output power, intensity, and pressure* — The manufacturer should be able to supply figures for the output power, intensity, and pressure amplitude related to the operating modes of the machine.

DAMAGE TO SCANNERS

The expense and complexity of real-time probes speak for themselves regarding careful handling. It is worth pointing out the cost of transducers to all new users.

Any plans to use a probe in a water-bath should be thoroughly checked out with the manufacturer. Probes often contain electronic components and electric motors. Immersion in water beyond specified limits may be dangerous or damaging.

In most environments, the air filters should be cleaned at least once a month; otherwise, components will be subject to undesirably high temperatures. The suitability of a machine for use in the presence of explosive anaesthetic gases should be confirmed.

Finally, it is reassuring to know that machines cannot be damaged by setting their controls in unusual positions. Damage to transducers is discussed further in Chapter 27.

CONTACT AND IMMERSION SCANNING

We have, so far, paid little attention to the means by which machines are coupled to the patient. The dominant factor in the design of any coupling method is the inability of ultrasound in the MHz frequency range to pass through air. The patient and the transducer must be linked by some means that excludes air. The two methods commonly employed are contact scanning and immersion scanning.

Contact scanning

As its name implies, in contact scanning the

transducer is held in direct contact with the skin of the patient. This method is particularly successful in abdominal examinations, in which the skin surface is compliant, and it is easy to maintain good contact with the transducer. A liberal coating of liquid such as arachis oil, or gel, is administered to the skin before the transducer is applied. If the motion of the transducer removes this fluid coupling medium, it should immediately be replaced. It is easy to show experimentally that even the thinnest film of air is an impenetrable barrier to ultrasound. The type of coupling liquid is unimportant since it is a very thin layer and does not attenuate the transmitted ultrasound.

Contact scanning is usually the method of first choice as it allows the most flexible scanning procedure. Owing to its convenience, it sometimes finds application in less than ideal situations. An example of this is head scanning, in which the proximity of bone to the surface of the skin makes contact difficult. The orbit of a closed eye can be studied by contact scanning.

Immersion scanning (water-bath scanning)

Where the contact between the transducer and the patient is difficult, immersion scanning is employed. Here the transducer is coupled acoustically to the patient via a water-bath (Fig. 13.11). The water may be in direct contact with the skin or held in a thin plastic or rubber bag that is coupled to the skin with oil. Immersion scanning finds application in scanning the eye, breast, head, thyroid, and abdomen. Motorized scanning is much more readily achieved with an immersion technique since there is no friction between the patient and the transducer.

The main difficulty in immersion scanning is the management of quantities of water. In addition, with normal transducers, sensitivity and resolution are slightly degraded, as the tissue structures are further removed from the transducer than in contact scanning. Two or three commercial instruments are designed for immersion scanning and do not suffer from these difficulties. Contact scanners are easily converted to immersion scanners by the addition of a water-bath. Before using a contact scanner with a water-bath, advice should be sought from the manufacturers as to the possibility of electric hazard or of corrosion in the transducer.

There is one design criterion that must be met in the construction of a water-bath; this arises from the strong, multiple-reflection artefacts in the water layer between the transducer and the skin. Absorption in water is negligible, and an ultrasonic pulse can be reflected backward and forward many times in the water layer. This is known as 'reverberation' or 'multiple reflection'. To keep the reverberation echoes clear of those from the tissue, one must ensure that the depth of the water (d_w) is greater than the depth of the surfaces of interest inside the tissue (d_s) (Fig. 13.11). This becomes clear when the expected positions of

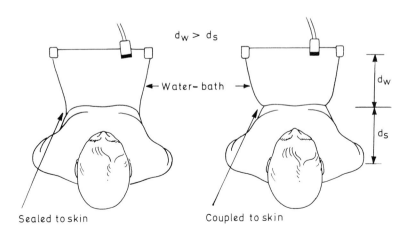

Fig. 13.11 Water-bath coupling techniques.

reverberations are deduced. The multiple-reflection artefact is easily identified because the first reverberation echo is twice as far from the transmission pulse as is the water/skin interface echo.

In eye scanning, the depth of the water-bath is typically 6 cm, whereas in abdominal work it may be 20 cm. The latter represents a considerable weight of water. If the first centimetre of depth of tissue is not of great relevance, it is possible to use a very shallow bath of oil, for example, castor oil. The transducer is held within a few millimetres of the skin, and the reverberation echoes die out quickly as a result of absorption in the oil.

Small-parts scanners designed for imaging superficial structures often incorporate a water-bath of a depth determined by the above criteria.

Stand-off gel

Silicone gel material has been marketed by several companies as a stand-off material for ultrasonic scanners. It has ultrasonic properties similar to those of tissue, though it can be more attenuating at high frequencies. A layer of this material can be conveniently interposed between the transducer and the skin surface. Good contact is obtained, and the attenuation of the gel is such that multiple reflections in the stand-off layer are not a problem.

SUMMARY

Practical points for the production and reproduction of scans were discussed.

1. The importance of the sensitivity controls — suppression, frequency, gain, intensity (power), TGC — was emphasized, and the collective use explained.

2. Physical factors which influence the interpretation of images were listed; 12 examples were presented of factors which contribute to pattern recognition.

3. A simple scheme for labelling the plane of scan was included, as were 10 items for the specification of a technique.

4. The versatility of real-time scanning was shown by noting how it could be combined with other procedures such as M-mode, stop-action recording, Doppler methods, and biopsy.

5. In view of the very extensive range of scanners, a best-buy check list was presented.

6. A comparison of immersion and contact scanning was made.

REFERENCES

Wainstock M A 1976 A method for obtaining water tight seals during ultrasonic scans of the eye. JCU 4: 439

Warren P S, Garrett W J, Kossoff G 1978 The liquid-filled stomach — an ultrasonic window to the upper abdomen. JCU 6: 315–320

Ziskin M C, Bonakdarpour A , Weinstein D P et al 1972 Contrast agents for diagnostic ultrasound. Investigative Radiology 7: 500–505

14. B-scan instruments, performance and use

This brief chapter is largely of historical interest. It can be omitted and read at leisure. It is of some relevance since much of the knowledge on which real-time B-scanners are based was acquired through work on B-scanners. Also many of the established clinical techniques were developed using this older type of machine.

B-scan instruments, in which the transducer is moved relatively slowly by hand or motor drive, were the main type of scanner in the 1970s. They have now been largely superseded by real-time B-scanners. However, since they offer a large field of view and a variable scanning action, they will be briefly considered in this chapter. As usual, the nomenclature has been determined by popular usage rather than by an organized consensus. In this text, a B-scanner is a slow-scan device,

whereas a real-time B-scanner generates more than 5 frames per second. B-scan units, capable of generating high-quality images from single sweeps of the ultrasound beam, preceded the development of real-time B-scanners based on a similar scanning action.

Like real-time scanners, B-scanners generate an image by detecting echoes from a pulsed ultrasonic beam which is swept in a plane through the tissues. The transducer, usually a single-element device, is moved by hand over the skin of the patient. A mechanical gantry supports the transducer, whose orientation is continuously measured. This allows the lines of echo spots to be located in the correct position on the display (Fig. 14.1). The mechanical gantry is designed to permit the beam to be swept through a large area

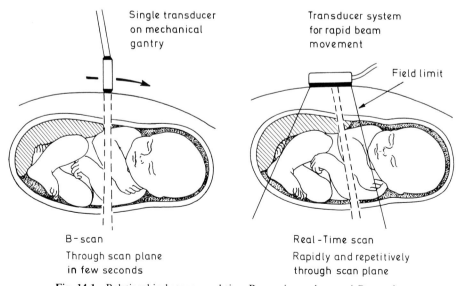

Fig. 14.1 Relationship between real-time B-scanning and manual B-scanning.

(e.g. 30 × 20 cm) and also to enable the operator to perform a variable scanning action. During the scan, structures may be examined from several directions, and the echoes are then superimposed in the image. Constructing the image from echoes gathered from different directions is called 'compound scanning', in contrast to the simple, single-direction scans of most real-time B-scan instruments. The scan time is relatively long; a few seconds are required to complete each image. As for real-time B-scanning, narrow focused beams give good resolution. Indeed, virtually all of the considerations which influence the operation of a real-time unit are of direct relevance for manual B-scanning. B-scanners require skilled manipulation to produce the best results.

B-SCAN EQUIPMENT

All compound B-scan instruments have the same basic structure, although individual commercial units each have their own characteristics.

In compound B-scanning, the ultrasound beam must sweep freely in a plane, and, at the same time, the line of echoes should move in a related manner on the display screen. To achieve this, the instrument must carry out continuous electronic measurement of the direction of the ultrasonic beam. Measurement of the vertical and horizontal positions of the transducer, as well as of its angle of rotation from a fixed position, gives the direction of the ultrasonic beam. The electric voltages produced by the measuring devices are used to control the direction of the line of echo spots on the display screen.

An ultrasonic B-scan instrument consists of four parts:

1. A mechanical system to support the transducer and allow it the necessary freedom of action

2. A registration system to record continuously the direction of the ultrasonic beam

3. An electronic system to generate and process the echoes

4. A display, storage, and recording system suitable for two-dimensional images.

A block diagram of a B-scanner is shown in Figure 14.2. A B-scan machine gantry is shown in Figure 14.3.

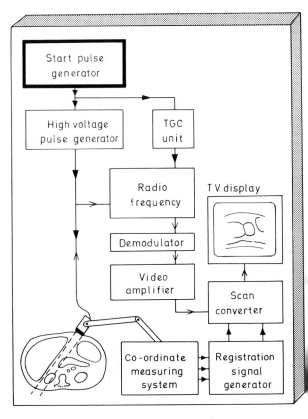

Fig. 14.2   Block diagram of a B-scan instrument.

Mechanical system

The most common type of mechanics has the transducer mounted such that it can rotate through a large angle on the extremity of two hinged arms (Fig. 14.4a). Another approach is to support the transducer in such a way that it can rotate and move vertically and horizontally on an arrangement of rods and bearings (Fig. 14.4b). Both mechanisms allow free movement of the transducer in the plane of scan. To change the plane of scan, one usually has to manoeuvre the transducer and a large part of the mechanics. B-scan machines are sometimes partly motorized to assist with larger movements of the mechanical system or to permit stepping of the plane of scan through a sequence of parallel sections.

Registration system

The beam position-measuring process is often performed by devices called 'potentiometers' which

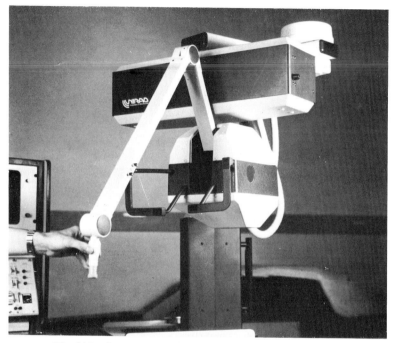

Fig. 14.3 Common type of mechanical gantry for a B-scanner.

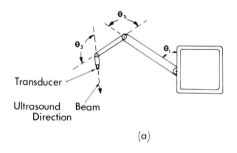

(a)

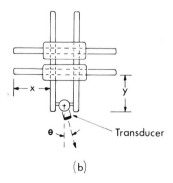

(b)

Fig. 14.4 Two types of mechanical system designed to allow freedom of movement of the transducer in the scan plane.

are attached to the system and whose electrical resistance depends on the position of the transducer. This resistance changes with the movement of the transducer so that voltage signals, which are a measure of position, can be generated. 'Linear' potentiometers are used to measure linear movements; 'sine/cosine' potentiometers, to measure angular changes. Position and angle measurement is also performed by devices based on optical and magnetic sensors.

Electronic system

The electronic system for the generation and detection of echoes is similar to that described for A-scanning and real-time B-scanning; the basic methods of generating and processing the echo signals are the same (Fig. 14.2).

Storage, display, and recording systems

The scan converter for a B-scan image is generally larger than that found in real-time units since larger fields of view have to be accommodated. Typically, an array of 512 × 512 pixels is adequate. In a B-scan image, each line of echoes is individually generated, since there is sufficient time available, and there is no need to increase the line density by inserting artificial ones. The display and recording devices are identical to those found on real-time instruments.

USING B-SCANNERS

The practicalities of using B-scanners have much in common with those described in Chapters 12 and 13 for real-time B-scan instruments. Resolution, the effect of sensitivity controls, measurement, and the interpretation of images are very similar. The main difference lies with the scanning techniques.

The scanning gantry is adjusted in such a way that a scan can be performed through the tissues to be studied. Normally, the initial plane of scan passes centrally through the tissue; for example, a vertical plane parallel to the longitudinal axis of the abdomen. The ultrasonic beam is then directed into the centre of the area to be scanned. The line of echo spots is electronically centralized on the display screen. A few scans are then performed so that a suitable scale of display can be selected (the largest that can accommodate the whole B-scan image).

The majority of scanning actions employed in clinical use are simple contact scans in which the ultrasonic beam is quickly swept once through the scan plane; the time for a scan is typically 1 or 2 seconds. A grey-tone image is produced by collecting scattered and specularly reflected ultrasound from interfaces within the body. During this simple type of scan, a cardiac impulse or respiratory motion will move the tissues; however, these effects are minimal since the technique does not depend on the accurate superposition of echo data from many beam directions. Suspension of respiration does prevent large tissue movements. Note that in this scanning technique, each tissue is interrogated from one beam direction, and some large surfaces may, therefore, not appear with their expected prominence.

A greater amount of ultrasonic information is obtained by moving the transducer over the surface of the body and rocking it through a large angle, for example, 60°, at points separated by 2 or 3 cm. The time taken for such a scan is typically 10 seconds. During the scan, it is important to maintain, continuously, good contact with the skin. A considerable drawback of this scanning technique is the long duration and the associated image degradation caused by the patient moving.

Another variation of scanning action is one in which particular structures or interfaces are imaged as completely as possible. The scanning action employed here may greatly overemphasize a fairly small area by viewing it from many directions.

CLASSIFICATION OF SCANNING ACTIONS

No standard terminology exists, and since a large number of scanning actions are possible, it is difficult to devise a labelling method to cover all eventualities. We will consider only a limited classification.

Four types of simple scanning modes can be assigned the labels shown in Figure 14.5. The term 'simple' is applied to scans in which, for the most part, the ultrasound beam passes through each area of tissue only once.

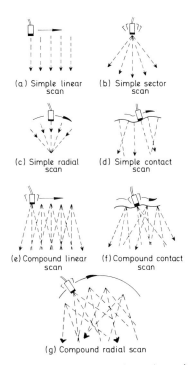

(a) Simple linear scan   (b) Simple sector scan

(c) Simple radial scan   (d) Simple contact scan

(e) Compound linear scan   (f) Compound contact scan

(g) Compound radial scan

Fig. 14.5   A classification of scanning actions.

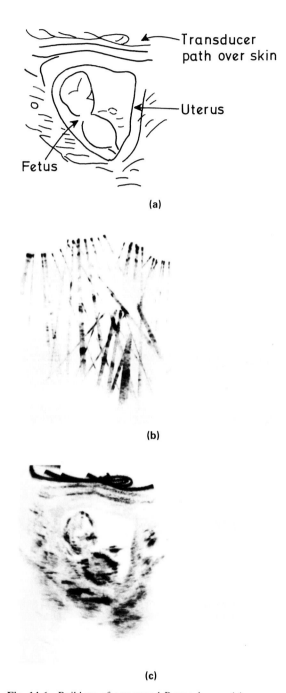

(a)

(b)

(c)

Fig. 14.6 Build-up of compound B-scan image. (**a**) Structures scanned, (**b**) sample lines of echoes, (**c**) complete image.

To perform a more thorough scan, a combination of some of the above scanning motions can be used so that tissues can be viewed from several directions. Echoes from a target are detected from a number of directions of the ultrasonic beam and are combined in the scan converter. The image is built up, therefore, by compounding many sets of echo patterns. Scanning involving combinations of simple modes is called 'compound scanning'. The most common types of compound scan involve adding sector scans, that is, a rocking action, to a simple linear scan or a simple contact scan (Fig. 14.5). Compound linear scans are common in water-bath techniques.

Simple contact scans are effective in abdominal examinations because they may be completed before respiratory movements degrade the image. Compound contact scanning collects most echo information and is also of value, its main deficiency being that it takes longer than simple scanning to perform. A compound scan image is presented in Figure 14.6.

SUMMARY

B-scan machines still have some interesting features, but their interest is largely historical. They were shown to consist of four parts — mechanics, a registration system, an echo-generation system, and display units. The versatility of B-scanners was seen in the different scanning actions.

REFERENCES

Brown T G 1967 Visualisation of soft tissues in two and three dimensions — limitations and development. Ultrasonics 5: 118–124
Coleman D J, Konig W F, Katz L 1969 A hand-operated, ultrasound scan system for ophthalmic evaluation. Am J Ophthalmol 68: 256–263
Holm H H, Northeved A 1968 An ultrasonic scanning apparatus for use in medical diagnosis. Acta Chir Scand 134: 177–181
Kossoff G: 1972 Improved techniques in ultrasonic cross-sectional echography. Ultrasonics 10: 221–227

15. Artefacts in echo images

An artefact in an ultrasonic echo image is a pattern of echoes which does not correspond to the structures scanned. Like other imaging techniques, ultrasonic imaging may produce erroneous results owing to artefacts. While artefacts are not a major problem, it is essential to be aware of them and, if possible, to have an explanation of their origin. The examples below are not exhaustive and, doubtless, readers will be able to add some from their own experience.

PROPAGATION ARTEFACTS

This type of artefact arises as a result of effects which influence ultrasonic pulses as they pass through tissue.

Multiple reflection (reverberation)

It is quite common for an echo to reach the transducer by an indirect path as a result of its being reflected more than once. This usually makes the echo return to the transducer at a time later than that corresponding to the direct go–return time of the surface which first produced it. Artefact echoes caused by this process are often weak and difficult to identify, but some are very prominent. This type of artefact is particularly important since the spurious echoes may be misinterpreted as coming from actual tissue structures.

Figure 15.1a illustrates an artefact echo which is fairly common in practice and which is generated when a strongly reflecting surface lies approximately parallel to the transducer face. The first genuine echo from the surface is located at the correct depth in the image. However, when this genuine echo strikes the transducer face, part of its energy is reflected back into the tissue and travels again towards the surface where the artefact echo is produced. This echo is also detected by the transducer and is presented on the display at twice the depth of the genuine echo. The time delay of the artefact echo after the instant of transmission is obviously twice that of the genuine echo. This multiple reflection process may not fade out after the arrival of the artefact echo, since some of its energy may be reflected from the transducer back into the tissue, giving rise to a second artefact, and so on until the artefact signals become too weak to be detected. Examples of this artefact are multiple reflection in layers between the transducer and muscle, the transducer and the anterior bladder wall, the transducer and bowel gas, and the transducer and the anterior fetal skull. In immersion scanning or with transducer assemblies which use a stand-off device, this manifestation of multiple reflections is a common problem, since ultrasound may readily bounce around in the layer between the transducer and the skin.

In addition to reverberation in superficial tissue layers, multiple reflection may take place inside a deeper layer, giving rise to additional artefact echoes after the two direct ones from the boundaries of the layer. Reflection at these boundaries needs to be fairly strong for the artefact echoes to be observed. Examples of this artefact can be seen in images of the lens of the eye, a layer of bone or fetal skull, the total width of a fetal head, and the blood-filled chambers of the heart.

Figure 15.1b is an example of reverberation in a small structure which does not necessarily consist of parallel surfaces. Many reflections may occur, producing many indistinct echoes in a long tail

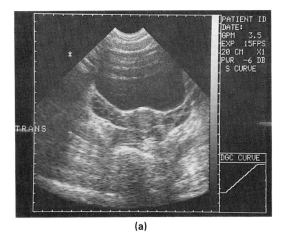

(a)

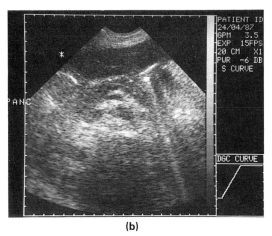

(b)

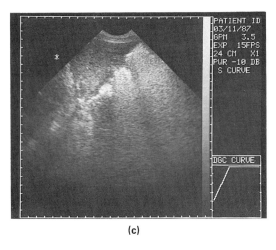

(c)

Fig. 15.1 (a) Multiple reflection echoes in the bladder, (b) multiple reflection in small structures causing a line of echoes down the image, (c) multiple reflection in gas, obscuring deep regions of the image.

after the initial echo. This is sometimes called the 'comet' artefact. It can be seen at the bevelled end or body of a biopsy needle, below small collections of gas and liquid, and associated with tiny crystals in the gall bladder. This artefact can occur on a large scale when an ultrasound beam interacts with bowel or lung gas, obscuring virtually all of the image (Fig. 15.1c).

Echoes returning to the transducer by an elongated route could cause a major boundary to be presented at the wrong depth, but such echoes are more likely to contribute to a background signal level, which may appear in liquid-filled vessels and ducts in the image.

It is worth noting that if the thickness of the layer in which the multiple reflections occur is changing, the artefact echoes move more quickly than the genuine echoes, since the total path of the artefact pulses changes more.

Shadowing

If a transmitted ultrasonic pulse passes through a highly absorbing layer or through a strongly reflecting interface, it is greatly attenuated. It is then capable of producing only weak echoes at subsequent interfaces. In turn, the weak echoes must cross the attenuating structures before reaching the transducer (Fig. 15.2a). An ultrasonic beam may also be weakened and dispersed by refraction and diffraction if it passes along a tissue boundary, for example, at the edge of a cyst or the fetal body (Fig. 15.2b). Echoes from deeper structures are then very weak and may not be detected. At the edge of the gall bladder this artefact could be mistaken for the shadow cast by a small gallstone.

Bone and pockets of gas are prime examples of strongly absorbing and reflecting structures. Shadows created by the ribs, the skull, the pelvis, or the spinal column make it difficult to image structures beyond them. A barium contrast agent in the abdomen also has strongly attenuating properties. Occasionally, shadowing can produce diagnostic information; for example, in the case of gallstones or some types of tumour masses (Fig. 15.2c). It is possible to compensate for the effect of shadowing, to some extent, by careful adjustment of the TGC.

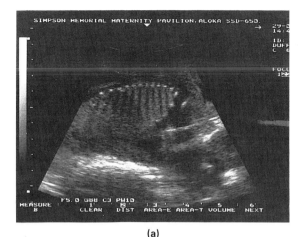

(a)

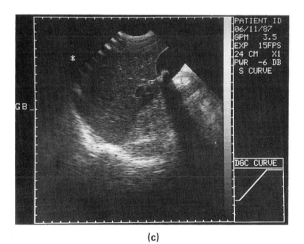

(b)

(c)

Fig. 15.2 (a) Shadowing at fetal ribs, (b) shadowing at edge of structure, (c) shadowing by gallstones.

Enhancement

Enhancement is the converse of shadowing. When the transmitted pulse and echoes pass through a weakly attenuating region, strong echoes are received from structures beyond it (Fig. 15.2c). This converse of shadowing is often regarded as advantageous; for example, in aiding diagnosis of early pregnancy through a full bladder, scanning the orbit of the eye, or examining heart valves through chambers filled with blood. Indeed, the observation of large-amplitude echoes beyond an echo-free region is used as a means of diagnosing cysts, pericardial effusions, etc. However, enhancement is basically an artefact, and it can give rise to an unbalanced image of, for example, fetal anatomy through different depths of amniotic fluid.

Refraction

Deviation of an ultrasonic beam by refraction at a tissue interface where the velocity of sound changes was discussed in Chapter 4. Refraction is most troublesome at a bone/soft-tissue interface, where deviations as large as 20° can arise, and, hence, the image is degraded. This phenomenon has also been invoked to explain one gestation sac's appearing as two. At the start of the scan, the sac is imaged directly; further on during the scan sweep it is imaged again by the beam's being deviated towards it by a wedge-shaped muscle layer. Refraction at the lens of the eye can cause irregular bumps to appear in the image of the retina (Fig. 15.3).

Specular reflection

We noted earlier that when an ultrasound beam intercepts a smooth surface at an angle, most of the beam is reflected away from the transducer, and either no echo or a very weak one may be detected. This may result in a major boundary's being absent or appearing weakly in an image. Examples of this problem are the failures to image parts of organ boundaries or the midline structure of the fetal brain (Fig. 15.4). As a means of avoiding this problem, it is common practice to try to direct the beam perpendicularly to the surface.

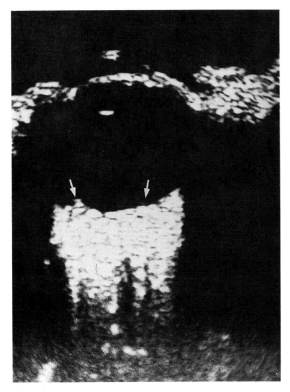

Fig. 15.3 Irregularities in image of retina caused by refraction in lens (courtesy of Restori M).

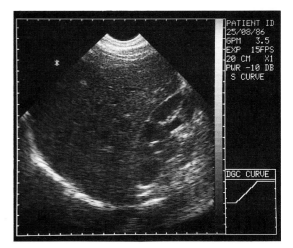

Fig. 15.4 Specular reflection from kidney surface; echoes from surface are stronger at near-perpendicular incidence.

This usually solves the problem, but it should be remembered that to place a beam exactly perpendicular to a surface is quite difficult, since it is a problem in three-dimensional space and not in a two-dimensional plane. This artefact accounts for the large variations in amplitude which are often observed in the echo from a moving surface.

Speckle

In Chapter 12, the physical explanation of the speckled appearance of organ parenchyma was given in the discussion of contrast resolution. The appearance of the speckle pattern depends on the characteristics of the scattering centres in the tissue, the ultrasonic pulse shape, and the signal processing in the machine. Although with the same machine comparisons can be made among patients and among disease states, the pattern is an artefact since it does not truly depict tissue structure (Fig. 15.5).

The difference between true structure and speckle pattern is emphasized when the structure moves. The motion of the speckle may not be related to that of the structure. In an extreme case, it can be in exactly the opposite direction. Computer-processing techniques may be used to smooth speckle without blurring the edges of genuine structures.

Lack of coupling agent

Should the interface between the transducer and the skin lack sufficient liquid to expel all of the air, difficulty will be experienced in detecting echoes (Fig. 15.6). An extremely thin film of air can eliminate all echoes. During scanning, the skin surface may gradually be wiped dry, resulting in diminution of the echoes. With a strongly curved mechanical transducer, air at part of the face can cause reverberations in the transducer assembly (Fig. 15.6). Slightly increased pressure on the skin surface may reduce this artefact.

In A-scanning of the head, it is obviously important to expel air completely from the hair. Similarly, in water-bath scanning in which the water is supported in a container, it is important to ensure good coupling between the base of the container and the skin over the entire area of interest.

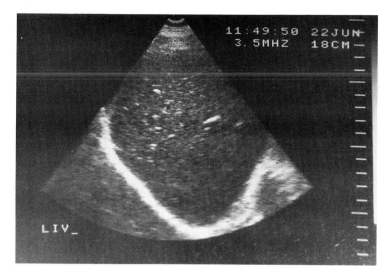

Fig. 15.5 Speckle pattern in image of parenchyma of liver. Echoes beyond the diaphragm are due to the mirror artefact.

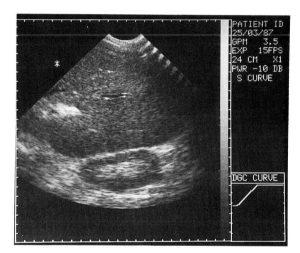

Fig. 15.6 Lack-of-coupling-agent artefact. Regular echoes on right side of image are produced when the window of the rotating transducer has left the skin. Lack of echoes next to regular echoes occurs as a result of poor contact between the window and the skin.

High- or low-velocity layer

When a pulse passes through a layer in which the velocity of sound is substantially different from the soft-tissue average of 1540 m/s, an error results in the depth registration of echoes from reflectors beyond the layer. The most common example of a high-velocity material is bone, in which the velocity is 3500 m/s. A small error (e.g. 0.3 mm)

in positioning the echo from the retina can arise because of the higher velocity of sound in the lens. This artefact is not particularly important in diagnostic ultrasonics since most soft tissues have velocities close to the average value.

Mirror artefact

If a strong smooth reflector is in the proximity of a structure being scanned, a second, mirror image of the structure may be observed. This is caused by sound scattering from the structure to the smooth reflector and then back to the transducer. The most common example of this is when a second image of the liver tissue pattern is observed in the lungs on the wrong side of the diaphragm which has acted as a smooth reflector to generate the artefact (Fig. 15.5).

BEAM-SHAPE ARTEFACTS

This type of artefact arises because the beam is not ideally narrow and uniform along all of its length, and the transmitted pulse has a finite length.

Pulse length

Any ultrasonic pulse has a finite length, typically

2 or 3 wavelengths. The echo signal from a thin-tissue interface is depicted on the display screen as a line of finite width. If the tissue interface is a strong reflector, it may appear quite wide in the image. We noted in Chapter 12 that this artefact determines the axial resolution of an imaging system.

Beam width

The main effect of the width of an ultrasonic beam in imaging is to make a point target appear as a short line. This occurs because echoes are received from the target for all of the time that it is in the scanning beam. Similarly, a structure may appear extended in an image as a result of the beam-width artefact; this can often be seen at the end of a needle, a catheter, or a fetal bone. Reduction of the sensitivity of the scanner decreases the effective beam width and therefore helps in the identification of end points. It is also important to remember that the width of the beam out of the plane of scan means that echoes are received from a tissue layer of finite thickness (Fig. 15.7).

Since the width of a beam varies along its length, the echo lines in the image also vary. Quite large differences in line length can be seen throughout the image; for instance, away from the focus, a point target may produce a length 3 or 4 times that at the focus.

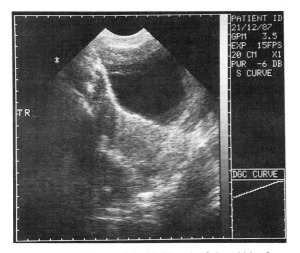

Fig. 15.7 At the base of the bladder, the finite width of the ultrasound beam causes echoes from the side wall to be included in the image.

Focusing

Echoes generated at the focus of the beam may be larger than those produced in neighbouring regions, since the transmitted wave amplitude is larger at the focus (Fig. 13.9). A bright band of echoes across an image results from this artefact. Compensation for this artefact may be accomplished by adjustment of the TGC. This artefact should be distinguished from one of like appearance arising from badly set up TGC.

Side-lobes and grating-lobes

During the discussion of beam generation in Chapter 5, we saw that, apart from the main ultrasonic beam from a transducer, side-lobes and grating-lobes are also generated. These lobes can produce echoes which may be recorded in the image. The most obvious candidates for detection by side-lobes or grating-lobes are bone and gas, but normal soft tissues are also involved, especially near the transducer. The echoes from side-lobes are registered in the image along the direction of the main beam, since the machine assumes that all echoes are produced from interfaces on the axis of the beam (Fig. 15.8).

Much of the effort in array design has been aimed at reducing the size of the grating-lobes. They have been a particular problem in phased arrays for which the grating-lobes are increased when the main beam is deflected to the side of the sector. One of the most common examples of grating-lobe artefact is the detection of off-axis heart wall when the main beam is within a chamber. The gas next to the diaphragm can also generate large artefactual echoes in a liver image. Since grating-lobes from an array are normally stronger than side-lobes from a single crystal, they can give rise to artefacts at greater depth in the image.

Beam degradation

Refraction, diffraction, attenuation, scattering, reflection, and non-linear propagation degrade the shape of an ultrasonic beam in tissue. The degree of degradation may be slight or considerable. It is difficult to assess how much a beam is degraded in any particular situation, since in-vivo measure-

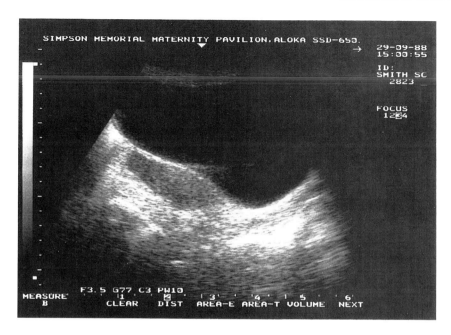

Fig. 15.8   At the base of the bladder, a strong echo signal, generated by a side-lobe, extends into the image of liquid. Echoes produced by side-lobes are located along the direction of the main beam at each instant.

ments cannot be readily made. From the limited evidence available, it appears that even when good-quality images, say, of the abdomen, are observed, the degradation of the beam from that plotted in a water-tank is probably quite large. In the extreme case, the spurious echoes and indistinct tissue boundaries resulting from the beam-degradation artefact render the image useless. The explanations for extreme degradation in a small percentage of patients have not been fully confirmed. They are sometimes related to fat layers or tissues of increased rigidity and density ('the hard-body problem').

Transducer defects

Occasionally, spurious echo signals can result from ultrasound's being transmitted within the body of the transducer or directly among the elements of an array. These signals may be observed close to the transmission signal when the transducer is held in the air. It is also possible for the main beam to be asymmetrical if there is a defect in the piezoelectric element or in the way it is mounted. A poor electrical connection to the element can generate noise signals. A non-functioning element causes a low-echo region along a few scan lines in the image from a linear array, and degradation of the beam from a phased array. Transducer defects are not a common problem, but they should be suspected if a persistent artefact is seen in the image. They can be identified with reasonable certainty by changing the transducer or by causing the tissues to move and observing the signals which remain static.

ELECTRONIC ARTEFACTS

Since the electronic system has a very strong influence on the echo signals, the possibility of creating artefacts is also large.

Poor TGC adjustment

Just as TGC can produce well-balanced images by applying appropriate amplification to the echoes from each depth, it can cause unbalanced ones if it is poorly adjusted. It is virtually impossible to set up TGC perfectly, especially if the beam sweeps through pockets of liquid. Structures

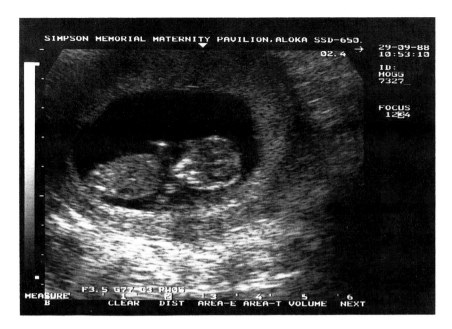

Fig. 15.9 Echoes from deep structures are presented at too high a level as a result of the TGC not allowing for the low attenuation in liquid.

beyond pockets of liquid are often presented as saturated echoes unless steps are taken to adjust the TGC in that region (Fig. 15.9). Likewise, structures beyond attenuating layers are often represented by echoes which are relatively weak. In practice, the imaging of subtle changes in tissue reflectivity is most affected by poor TGC, for example, at the pyramids in the kidney, or at the body of the pancreas.

In M-scanning, carefully adjusted TGC will help to improve the completeness of traces of fast-moving reflectors. The changing orientation of a heart valve can make the amplitude of the echo fluctuate greatly and make it difficult to accommodate with TGC. This is the reason that the TGC controls, consisting of a line of knobs, each of which influences a particular, small depth range, first appeared in cardiac machines.

Automatic TGC

The artefacts of ATGC have not been extensively studied. However, in a well-designed system, they are not particularly prominent. One artefact which has been noted is the introduction of noise in images of large fluid-filled structures (Fig. 15.10). If

there are very few echoes in the region which the machine is using to determine the average echo level prior to adjusting the gain, a high gain will be set, and, hence, weak noise signals will be recorded. The design of the ATGC can be made to allow for this situation, and the gain rise is then limited. In practice, this is not a serious artefact.

Ring-down space (transducer dead space)

The receiver cannot handle echoes during the short time that the transducer is vibrating as a result of the excitation pulse. Tissue next to the transducer face cannot, therefore, be imaged. In modern transducers of 3.5 or 5 MHz this space is quite small, e.g. 5 mm.

Electronic noise

When the gain of the receiving amplifier is high, for instance, when the TGC has reached its maximum at a large range, many small signals may be observed on an ultrasonic display of any type. On an A-scan, they are sometimes called 'grass'; on B-mode, they show as a fine uniform pattern of spots (Fig. 15.11). These noise signals are

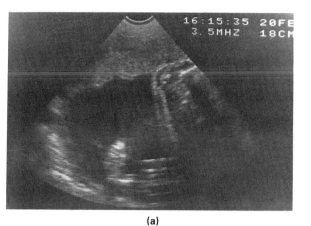

(a)

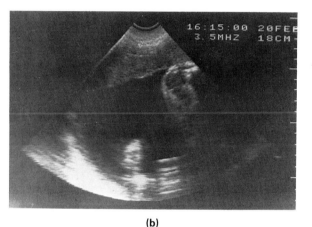

(b)

Fig. 15.10 (a) Artefact noise signals in liquid caused by simple automatic TGC not recognizing liquid, (b) manual TGC presenting liquid as clear structure, but saturating echo signals from deep tissues (courtesy of Pye S).

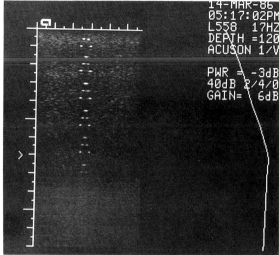

Fig. 15.11 Weak uniform signals at depths beyond targets as a result of electronic noise.

generated within the electronics and are not echoes. Electronic noise limits the smallness of an echo which can be detected.

Misregistration

An imaging instrument must be able to register echo signals accurately at their correct positions. Should a fault develop in the range-calculating electronics or the beam position-measuring system, echoes will not register in their correct positions. This fault is most serious and causes image blurring if it occurs in a compound scanner. For example, a small point target scanned from three different directions might be displayed as three separately located echoes rather than as three superimposed echoes. In the simple scans normally performed by real-time B-scanners, misregistration results in image distortion rather than image blurring.

Range ambiguity

If a machine operates at a very high pulse-repetition rate, as is sometimes done in scanning superficial tissues with a high line density, the deep echoes from one transmission may still be being received when the next pulse is transmitted (Fig. 15.12). The display electronics treat the deep echoes from the first pulse as though they were produced by the second pulse, and they therefore appear superficially in the image (Fig. 15.13). Since multiple-reflection echoes in a water-bath often last for a considerable time after the instant of transmission, they may also be located superficially.

SCAN-CONVERTER ARTEFACTS

Pixel visibility

If the scan-converter memory is too small for the image to be stored, or if the echoes are not digitized to a sufficient number of bits, the pixels

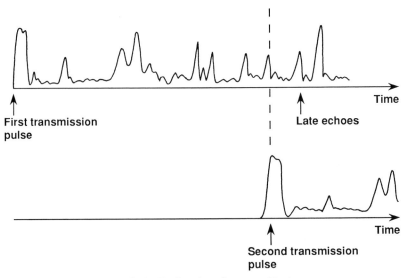

Fig. 15.12   Explanation of range ambiguity.

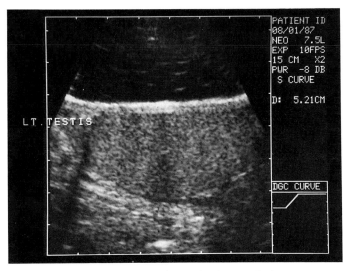

Fig. 15.13   Echoes in superficial regions, i.e. in water-bath, caused by range ambiguity (courtesy Wild S R).

will be visible in the image. This was a common artefact in early scan converters.

Blank pixels

When a sector-shaped image is stored in a rectangular pixel array, not all of the array elements lie on a scan line, especially at depths where the scan lines have spread out. Manufacturers overcome this problem by using the echo data in neighbour-ing pixels to generate a value for the blank one. Commonly, the average of the immediate neighbours is used. Some early scan converters did not perform this task well, and, as a result, some pixels were left blank.

Image processing

No way of presenting echoes in an ultrasound image can claim to be more correct than another.

Perhaps the closest representation of the reflectivity of tissues is achieved in an image in which the speckle has been averaged out, but even this may blur tissue boundaries. All presentations of echoes and image processing are, to some extent, artefactual and are the product of the judgement and opinions of the designer; for example, the allocation of grey shades to echo amplitudes, or the degree of edge enhancement employed (Fig. 15.14). To accommodate these necessary, but somewhat arbitrary, design decisions, we must relate the appearance of structures in an image to experience in clinical usage with each machine.

Lag

A common facility is to compose the image from echo information gathered over several scan frames. If more than about 5 frames are used to provide data for each image, lag (persistence) is seen in the image, since the data for the 1st and 5th frames may correspond to slightly different scan planes. This lag may be acceptable if summing data over several frames helps to reduce the noise in the image.

DISPLAY AND RECORDING ARTEFACTS

Geometric distortion

This artefact is most likely to arise from a fault in the time-to-distance electronics in the scanner or from a defect in the TV monitor (Fig. 15.15). It is readily checked by scanning a regular grid of

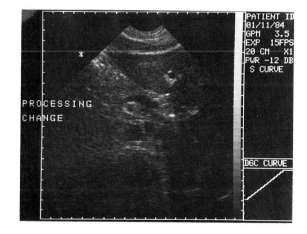

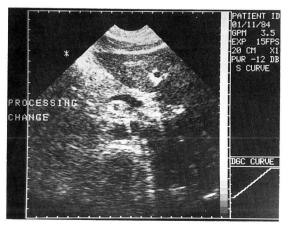

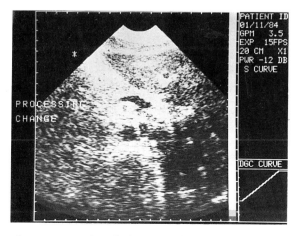

Fig. 15.14 Influence of image processing on presentation of echoes.

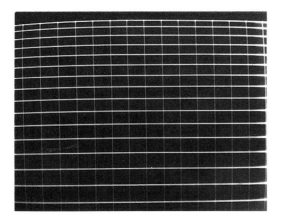

Fig. 15.15   Display distortion of regular grid pattern.

wires (App. 1). Large distortions can be present in an image without the operator's being fully aware of them. Measurements made from distorted images may have large errors.

Saturation

To preserve the information in weak echoes, the instrument often compresses large amplitude echoes into a few bright-grey shades. This is essentially an artefact which may obscure some useful information. It is inescapable as a result of the limited dynamic range of the display screens. This artefact can be removed at the expense of the weak echoes by reducing the sensitivity of the scanner.

Film exposure

The optimum exposure of a film is dependent, to some extent, on personal preference for a particular type of image, for example, high or low contrast. Like the display screen, the film can accommodate only a limited range of echo magnitudes. Film, therefore, must introduce quite a considerable number of artefacts in the recording of echoes.

Low frame rate

A low frame rate results in a fast-moving reflector's being presented at separate points along its path. For an example, consider a mitral valve leaflet that moves 3 cm in 160 ms during its opening flick. With a frame rate of 25/s, the time interval for each frame is 40 ms, and the tip of the valve leaflet is detected only at three or four distinct positions. The result is to depict fast-moving structures as proceeding in a series of jumps. In addition, different regions in the scan sweep are interrogated ultrasonically at different times; it could take the ultrasound beam 15 ms to sweep over the mitral valve, during which time the tip of the valve could move 5 mm. The image of the valve action is therefore slightly distorted.

Low line density

The line density in the image produced by a sector scanner decreases with depth and contributes to the degradation of the image quality with depth.

SUMMARY

Examples of artefacts in B-scan images were listed and classified under five headings.

1. Nine examples were presented of propagation artefacts.
2. Six examples were quoted of beam-shape artefacts.
3. Six examples were given of electronic artefacts.
4. Four scan-converter artefacts were presented.
5. Five display and recording artefacts were considered.

REFERENCES

Kremkau F W, Taylor K J W 1986 Artefacts in ultrasound imaging. J Ultrasound Medicine 5: 227–237
Sanders R C 1986 Atlas of ultrasonographic artefacts and variants. Wolfe Medical, London.

16. M-scan instruments, performance and use

The M-scan was considered in Chapter 2; it will now be considered more fully. During ultrasonic scanning, echo pulses are received at the transducer very soon after the instant of transmission. Even echoes produced by deep-lying tissue interfaces are received within 0.5 ms. It is, therefore, possible to follow rapid motion of a structure by detecting an echo from it at closely spaced times. A common technique for doing so is called 'M-scanning' (motion scanning); the terms 'time-motion scanning' (T-M scanning), 'time-position scanning' (T-P scanning), 'echocardiography', and 'ultrasonic cardiography' (UCG) are alternatives. The result produced by this technique is a trace of position versus time for each interface detected. As might be expected, M-scanning is employed primarily to study the action of the adult heart, but is also used to study blood vessels and fetal hearts. Other possible areas of application are moving structures in the orbit of the eye or in the brain, pharyngeal walls, fetal breathing, and stomach contractions.

The M-scan mode is normally a feature of real-time B-scanners, but stand-alone M-scan units are also found. M-scanning was the central ultrasonic technique of cardiology for many years. This chapter could be omitted in an initial study.

PRINCIPLE OF M-SCANNING

The process of transmitting an ultrasonic pulse and detecting echoes in M-scanning is the same as for imaging. Indeed, M-scanning is merely another way of presenting the echo information (Fig. 16.1).

In M-scanning a transducer is coupled to the skin and the ultrasonic beam directed toward the

moving tissue interfaces. The echo pattern is presented on a display scope as a line of echo spots that sweeps at a uniform speed of a few centimetres per second across the screen. Echo spots from static structures trace out straight lines on the screen, whereas those from moving structures produce fluctuating recordings that show their changing positions with time (Fig. 2.12). It can be

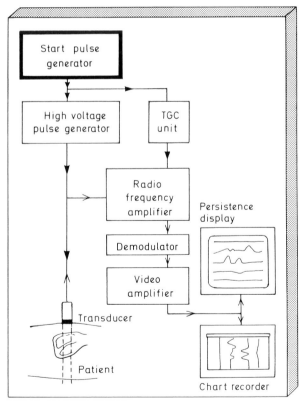

Fig. 16.1 Block of the functional units of an M-scan system.

seen that the motions of several structures are depicted simultaneously. By repetitively sweeping the line of echoes across the screen, a new pattern continually replaces the old one.

An important point to remember is that the ultrasonic beam is held fixed while the motion of structures of interest is being depicted. The record produced is therefore one of the motion of structures along one line through the tissues, although this line is selected after an initial search. In this respect, M-scanning is similar to A-scanning. However, characteristic motions, for instance, those of heart valves and chamber walls, aid identification of anatomy.

Only a limited time span can be accommodated when a trace is shown on a screen. The trace on the display screen can be photographed to provide a record. Expansion of the technique is possible by the inclusion of a fibre-optic chart recorder in the system; this is essential for cardiac examinations. With this type of recorder, the complete M trace can be recorded over a longer time span (Fig. 16.2).

M-SCAN INSTRUMENTS

M-scan units consist of circuitry to transmit and receive pulsed ultrasound, with extra provision to feed the echo signals to a display module and a fibre-optic chart recorder. The sensitivity con-

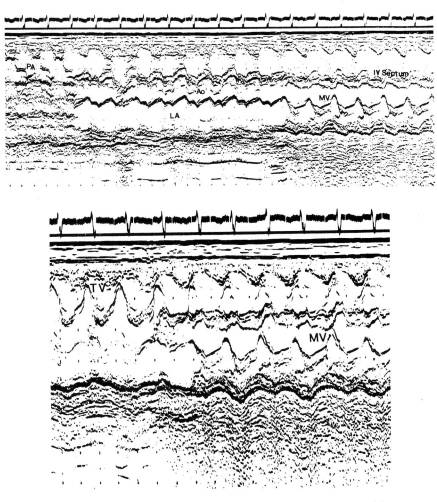

Fig. 16.2   M-mode traces of the heart of a child (courtesy of Godman M).

trols are the same as for A-, B-, and real-time B-scan instruments, and are manipulated as described in Chapter 7. The display controls for each output are more or less self-explanatory.

With an electronic memory display, which may make use of the scan converter memory or be completely independent, the scroll mode of writing the M trace is an option. In this mode, the new lines of echo information appear on one side of the screen and are slowly moved across it. Thus, the whole M-mode pattern moves across the screen while new echo lines are continually added at one side. This should be distinguished from the M-mode presentation technique in which new information is put into the line of echoes as it moves across the screen (Fig. 16.3). An advantage of the scroll presentation is that when a good recording is seen on the screen, the trace is frozen and may be viewed indefinitely.

A requirement of a transducer for cardiac examinations is that its dimensions should be small enough for it to fit conveniently between the ribs. For adults 2–3 MHz ultrasound is employed; for paediatric application, 5–7 MHz. Focusing in single-element transducers is normally arranged to be at the depth of the mitral valve; around 7 cm deep in adults.

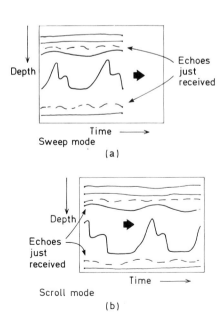

Fig. 16.3 Presentation of M-scan on a display screen.

Time-gain compensation (TGC, swept gain)

Standard TGC controls are found on cardiac systems; AGC is also utilized. Common in cardiac work is the type of compensation for attenuation with depth which provides individual controls to govern the gain corresponding to each small range in depth (Ch. 7). Great flexibility is possible for the change of gain with depth. The reasoning behind this approach is that within the heart, high sensitivity is required in the region of valves and lower sensitivity near walls. In addition, the heart with its chambers of blood bounded by muscle does not attenuate an ultrasonic beam uniformly with depth.

Sweep trigger

The sweep trigger starts the generation of the M-mode pattern on the screen. Typically, the sweep is performed continuously. This is called a 'free-run' mode. It is also possible to trigger the sweep by some external signal, for example, by an ECG or pressure waveform. This is a simple matter, but it is rarely done in practice.

Sweep-speed selection

The optimal speed depends on the application and the particular motion under study. For example, it may be desired to use the whole screen to record one heart cycle so that details of a valve motion are clearly presented. At the other extreme, the object may be to record many cycles so that heart rate is measurable. A control is, therefore, available to adjust the sweep speed from high values, for example, 50 cm/s, to low values, for example, 0.2 cm/s. Note that too low a speed can obscure detail.

Paper speed in a chart recorder is equivalent to sweep speed on the screen. Paper speeds in the range 1–200 mm/s are usually offered.

Electronic gating

Electronic gating of specific echoes from the echo train is used in selecting a small group of echoes to fill the whole width of the recording medium. The technique improves accuracy in measuring the range of movement of heart walls, etc.

Physiologic signal inputs

It is invaluable to be able to record other physiologic signals along with the ultrasonic echoes. Inputs to the ultrasonic instrument should be available to permit this combined display. Routinely, the ECG is recorded with an M-scan trace. To attempt to display more than two physiologic signals on the same screen as the ultrasonic information may be impractical because of the limited space. This limitation is one of the reasons for using chart recorders.

CHART RECORDERS

On first impression the problems of recording the trace of an interface seem no different from those associated with other signals such as an ECG. The situation is, however, more complex since each trace is built up from very short duration echoes received at a rate of about 1000/s. In addition, it is desirable to be able to record simultaneously traces from a number of reflecting interfaces.

Fibre-optic chart recorder (line-scan recorder)

A special type of cathode-ray tube recorder allows the complete echo pattern to be recorded on paper. The special feature is that part of the glass display screen is replaced by a plate comprising many thousands of short fibre-optic light guides placed side by side. These optical fibres are similar to those found in endoscopes. The phosphor of the CRT is deposited on one side of the strip of optical fibres so that a line of bright echo spots on the phosphor can be transferred to the outside of the tube without loss of definition (Fig. 16.4).

During the ultrasonic examination, the recording paper is moved past the outside of the fibre plate at an appropriate speed. The echo spots, situated on a fixed line along the outside of the fibre plate, produce a trace on the paper. For immediate viewing, paper sensitive to ultraviolet light allows the result to be studied in a few seconds. A higher contrast record is produced with paper that is passed through a thermal processor. Some instruments use paper that can be developed in an automatic, X-ray film processor. The slight delay of this method is often acceptable. In Chapter 26, recording techniques are discussed further.

A typical fibre-optic CRT recorder handles four other channels of information simultaneously with the ultrasonic data. The additional signals are fed

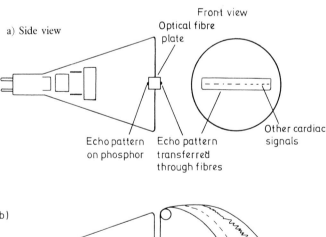

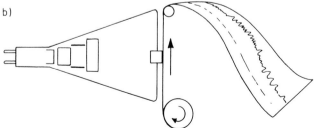

Fig. 16.4   Schematic diagram of a fibre-optic chart recorder.

to the CRT and appear as moving bright spots next to the line of echoes. The recorder deals with all this information at the same time by rapidly sampling all input signals. This technique of using one display to present, simultaneously, several sets of signals is called 'multiplexing'.

Electrical safety

This discussion of recording techniques brings out the fact that several different instruments may be linked to the patient at any one time. Precautions such as ensuring that the instruments have a common earth should be taken to avoid electrical hazards; it is advisable to have any arrangement of instruments checked from this standpoint. Ultrasonic instruments present no special electrical safety problems.

INITIAL PROCEDURE FOR M-SCANNING

We will now consider briefly the procedure involved in M-scanning of heart structures with a real-time B-scan system. The approach is similar to that of other scanning techniques.

Before the examination of the patient, the operator should check the instrument controls for suitability of baseline settings. As in the methods of previous chapters, the sensitivity controls are particularly important (Ch. 7). The scale of display, brilliance, and camera adjustment should also be optimized. When the M-mode facility is selected, the pulse repetition frequency (PRF) along the chosen line should be high (typically 600 pulses/s). This ensures that echoes are received from fast-moving structures at all positions in their motion. For example, a valve cusp moving at a speed of 300 mm/s sends back an echo after each 0.5 mm change in its position if the PRF is 600 pulses/s. A high PRF also assists the recording techniques by producing bright echo spots. The PRF is normally set automatically when the M-mode facility of a real-time imaging system is selected.

After the instrument controls have been checked, the transducer is applied to the chest at an appropriate rib space for imaging the heart. Difficulty in detecting moving heart structures usually means that bone or lung has intercepted the beam.

Typically, a 3 MHz transducer is used in heart scanning, and its size is such as to fit between adult rib spaces; for example, a width of 1.5 cm. For infants, a 5 MHz probe is commonly employed, and the rib problem is ignored as a result of the reduced attenuation experienced in cartilage. A coupling medium of the gel type is most suitable for heart examinations because it allows manipulation of the transducer without loss of contact.

To generate an M-scan, we activate the M-mode facility and manipulate a control to select the desired M-scan beam direction through the displayed anatomy. This direction is indicated by increased brightness of the scan line selected. The M-scan trace is then observed as it is repetitively generated on the screen. Final optimization of the M-scan is arranged by altering the selected direction while the characteristics of the trace are examined. Selection of a trace shape for recording is essentially a pattern-recognition process in which the trace is compared with those in the scientific literature or those encountered previously. In unusual situations, however, one must solve the problem of deducing the trace shape that results from the interception of a fixed beam and the moving cardiac structures. Once the operator ascertains the optimum beam path, the recorder is activated. In some instances, the M-scan direction may be systematically moved to intercept neighbouring structures during the recording (Fig. 2.13).

The ECG waveform is recorded either in a space reserved for it at the side of the trace, or in some echo-free region.

Application of the M-mode in fields other than cardiology also involves prior use of an ultrasonic-imaging technique. In the early detection of fetal heart beats, the thorax of the fetus is identified on a real-time B-scan image.

Production of recordings

To record complete and meaningful M-scan traces, one must optimize the instrument controls while relating the observed echo patterns to cardiac anatomy. It is always worthwhile to check that weak and fast-moving echoes are, in fact, being recorded on the chart paper. Each application may require particular settings of the brilliance control to ensure optimum trace quality. The concepts associated with grey-shade imaging are also important for M-traces. The echo-amplitude dynamic range from heart tissues, 30 dB (32–1), is compressed to suit the recording technique, and the compressed echo amplitudes are directly related to shades of grey in the recording. With ultraviolet-light recording paper, as used in fibre-optic chart recorders, up to 5 shades can be distinguished. Other papers requiring thermal processing or photographic development produce 7 or 8 shades of grey. Grey tones assist in the identification of structures in a trace, particularly the muscle of heart walls.

As mentioned earlier, the sweep speed of the line of echo dots or the chart-paper speed should be adjusted to show the required amount of detail. Similarly, the range of depth displayed on the recording device should be such as to make the best use of the space available. Proper setting up of sweep speed and display range makes the measurement of range of movement and of gradients from the recordings more accurate. Figure 16.5a shows an M-mode trace from a system set up to record fast cardiac actions, while Figure 16.5b shows it arranged to record slow stomach contractions.

Although the sensitivity controls have been previously set up to baseline positions, it may be helpful during the search process to manipulate one of them occasionally, for example, the overall gain, as this helps to display particular structures clearly. For instance, when pursuing a particularly elusive structure, one may find it advisable to adjust the gain to suit only this structure and sacrifice the echo information from other areas. A complete trace is obtained only when the echo of interest is maintained above a certain minimum amplitude throughout the cardiac cycle. This is often difficult because the directions of the ultrasonic beam into the heart are limited by bone and lung. Occasionally, moving the patient on to the left or right side may move the heart and help the detection and recording of moving surfaces.

The adjustment of TGC in heart studies is

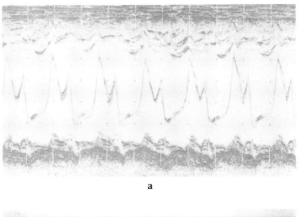

a

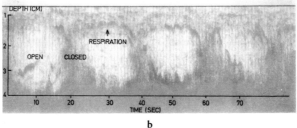

b

Fig. 16.5 (a) M-scan of heart-valve motion. Regular arrays of spots are separated in time by 0.5 s and depth by 1 cm. (b) M-scan of contractions of the antrum of the stomach.

governed more by the need to detect particular structures than the need to compensate for attenuation. An instance of this is in mitral valve studies, where the initial gain is held low for 2 or 3 cm to prevent the chest wall echoes overloading the display. The slope is then made high, for example, 10 dB/cm with 3 MHz ultrasound, so that the sensitivity is high throughout the range where the mitral valve is observed.

Having obtained a good, clear echo pattern, the operator should record it over a number of heart cycles. This allows variations in the traces caused by respiration and patient movement to be taken into account.

CALIBRATION OF TRACES

In M-scanning, it is particularly important to be able to specify both range and time calibration for each scan. This calibration is most convenient if markers appear automatically on each photographic print or chart record. Without such calibration, the value of the method is diminished, because measurements of displacements and speeds of movement cannot be made absolutely.

Range calibration

Depth calibration is usually presented as a line of spots whose separation is exactly known in millimetres (e.g. 10 mm). Because the lines of spots are repeated at regular time intervals (e.g. 0.5 s), the space between any two lines gives the time-scale calibration (Fig. 16.2). In the various applications of M-scanning, ranges of movement from 60 mm to less than 1 mm have to be measured. For example, the range of movement of the mitral valve cusp in an adult could be 60 mm, whereas the range of movement of fetal heart structures may be only 1 or 2 mm.

It is obvious that the range calibration of a trace should be accurate to within 0.5 mm.

Time calibration

M-scan instruments should be capable of calibrating the time axis to an accuracy of 0.01 s. The range of sweep or paper speeds required of an instrument is from 200 to 2 mm/s.

RESOLUTION IN M-SCANNING

The axial, lateral, and contrast resolutions attainable in M-scanning are the same as those quoted for real-time B-scanning in Chapter 12. All detected structures do not necessarily lie along a line through the heart, but, rather, within a beam of finite width.

The measurement of time can be made with good temporal resolution. For example, if the pulse repetition frequency is 1000, the position of a reflector can be sampled at 1/1000-second time intervals, i.e. 1 ms intervals.

LIMITATIONS OF M-SCANNING

The basic limitations are as follows:

1. Traces are recorded along only one line at a time. With complex motions, this can make measurement difficult.

2. The identification of the sources of the echoes can be difficult.

3. The interpretation of traces obtained from complex motions is not easy.

4. In cardiac scanning, the access to the heart with an ultrasonic beam is limited by lung and bone. This can create problems in detecting structures of interest.

5. Movement of structures increases the problems of setting up the sensitivity controls to optimize the echo magnitudes.

ARTEFACTS IN M-SCANNING

Many of the artefacts in M-scanning are like those discussed for imaging in Chapter 15. However, moving structures produce characteristic traces that help artefacts to be identified. A few of the more relevant artefacts will now be recalled and their significance in M-scan work indicated.

Misleading trace shapes

The interpretation of M-scan traces should always be made with caution. Obviously, for a structure moving in a complex manner within a fixed beam, misleading traces could be generated. This could be a result of the motion of the structure across the beam or of echoes being detected from different parts of the structure at different times in the cardiac cycle.

Effect of beam width

As in an A-scan pattern, two neighbouring surfaces can appear to be one behind the other because of the finite width of the ultrasonic beam. Care should be taken in interpreting the distance between two echoes as heart wall or valve thickness.

Shadowing and enhancement

If echoes from within the heart are detected only weakly, it is possible that part of the ultrasonic beam is being attenuated by lung or bone. Enhancement of echo amplitudes occurs continually in heart examinations because blood exhibits low attenuation. This is helpful in detecting weak echoes such as those from valves.

Multiple reflection (reverberation)

This phenomenon can readily occur in the fluid-filled chambers of the heart. At high sensitivity, a reverberation between the transducer and the posterior wall of the left ventricle is seen as a moving echo beyond the genuine heart signals. Another example is that between the transducer and the anterior wall of the heart when a pericardial effusion is present. The range of movement of the reverberant-echo trace is twice that of the genuine heart-wall echo because the change in the tissue thickness has twice the effect on the path length of the double-reflection echo.

Electronic processing

Artefacts resulting from electronic processing are similar to those studied for imaging. Adjustment of the TGC is difficult because of the motion of the structures as well as the combination of fluid-filled chambers and strong reflecting boundaries.

High- or low-velocity layers

The effect of a non-average-velocity layer on the range calibration is usually important only for

bone layers. We have already noted that attenuation in bone makes it undesirable to transmit the ultrasonic beam through it into the heart. An exception is in the case of young infants, whose bone is less attenuating.

Trace-sample rate

The PRF determines the rate at which the echo lines are gathered to form the M-scan trace. If it is too low, the sharp points in the trace will be rounded and the trace will not truly represent the motion of the reflector. In adult and fetal heart work, it is reasonable to gather echo lines at 1 ms intervals; in other words, a PRF of around 1 kHz is required.

Prosthetic materials

The materials used in prostheses may have acoustic characteristics very different from those of blood or soft tissue; for example, the high acoustic impedance and low attenuation of steel or the very smooth surfaces of valve flaps. The velocity of sound in non-biological materials is usually very different from that of tissue.

Drop-out

The angle of a moving tissue boundary in relation to an ultrasound beam often changes markedly with related large changes in the echo size. Drop-out (gaps) therefore appears in the M-scan trace. This problem may be helped by arranging high gain at the tissue depth corresponding to the missing structure.

Edge enhancement

As a means of providing crisp traces, the leading edges of echoes can be emphasized electronically and the tails suppressed. A clear space may then be present below the leading edge. Obviously, this should not be interpreted as an echo-free space. This artefact emphasizes the need to be thoroughly acquainted with the performance of the machine on normal persons and, if possible, with any special signal processing which may be incorporated in it.

INTERPRETATION OF M-SCAN TRACES

The interpretation of traces has to be made with a full awareness of the limitation of the technique. There are one or two additional points of interest. One should note that motion may make the echo amplitude from a specific structure vary through a range of 30–40 dB. In other words, a strong echo received at one point in the cardiac cycle may be very weak at a later stage as a result of the reflector's either changing its orientation or moving out of the beam.

Note that very small tissue movements often result in pulsations in the echo amplitudes that in turn, produce varying shades of grey in a photograph or paper-chart record. These variations in grey shade may make the small movements detectable. The record from a fetal heart in early pregnancy is often of this type (Fig. 2.14).

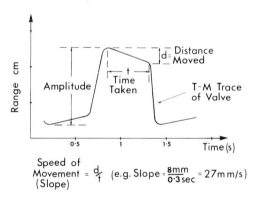

Fig. 16.6 Example of measurement from an M-scan trace.

MEASUREMENT FROM M-SCAN TRACES

From a trace of a single structure, two quantities can be measured, distance and time. Most often, it is the movements of heart valves that are quantified in this manner. Figure 16.6 indicates the ways in which range of movement, and rate of movement are obtained from the trace. From the movements of several surfaces recorded simultaneously, it is possible to measure the distances among the surfaces, and how they change. A common example of this is the measurement of the distance between the wall of the left ventricle and the interventricular septum of the heart. Having made such measurements and some assumptions, we can calculate the ejection fraction, the velocity of circumferential fibre shortening, and the stroke volume, although the error involved may be unacceptably high.

Deductions about the strengths of echoes may be made from a recording, in order, for example, to estimate the degree of calcification of a valve. It is important to do this only when the sensitivity is at a well-established baseline setting.

As with other scanning methods, the main source of error in measurement is in the uncertainty regarding the particular dimension that has been recorded. For instance, it is difficult to know if the recorded echo comes from the free end of a valve or from a neighbouring part. Error in the measurement of range from a trace is typically ± 2 mm at 3 MHz, and ± 1 mm at 5 MHz.

Error in the measurement of time arises from uncertainty as to the exact point on the trace from which to take a reading. For cardiac examination, this error is likely to be ± 10 ms.

M-SCAN PLUS DOPPLER

Simultaneous presentation of an M-scan trace showing tissue motion and a Doppler sonogram of associated blood flow is of value in some examinations. Further discussion of this modality is postponed until Chapter 20 when Doppler techniques will have been studied more fully.

SUMMARY

The M-mode was seen to be still an important feature of cardiac systems since it presented long recordings of structure position versus time. The method of echo generation was seen to be similar to that of A-scan and real-time B-scan imaging. The techniques also have resolution factors, artefacts, and sensitivity controls in common. Fibre-optic chart recorders were demonstrated to be particularly suited to M-scanning. Measurement of distance, velocity, and acceleration can be made from calibrated recordings.

17. Miscellaneous pulsed-echo imaging scanners

In this chapter, some echo-imaging systems with distinctive characteristics will be discussed in more detail. A few of these represent techniques that are not widely applied, but these systems do indicate the variations possible in the design of ultrasonic scanners. The selection of devices for inclusion proved difficult since many experimental systems exist. This chapter could be omitted in an initial study.

UI OCTOSON

A machine of particular interest is called the 'Octoson' because its transducer assembly consists of eight focused crystals. The crystals have an operating frequency of 3 MHz and diameters of 7 cm. Large diameters, that is, apertures, are employed to give good focusing and high sensitivity. The structure of the machine is shown diagrammatically in Figure 17.1.

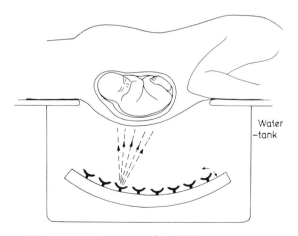

Fig. 17.1 Basic structure of the UI Octoson scanner.

The transducers are immersed in a water-bath and scan the patient from below. Normally, the patient lies on a thin plastic membrane with acoustic coupling by a gel. For some applications, such as breast scanning, part of the patient is immersed directly. The eight transducers move on the arc of a circle and each performs an oscillating action during this motion. The sector angle of the oscillatory action is adjustable up to 66°. Each transducer, in turn, transmits a pulse of ultrasound and receives a train of echoes. This continues throughout the duration of the compound scan, which is typically 2 s. The number of transducers in operation varies from all eight to only one. With one transducer functioning, simple scans are performed at a rate of 4/s.

A high degree of freedom of movement is permitted by the mechanical system supporting the transducers. One may select longitudinal, transverse, and oblique scan planes through the patient. In each position, the scan plane can be tilted. The depth of the beam focus within the patient is altered by changing the distance of the transducer array from the membrane. Small changes in the position of the plane of scan are possible in steps of 1–20 mm. Alteration of the plane of scan may be placed under microprocessor control, whereby the instrument produces images in a sequence of scan planes. This, combined with the motorized transducer movement, results in a highly automated system that provides reproducible results. A picture of the machine is shown in Figure 17.2.

This machine has been employed very successfully in paediatrics because it does not disturb the patient. It is also applied in fields such as obstetrics and gynaecology, where it has produced

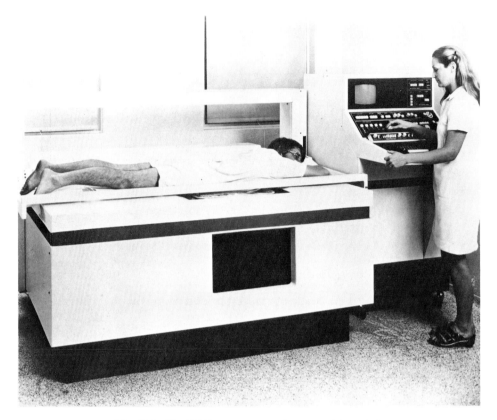

Fig. 17.2 The UI Octoson scanner (courtesy of Ausonics).

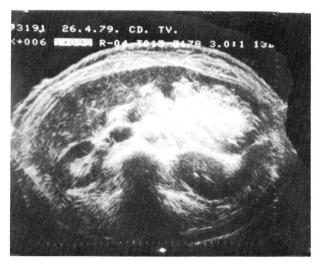

Fig. 17.3 Image from UI Octoson scanner (courtesy of
Kossoff G).

detailed images of internal fetal anatomy. Access to the pelvis and high-upper abdomen is somewhat limited by the presence of bone. The maximum acoustic output power is 1.2 mW, which is relatively low. High-quality, grey-tone images are produced by this instrument (Fig. 17.3).

BREAST SCANNER

The first ultrasonic B-scans were of the breast. The technique, however, has not become widespread because the detection of small lesions is difficult. Development is still continuing in the field of ultrasonic breast imaging. The mobility of the organ has usually dictated that it be scanned with a water-bath scanner in which the breast is immersed from the top. Ultrasound of a frequency of 5–10 MHz provides sufficient penetration for the examination of these superficial tissues. An example of the type of machine which has been marketed is shown in Figure 17.4.

In this machine, three large-diameter transducers are mounted on a wheel at the bottom of the tank. The wheel rotates to perform a sector scan of the breast. As a means to optimize resolution, the focal zone of each transducer is at a different range, and echo signals from the appropriate range are electronically selected for display as each transducer beam sweeps through the field of view. The image is formed in 1 s. A second identical transducer wheel may be activated to interrogate the tissues from a second direction and provide some compounding of the echo signals in the image.

Parallel planes of scan are produced at separations of 2 mm. The operator can select any scan plane by moving the mechanical system supporting the transducer wheels. The sequence of scans is under computer control, and in an examination 100 images may be produced.

On a test object, structures with dimensions of 2 mm are resolved with this scanner. Figure 17.5 is a breast-scan image from this commercial scanner.

Conventional real-time B-scanners also find increasing application in breast imaging. They are able to contribute to the diagnosis of some disease states and assist with aspiration techniques.

THREE DIMENSIONAL SCANNING

The images we have considered, so far, have been made by scanning an ultrasonic beam in a two-dimensional plane. It is perfectly feasible to allow the ultrasonic beam freedom of action in three dimensions in order that echo information is obtained throughout the volume of the tissues. There are two problems associated with this and other

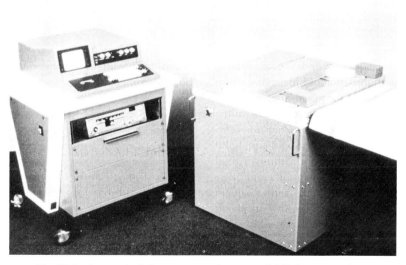

Fig. 17.4 A water-bath breast scanner (courtesy of Life Instruments).

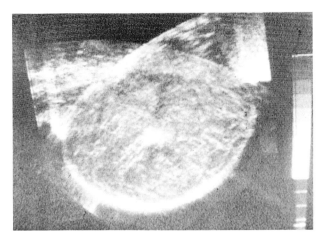

Fig. 17.5 Image from a water-bath breast scanner showing a small focal lesion (courtesy of Life Instruments).

methods of three-dimensional ultrasonic imaging. One is to store the large amount of ultrasonic information, and the other, bigger problem is to display it. Means exist for presenting three-dimensional images; however, because the echo density in ultrasonic imaging is high, the echo spots of anterior structures obscure those from posterior ones. A partial solution to this problem is to display, in rapid succession, two-dimensional images of neighbouring sections through the tissue volume.

Theoretically, echo data from three-dimensional scanning can be stored in a very large digital scan converter, and any two-dimensional section can be displayed on demand. This is now available though it is still expensive.

Searching with a real-time B-scanner gives an appreciation of three-dimensional structures. In the future, any dedicated 3-D scanner will have to offer more than can be achieved with this established technique.

C-SCANNING (CONSTANT-DEPTH SCANNING)

C-scanning is a technique for producing a two-dimensional ultrasonic image of structures lying in a plane at a specific depth within the body (Fig. 17.6). Usually a water-bath is employed to link the transducer and the patient. The transducer is made to move along a succession of closely spaced

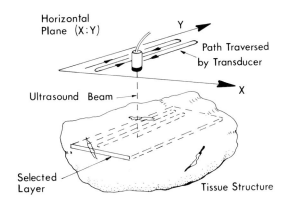

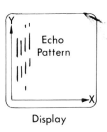

Fig. 17.6 The principle of C-scanning. Echoes received from a selected horizontal layer are displayed as bright spots at the appropriate points on the screen.

parallel lines in a horizontal plane, that is, in a raster movement. At adjacent points in its motion, an ultrasonic pulse is propagated into the body, and the echoes received are gated so that only echoes generated at a preselected depth within the body are accepted. In this way, a thin horizontal layer within the body is examined.

At each point where an echo is detected from the selected layer, a grey-tone spot is presented on the display. Thus, a two-dimensional image is obtained of interfaces in the tissue layer that have reflected detectable echoes. This type of scanning produces a horizontal ultrasonic tomogram, whereas normally, in ultrasonic imaging, the tomogram planes are orientated more vertically.

C-scan systems that do not require an immersion technique are also feasible. For instance, it is possible to compensate electronically for the rise and fall of the transducer as it performs a raster movement pattern in contact with the patient. It is also possible to do a C-scan by placing the transducer at one point on the skin and then manipulating it in such a way that the beam performs an ever-increasing conical scan. Again, echoes from a layer are selected by gating and by electronically allowing for the angle of the beam to the vertical.

Judgement of the value of C-scanning, at this stage, is perhaps premature as the technique has not been applied extensively. One advantage is the high resolution that can be achieved. The layer selected can be made thin (1 or 2 mm) by reducing the time during which the gate is open. In addition, the ultrasonic beam width can be decreased by focusing it at the required depth to give a good lateral resolution. Problems associated with TGC

may also be reduced because the operator need only concentrate on the layer of interest.

CIRCUMFERENTIAL SCANNER

Circumferential scanning requires that the structure examined be wholly or partly immersed in water. A transducer is then moved in a circular path round it. This technique has been applied to limb and head scanning. As the transducer progresses round its path, it is rocked in the plane of scan, resulting in a very thorough scan of the tissues. High-quality images of sections through the leg have been produced by a circumferential scanner consisting of six linear arrays pointing towards the centre of the limb. Circumferential scanning has not been widely applied.

SUMMARY

Five examples of slightly unusual scanners were presented. These showed that ultrasonic scanning can be tailored to special needs.

REFERENCES

Jellins J, Kossoff G 1973 Velocity compensation in water-coupled breast echography. Ultrasonics 11: 223–226
McCready V R, Hill C R 1971 A constant depth ultrasonic scanner. Brit J Radiol 44: 747–750
Makow D M, Real R R 1965 Immersion ultrasonic brain examination — 360° compound scan. Ultrasonics 3: 75–80

18. Detection of motion by the Doppler effect

Our studies of Doppler techniques will be assisted by a brief review of some aspects of haemodynamics.

HAEMODYNAMICS

Doppler blood flow instruments are the most powerful non-invasive tools we have for obtaining information about the velocities of blood in the body. Most value is gleaned from them by the user with a good working knowledge of haemodynamics. However, knowledge of a few basic concepts allows some clinically valuable techniques to be implemented. This is true of established techniques. When new techniques are being developed, it is essential to consider the haemodynamics of the situation in more detail. In particular, it is important to remember that both upstream and downstream conditions influence the result obtained at a particular vascular site. Doppler methods have been successful where the haemodynamics can be simply described. Problems still exist in their application to more complex situations; for example, in the lower limbs when flow is influenced by proximal disease, distal disease, and collateral vessels. Further reading on haemodynamics related to Doppler techniques is listed in the references.

Doppler instruments are most commonly employed to study flow in arteries where the shape of the pulsatile-velocity waveform can be related to disease of the vessels or of the tissue to be supplied. Venous flow is slow and influenced by pressure from surrounding tissues and respiration. Deep-vein thrombosis is a condition studied by Doppler techniques.

Steady flow

In a steady-flow pattern, blood moves along the vessel at a constant speed. As a result of the frictional drag of the vessel wall and the viscosity of the blood, fluid at the centre of the vessel travels faster than that closer to the wall. This type of flow is most likely to be found in veins, provided that it is not influenced by respiration.

Pulsed flow

When the left ventricle of the heart contracts, a bolus of blood is accelerated into the aorta. A pressure rise is therefore created at the entrance of the aorta. The pressure rise then travels as a pulsed wave along the aorta and into the smaller arteries and arterioles. As the pulsed-pressure wave front reaches each point, the blood at that point is set in motion down the vessel (Fig. 18.1). The initial

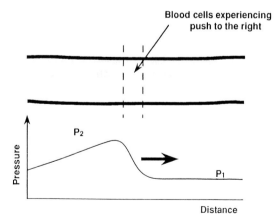

Fig. 18.1 Pressure pulse generated by the heart travelling along an artery and causing motion of blood.

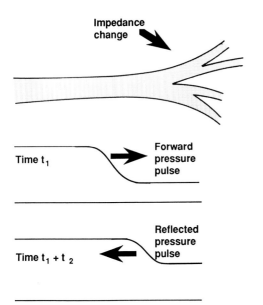

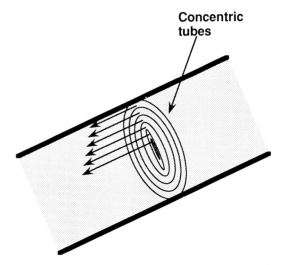

Fig. 18.3 Laminar flow in a vessel; the blood cells travel parallel to the walls.

Fig. 18.2 Reflection of a pressure pulse at an impedance change in the arteries.

injection of blood also stretches the aorta, which then shrinks and maintains some blood flow after the pressure wave front has passed. The initial forward flow may be reduced or reversed as a result of reflection of the pressure wave from the arterioles (Fig. 18.2). The reverse flow caused by the reflected wave is most easily seen in arteries, such as the femoral, which are near the arterioles. The reflected wave becomes attenuated by the time it reaches the aorta. It is useful to distinguish the velocity of the blood cells from that of the pressure wave. The pressure wave front travels along the aorta at a speed of around 5 m/s, whereas the blood velocity fluctuates from near 0 to 1 m/s.

Laminar flow

In a vessel where the blood velocity changes smoothly from low values near the wall to higher values in the centre, the blood volume can be considered as cylindrical layers which move relative to one another (Fig. 18.3). This is known as laminar flow. It can exist for both steady and pulsed patterns of flow in arteries and veins.

Disturbed flow

A change in the shape of a vessel, for example, a bifurcation, or a structure within the vessel, such as a stenosis, can cause the flow to be disturbed. In this situation, localized or moving vortices (whirlpools) of blood may be generated. Disturbed flow is found in both normal and diseased vessels.

Turbulence

As velocity is increased, a point is reached where steady flow becomes unstable, and blood particles move in an erratic fashion as they pass along the vessel. The onset of this turbulent flow occurs at a fairly well-defined velocity for each flow pattern and vascular structure. Turbulence is most often encountered in high-speed jets associated with stenosed vessels and heart valves. Later it will be seen that considerable care has to be exercised when a Doppler unit is used to identify turbulence.

Velocity profile

The velocities which exist at any instant across a vessel may be plotted to provide a velocity profile, e.g. a parabolic or plug profile (Fig. 18.4). The former is commonly encountered in steady flow;

Plug flow

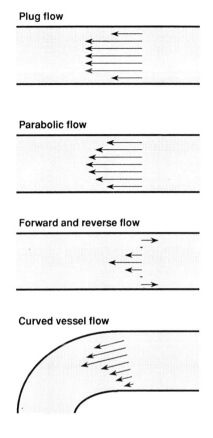

Parabolic flow

Forward and reverse flow

Curved vessel flow

Fig. 18.4 Common flow profiles in vessels

Stenosis

High velocities (e.g. 500 cm/s) may occur where a vessel or valve orifice is narrowed. The high velocity results since the blood-flow rate in ml/s in the narrow channel equals the flow rate in the larger diameter structures on either side of it (Fig. 18.5). The detection of abnormally high velocity is a common indicator of disease.

Flow in stenosis

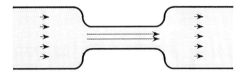

Fig. 18.5 Flow through a stenosis. The high speed in the narrow part makes the flow in ml/s the same in each portion of the vessel.

A stenosis will also dampen the pulse waveform as it passes through it. Sharp edges in the waveform can be seen to be smoothed.

It is worth noting that although a small stenosis will affect the velocities near it, the volume-flow rate will not be affected until the stenosis is quite severe, e.g. a 75% reduction in diameter.

Impedance

As a blood vessel decreases in diameter or becomes more rigid, it presents a greater impedance (resistance) to flow. Rigorous use of haemodynamic terminology would restrict 'impedance' to pulsatile flow and 'resistance' to steady flow, but this distinction is of little interest in practice.

Flow in a vessel is obviously affected by its impedance, but in many clinical studies it turns out that the impedance of the structures which the vessel supplies is of greater significance. For example, the impedance of the small arteries in the placenta is thought to influence the flow waveform in the umbilical artery. In normal circumstances, there is an increase in impedance where an artery meets the arterioles in the tissues to be supplied with blood. Part of the cardiac pressure pulse is reflected back along the artery and influences the blood flow (Fig. 18.2). This reflected pulse often

the latter where blood is accelerated into a vessel. An example of plug flow is that during early systole in the aorta. More complex profiles are encountered which vary throughout the cardiac cycle. Indeed, forward and reverse flow may occur simultaneously at different distances from the vessel wall when a reflected pressure pulse reverses the slow flow near the wall, but not the fast flow at the centre (Fig. 18.4). Alteration of the structure or curvature of a vessel further complicates the profile (Fig. 18.4). Doppler instruments exist which can record velocity at small steps across a vessel and present instantaneous velocity profiles. The profile obtained from any site depends on the position of the site in the vessel; in particular, how close it is to the entrance or exit of the vessel.

reduces diastolic blood flow, to some extent, and may cause reverse flow.

An abnormally high increase in the impedance at the end of a vessel causes a larger part of the cardiac pressure pulse to be reflected. In this situation, flow during diastole is often greatly reduced or reversed in direction. Reduced diastolic flow may be a strong indicator of disease in the structures supplied by the vessel.

If disease reduces the impedance mismatch at the end of the vessel, the reflected pulse is also reduced and, hence, diastolic flow is less affected. In this case, diastolic flow appears to be enhanced relative to the normal value. High diastolic flow indicates that the vessel is supplying a low-impedance structure.

The effect of the impedance of terminal vessels is most easily observed by noting the change in the brachial-artery velocity waveform when the fist is clenched and released (Fig. 18.6).

These results, which relate to flow in a healthy vessel terminated by an impedance change, cannot be applied to situations in which there is disease in the vessel itself. For example, a stenosis in a vessel may smooth out the pressure pulse and cause diastolic flow, even though there is an impedance change at the end of the vessel.

Pressure gradient

If the instantaneous maximum velocity of blood passing through an orifice from one chamber to another is measured (Fig. 18.7), the instantaneous pressure drop can be calculated using the following formula. In accordance with the practice in cardiac catheterization, the pressure drop is commonly referred to as the 'pressure gradient'.

$$p = 4v^2$$

where v is the instantaneous maximum velocity in m/s, and p is the drop in blood pressure (mmHg).

For a velocity of 2 m/s in a jet through a diseased mitral valve, the pressure gradient is calculated to be 16 mmHg. If one allows for differences in technique, good agreement has been found between the results from this formula and those from direct measurement during catheterization. The formula was derived from a more complete equation known as the Bernoulli equa-

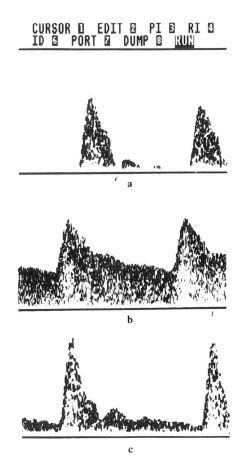

Fig. 18.6 Flow waveform in the radial artery. (**a**) Clenched fist presenting high impedance to flow; hence, reduced diastolic component; (**b**) post-clenching presenting low impedance and, hence, high diastolic component; (**c**) 5 minutes post-clenching, intermediate impedance, and normal pulsatile-flow pattern (courtesy Hoskins P)

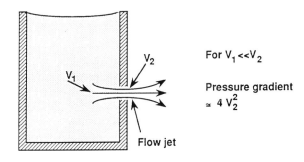

Fig. 18.7 Flow through an orifice from a chamber.

tion, which is an expression of the conservation of energy as the blood passes through the orifice.

It should be noted that this formula is valid only for blood passing through an orifice; it cannot be applied to calculate a pressure drop along an artery.

By measuring the time taken for the pressure gradient to fall to half of its peak value, i.e. for the velocity to reach v (peak)$/\sqrt{2}$, the area of the mitral valve orifice may be estimated using the formula:

$$\text{mitral valve area} = \text{MVA} = \frac{220 \text{ cm}^2}{t_{\frac{1}{2}}}$$

For example,
$t_{\frac{1}{2}} = 100$ ms
$\text{MVA} = 2.2$ cm^2

DETECTION OF MOTION BY THE DOPPLER EFFECT

So far, we have largely been concerned with diagnostic methods that make use of the amplitude of reflected ultrasound. Now we will consider techniques that exploit the shift in frequency of ultrasound when it is reflected from moving tissues. This frequency shift is an example of the Doppler effect. Diagnostic instruments designed to make use of the Doppler effect are highly sensitive, non-invasive, safe, and convenient for all concerned in their application. Many instruments have the added virtues of being small and inexpensive. Where results can be obtained with these basic instruments, it is usually a quick and simple process. More complex Doppler devices produce images of regions of blood flow or examine flow in detail at specific sites. For both these techniques, they are often linked with real-time B-scan instruments.

The coming together of ultrasonic Doppler and imaging technology has increased the power of diagnostic ultrasound. Blood flow can be measured quantitatively in well-defined vessels, or information on flow and its adjacent anatomy may be revealed.

As with pulse-echo imaging, knowledge of Doppler techniques can first be obtained by the study of simplified situations and then expanded by experience of applications and further study. Much of the knowledge acquired in the study of imaging is of direct value in Doppler applications. For example, the characteristics of ultrasound beams, the propagation of ultrasound in tissue, and the design of transducers are all relevant.

The Doppler effect

The Doppler effect is a change in the observed frequency of a wave because of motion of the source or the observer. By noting this change in frequency, the observer can deduce that movement is occurring.

An understanding of the Doppler effect can be obtained by considering the situation shown in Figure 18.8a. At first, let both the source and the observer be at rest and let the source emit a sound wave of frequency f_0. In this situation, the observer will detect a frequency of f_0. Now let the observer move toward the source with speed, u. Because of his motion, the observer meets each wave crest more quickly than he would if he were at rest. In other words, the observer detects more complete wavelengths per second; an increase in

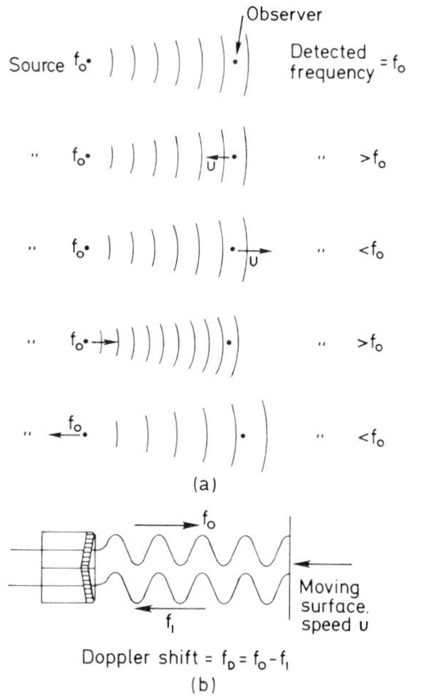

Fig. 18.8 (a) A Doppler shift in the frequency of the detected ultrasound caused by the motion of either the source or the observer. (b) A Doppler shift caused by reflection of the detected ultrasound from a moving target.

frequency. Similarly, when the observer is moving away from the source, each wavelength takes longer to pass than it would if he were at rest, so he detects fewer complete wavelengths per second; a decrease in frequency.

In the opposite situation, where the observer is at rest and the source is moving, a Doppler effect can also be observed (Fig. 18.8a). For instance, if the source is moving in the same direction as the propagated wave, it follows the wave crest that it has just emitted and so causes a reduction of the wavelength. The observer then detects an increased frequency corresponding to this reduction in wavelength. Similarly, when the source moves in the opposite direction from that of wave travel, a stretching of the wavelength occurs; a decrease in frequency.

Some clarification of nomenclature is advisable at this point. The term 'speed' is used when talking of the motion of an object without specifying its direction. To specify the 'velocity' of an object, we should give both the speed and the direction. In practice, there is usually no strict adherence to this terminology. If a velocity, u, is specified in a particular direction, then the component of that velocity, at an angle θ, is given by $u\cos\theta$ (Fig. 18.9). This latter quantity is used when an ultrasound beam intercepts a blood vessel at an angle to calculate the blood velocity component along the beam.

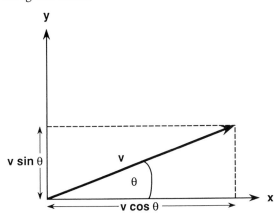

Velocity component in direction x = v_x = v cos θ
Velocity component in direction y = v_y = v sin θ

Fig. 18.9 A velocity in the direction of v can be regarded as being caused by two component velocities in the directions X and Y.

Doppler effect in diagnosis

The above examples illustrate how motion can change frequency. A simple way in which the Doppler effect is employed in diagnostic instruments is illustrated in Figure 18.8b. In this situation, a source and detector are placed at rest, side by side, and the source emits continuous wave ultrasound of frequency f_0. If this sound is reflected back to the detector by a surface moving at speed u toward the source, it will be found, on detection, to have a shift in frequency caused by the Doppler effect.

This Doppler effect can be considered as the combined result of the surface's meeting the waves more quickly than it would if it were at rest, and of its reducing the wavelength of the reflected waves by following after them. During the reflection process, the moving surface continually alters the phase of the reflected wave relative to the incident wave. This continual altering of the phase of the wave means that the wave cycle is completed more quickly and, therefore, that the frequency is increased. If the reflector is moving away from the source and detector, the changing phase on reflection results in a decrease in frequency.

In a diagnostic Doppler instrument, the source and detector may be respectively, a transmitting element and a receiving element, positioned next to each other in a hand-held probe. The reflecting surface is a moving interface within the body. Reflected ultrasound is, of course, also detected from static surfaces within the body, but it has not undergone a change in frequency. After the reflected ultrasound is received, the electronic system is able to distinguish between non-Doppler-shifted ultrasound from static surfaces and Doppler-shifted ultrasound from moving ones.

By noting whether the reflected ultrasound has a higher or lower frequency than that transmitted, one can tell the direction of motion of the reflecting surface, or, at least, the direction of the component of its velocity along the ultrasonic beam.

NUMERIC VALUES OF DOPPLER SHIFTS

If an ultrasonic wave of frequency f_0 is reflected by a surface moving with speed u in the same direction as the wave, it is easy to show that the change in frequency, that is, the Doppler shift f_D, is given approximately by

$$f_0 \text{ (transmitted)} - f_1 \text{ (reflected)} = f_D = f_0 \left(\frac{2u}{c}\right)$$

where c is, again, the speed of sound.

If the line of movement of the reflecting surface is at an angle, θ, to the transducer beam, then the Doppler shift, f_D, is given by

$$f_D = f_0 \left(\frac{2u \cos \theta}{c}\right)$$

where $u \cos \theta$ is merely the component of the velocity of the surface along the ultrasonic beam. Inserting numeric values into this formula produces an interesting result. Consider a typical case of blood flow in a superficial vessel:

Transmitted frequency, f_0, = 10 MHz
Velocity of sound in soft tissue, c, = 1540 m/s
Velocity of blood movement, u, = 30 cm/s

Angle between ultrasonic beam and direction of flow, θ, = 45°
The change in frequency on reflection is

$$\begin{aligned}
f_D &= f_0 \left(\frac{2u \cos \theta}{c}\right) \\
&= 10 \times 10^6 \times \left(\frac{2 \times 30}{154\,000}\right) \times \cos 45°
\end{aligned}$$

so,

$$f_D = 3896 \times \cos 45°$$

$$\cos 45° = 0.0707$$

Therefore,

$$f_D = 2754 \text{ Hz} = 2.75 \text{ kHz}$$

Consider a typical case of fetal heart detection:

$$\begin{aligned}
f_0 &= 2 \text{ MHz} \\
c &= 1540 \text{ m/s} \\
u &= 20 \text{ cm/s} \\
\theta &= 0° \\
f_D &= 2 \times 10^6 \times \left(\frac{2 \times 20}{154\,000}\right) \times \cos 0° \\
\cos 0° &= 1
\end{aligned}$$

Therefore

$$f_D = 519 \text{ Hz}$$

The shift in frequency in both of these examples turns out to be in the audible range. In an ultrasonic Doppler instrument, the electronics is designed to extract the shift in frequency, f_D. This is done by comparing the transmitted frequency and the reflected frequency, and then feeding a signal of frequency f_D to some output device. It is a happy coincidence that the numeric values of quantities such as frequency and velocity result in the shift in frequency, f_D, being in the audible range. Simple output devices such as a loudspeaker or earphones can thus be employed.

DETECTION OF DOPPLER-FREQUENCY SHIFT

Continuous-wave ultrasound (CW)

We have said that a continuous ultrasonic wave reflected from a moving surface experiences a continual changing of phase which results in a small shift in frequency, and that electronics can be designed to detect this shift and so produce a signal giving information about the motion. Recalling the discussion of wave phenomena in Chapter 5, we are able to appreciate how this frequency shift may be extracted, and how the characteristics of the sound emitted by the loudspeaker of a Doppler instrument arise.

Consider the simplest case of the transmitter and receiver crystals of a Doppler unit pointing at one surface moving toward them at a fixed velocity. Let the transmitter circuitry produce an electric excitation voltage of frequency f_0 and, hence, a corresponding ultrasonic wave of frequency f_0, and let the received Doppler-shifted ultrasound be of frequency f_1. The Doppler instrument converts the received ultrasonic wave into a corresponding electric signal of frequency f_1 and adds to it a reference signal of frequency f_0 from the transmitter circuitry. Therefore, two electric signals of neighbouring frequencies are being added together. In a manner analogous to the addition of two waves of neighbouring frequency, beats are formed as a result of electric signals becoming slowly in- and out-of-phase (Fig. 5.3, Fig. 18.10a). Just as in the case of ultrasonic waves, the beat frequency is

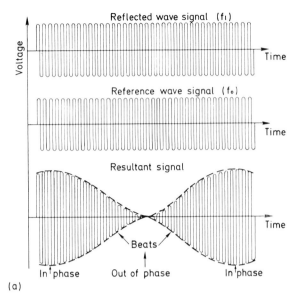

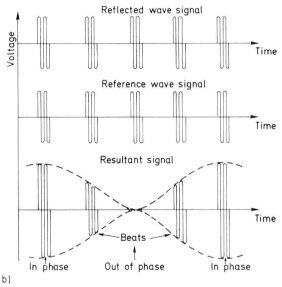

(a)

(b)

Fig. 18.10 (a) Mixing of two continuous signals of neighbouring frequencies with the production of a beat frequency, (b) mixing of two pulsed signals to produce a beat frequency.

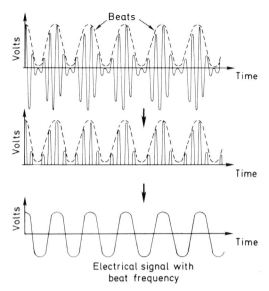

Fig. 18.11 A simple method of extracting the beat frequency.

From this example, it can be seen that a single surface moving at a fixed speed produces a single frequency at the output. In practice, there are many reflecting surfaces, and their speeds vary. The result is a complex signal at the output because of the addition of frequency components contributed by each moving surface. This complex output can be interpreted qualitatively by listening. High-pitched components in the audible sound are related to high speeds, whereas low-pitched components correspond to low speeds. Strong signals, that is, of high audible volume, correspond to strong echoes that have received a Doppler shift.

One should note that in Figure 18.10, for ease of graphic illustration, the frequencies f_0 and f_1 are only about 30 times the beat frequency, f_D; therefore, approximately 30 cycles of the higher-frequency signals are seen to contribute to one beat cycle. In practice, f_0 and f_1 are in the megahertz range, and f_D is in the kilohertz range, resulting in a few thousand high-frequency cycles per beat cycle.

Pulsed-wave ultrasound (PW)

If the transmitter excitation signals are applied to the crystal as cyclic pulses at regular intervals, then corresponding pulses of ultrasound are transmitted. For example, 10 cycle pulses can be

equal to the difference of the two frequencies ($f_0 - f_1$). Because the beat frequency, therefore, has the same value as the Doppler shift, it is extracted, and a signal with the Doppler shift frequency, $f_D = f_0 - f_1$, is obtained. In one approach to obtain a signal of this frequency, the electronics removes the negative parts of the resultant pulsating waveform and smoothes the positive parts (Fig. 18.11).

transmitted, separated by non-transmission intervals of a duration 20 times that of each pulse. Regularly spaced echoes are then received back from a reflector. If the reflector is moving, the changing of the phase in the pulsed-echo signal results in a frequency change. Just as the continuous-wave, Doppler-shifted signals produce beats when added to the reference oscillator signal, the pulsed echoes do the same (Fig. 18.10b). It can be seen from this figure that the pulse echoes are equivalent to samples of a continuous-wave signal and that with them it is possible to produce a signal at the beat frequency i.e. at the Doppler-shift frequency.

The pay-off for this added complexity is that since pulsed ultrasound is employed, the range of the moving target may be measured from the echo-return time, as well as from its speed from the Doppler shift. Note that in the above technique the range can be measured from one echo signal, whereas the Doppler shift determination requires the formation of a beat pattern with around 50 echoes in it.

As for the CW case, a group of reflectors moving with different velocities produces a range of Doppler-shift frequency components in the output signal.

Colour flow imaging

A pulsed beam of ultrasound is also employed in colour flow imaging to generate echo signals from regions of blood flow within the body. A Doppler shift is derived exactly as for PW Doppler at a large number of sample volumes along the beam (Fig. 18.10b, Fig. 18.12). However to build up an image in real-time the beam cannot dwell long in each direction. Typically the beam dwells long enough in each direction to collect 8 echoes from each sample volume. Note that this is much fewer than for the PW case, so in colour flow a short portion of Doppler shift signal is produced for each sample volume from a few echoes. Processing techniques have been developed to extract the Doppler shift frequency from each short portion of signal. Note that as usual, velocity can only be obtained from frequency if the angle between the beam and the flow direction is known. The direction of flow in each sample is detected and the corresponding image pixel is colour coded, e.g. red or blue depending on whether flow is toward or away from the transducer (see end of chapter). In practice for each beam direction flow velocity is extracted virtually simultaneously from about 100 sample volumes. Echoes are added into the

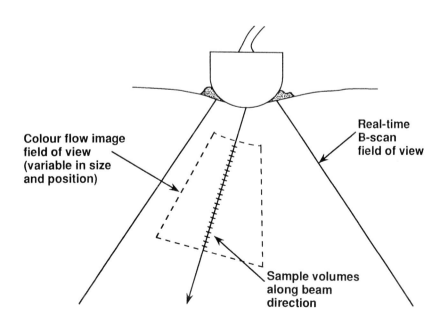

Fig. 18.12   Relation among sample volumes along scanning beam, colour flow image field of view and real-time B-scan field of view.

processing as soon as they are detected at each sample volume. This provides one line of velocity information for the colour flow image. The beam then moves on to collect echo data at the next line and so the image is built up.

A common way of processing each short portion of Doppler shift signal involves autocorrelation function processing (Ch. 6) to give an estimate of the Doppler shift frequency (velocity). These calculations are performed very quickly as the echoes are received from each sample volume. The autocorrelation function of a Doppler signal is related to its frequency spectrum and hence the Doppler shift frequency can be extracted from it. The more common Fourier frequency analysis is not used since the calculations would take too long and frequency calculated from a short portion of Doppler signal would be inaccurate.

The velocity estimate derived using a few echo signals and the autocorrelation technique is a cruder measure than that obtained by the conventional PW method using a large number of echoes, but it is obtained much more quickly. The estimate of velocity can be improved by using more echoes from each sample volume but this requires the line density, the frame rate or the field of view to be reduced. Using more echo signals also allows very low velocities to be estimated from slow changing (low frequency) Doppler shift signals.

In a blood vessel there may well be a range of cell velocities present within a sample volume. However the autocorrelation technique applied to a short portion of Doppler signal cannot produce the full spectrum of velocities; instead the average velocity and a statistical measure of the spread of velocities (the variance) are derived.

Detection of Doppler shifts in practice

A number of factors that influence detection in practice are worth considering. The importance of some factors is still being evaluated as the theory of Doppler units is developed further. These include, for example, the effect on the signal of scatterers moving in and out of the beam or the total effect of combining signals from many targets. Even though the theory of Doppler units, PW devices in particular, has still to be fully worked out, practical instruments are available

that have been experimentally shown to be good detectors of blood flow.

Blood-flow instruments must be extremely sensitive and capable of detecting weak signals from flowing blood in the presence of much stronger signals from static or pulsing tissues. The magnitude of the scattered signal from blood is typically 40 dB below that received from soft tissues. A 'wall effect' may be present when blood vessels are examined, resulting from the strong signal of the vessel wall masking the weaker signals from blood next to it. In many situations, although blood flow is obviously present in tissues, it is not detectable by present-day instruments. However, blood-flow signals may be detected even though the vessel is not clearly depicted; for instance, in the fetal brain or the renal artery of the neonate.

Pulsed-wave Doppler and colour-flow imaging instruments are limited in the upper blood velocity that they can measure. To produce the beat frequency from the detected echoes, one must have at least two sample echoes per beat-frequency cycle (Fig. 18.10b). In other words, the pulse-repetition frequency of the instrument must be at least twice the Doppler-shift frequency to be detected. The PRF is restricted by the time required to collect an echo from the target, however, and, hence, the maximum detectable Doppler shift is also restricted. Figure 18.13 illustrates how inadequate sampling of a signal means that it cannot be reproduced at a later time. This error in the production of the Doppler-shift signal is called 'aliasing'. It obviously gives an error in the measurement of velocity.

In practice, this means that the maximum target velocity, which can be measured, is limited by the PRF of the instrument. Recall the basic Doppler equation:

$$f_D = f_0 \ \frac{2u \cos \theta}{c}$$

i.e.

$$u = f_D \ \frac{c}{(2f_0 \cos \theta)}$$

put $u = u_{max}$ and $f_D = f_{D \ max} = \frac{PRF}{2}$

therefore,

$$u_{max} \quad = \frac{PRF}{2} \quad \frac{c}{(2f_0 \cos \theta)}$$

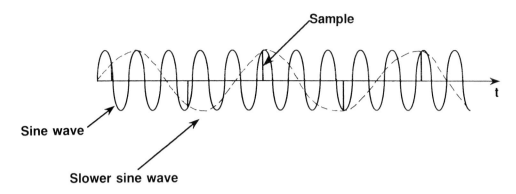

Fig. 18.13 Inadequate sampling of a signal (solid curve). Reconstructing the signal from the samples results in a lower-frequency signal being produced (dashed curve).

For example, for

$$f_0 = 5 \text{ MHz}$$
$$c = 1540 \text{ m/s}$$
$$\theta = 45° \text{ (cos } 45° = 0.707)$$
$$\text{PRF} = 5 \text{ kHz}$$

then

$$u_{max} = \frac{5 \times 10^3}{2} \quad \frac{1540}{2 \times 5 \times 10^6 \times 0.707}$$
$$= 54.5 \text{ cm/s}$$

This limitation is of most importance for deep blood vessels, which can be examined only at a low PRF and where pathology has resulted in high-speed blood flow (Table 18.1).

Table 18.1 Relationship between usable PRF and range. Maximum measurable velocity is calculated for a 5 MHz device and a beam-to-blood velocity angle of 45°

Range (cm)	Maximum PRF (kHz)	Maximum velocity (cm/s)
5	12	131
10	6	65
15	4	43
20	3	33

ANALYSIS OF DOPPLER SIGNALS

So far, we have concentrated on the synthesis of a complex Doppler signal by considering the addition of reflected or scattered signals from a number of moving targets. The most common example of this is the detection of blood flow where the Doppler signal is often heard as a complex sound consisting of very many contributions from moving red cells. The different frequencies, or notes in the audible signal, correspond to the different cell velocities.

It is possible to analyse the complex Doppler signal into its component frequencies and obtain more detailed information about the velocities of moving structures. Frequency analysis of signals was discussed in Chapter 6. By analysing consecutive portions of the Doppler signal a sonogram is produced showing how the velocities vary with time (Ch. 21). Analysers of value in blood-flow studies are considered along with other output devices later.

DETECTION OF DIRECTION OF MOVEMENT

We noted earlier that the frequency of reflected ultrasound is shifted upward or downward depending on whether the motion of the reflector is toward or away from the transducer. Thus, if 2 MHz ultrasound is reflected from an object travelling at 30 cm/s toward the transducer, it returns to the receiver with a frequency of 2.000 78 MHz, a shift of +0.000 78 MHz. If the object moves at 30 cm/s away from the transducer, the ultrasound returns with a frequency of 1.999 22 MHz, a shift of −0.000 78 MHz. Most Doppler instruments preserve this direction information. The very basic instruments record only the magnitude of the shift.

Directional Doppler instruments detect both the direction and speed of movement of the reflecting surface. Direction information is preserved electronically by separating the ultrasonic echo signals that are shifted up in frequency from those with a downward shift. The direction of flow for C W and P W Doppler units is detected using phase quadrature circuitry as described in Chapter 19. In colour flow imaging, the autocorrelation processing of quadrature signals (Ch. 6) derived from the Doppler signal provides directional information in addition to the mean velocity and the variance of the velocities.

SUMMARY

The basic ideas necessary for an understanding of Doppler blood-flow techniques were studied in this chapter. These techniques are the most powerful we have for obtaining information about blood flow.

1. Artery blood flow was seen to be caused by a pressure pulse generated by the heart. This pulse passes quickly along the arteries, giving an impulse to the blood cells.

2. In a brief discussion of haemodynamics, concepts of steady, pulsed, laminar, disturbed and turbulent flow were described.

3. The impedance of the supplied vascular bed was seen to have an important effect on the pulsatility of the flow waveform. This relationship is widely applied in diagnosis. End-diastolic flow was noted as being altered by high or low impedance at the arterioles.

4. The pressure drop at an orifice can be measured by application of a simple formula.

5. The Doppler effect on reflection from moving blood cells was studied and numerical values worked out.

6. Techniques for measuring the Doppler shift in CW, PW, and colour-flow imaging instruments were examined.

7. An important feature of Doppler instruments is the ability to detect direction of flow.

REFERENCES

Evans D H, McDicken W N, Skidmore R, Woodcock J P 1989 Doppler ultrasound: Physics, instrumentation and clinical applications. Wiley, Chichester, England
McDonald D A 1974 Blood flow in arteries. Edward Arnold, London

19. Basic Doppler instruments

In this chapter, basic continuous-wave (CW) and pulsed-wave (PW) instruments will be described. Subsequent chapters will contain descriptions of Doppler devices linked with real-time scanners, commonly known as 'duplex systems', and Doppler flow imaging instruments. A good understanding of the basic CW and PW instruments on their own will be very valuable when the larger systems are considered.

CONTINUOUS-WAVE DOPPLER INSTRUMENTS

The basic building blocks of a continuous-wave Doppler instrument are shown in Figure 19.1. The transducer generates and applies to one of its piezoelectric elements a continuously varying voltage of constant amplitude and of the required frequency, f_0. The applied voltage typically swings, as a sine wave, between +5 and −5 volts. Because the transmitting element is continually driven in the generation of a continuous wave of ultrasound, and because the excitation voltage would overload the receiver, a second element is used to detect the reflected ultrasound. This detected signal is amplified and mixed with part of the transmitter output to produce beats, as described in the previous chapter. The beat frequency, which is identical to the Doppler-shift frequency, is extracted in the demodulator and, after further amplification, is fed to an output device such as a loudspeaker. Since there are usually many moving surfaces, the Doppler signal is complex, being comprised of many frequency components. A filter is often placed before the audio amplifier to remove large low-frequency components such as those from slowly moving ves-

sel walls. This filter is called the 'wall-thump' filter. For example, in one blood-flow detector operating at 10 MHz, Doppler-shift frequencies below 200 Hz are removed by filtering. These low frequencies would detract from the operator's ability to hear clearly the higher frequencies from the blood corpuscles. The large amplitude of these

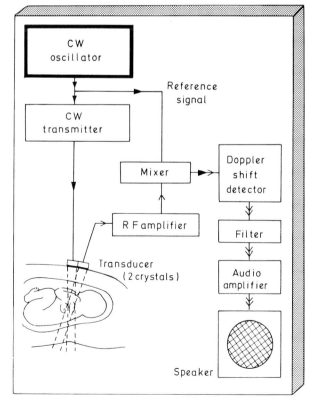

Fig. 19.1 Block diagram of a basic, continuous-wave (CW) Doppler instrument.

low-frequency signals would also upset the operation of subsequent processing circuitry. Fetal heart and blood flow instruments often filter out frequencies below 100 Hz.

We have already noted that basic CW Doppler instruments are small and inexpensive. The components in the block diagram can be reduced to dimensions that make the device about the size of a transistor radio. Doppler instruments are usually battery-powered; the batteries are either replaceable or rechargeable. Most instruments with rechargeable batteries should not be used on the patient while the charger is connected to the electricity supply.

Transducers in CW instruments

The shapes and configurations of piezoelectric-crystal or plastic elements in CW Doppler transducers vary considerably. Examples are illustrated in Figure 19.2a. Because the elements are required to generate or detect continuous-wave ultrasound efficiently, they have little or no damping material behind them; that is, they are air-backed. This makes them susceptible to

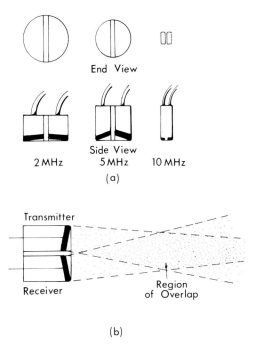

Fig. 19.2   The structure and simplified beam pattern of CW-Doppler transducers.

damage by misuse. With regard to impact or immersion in water, one should note that an electronic amplifier may be located close to the transducer, in the hand-held part of the instrument. There is often a plastic layer in front of the elements that provides protection and that acts, to some extent, as an acoustic matching layer between solid crystals and the soft tissue (see Ch. 27). As with pulsed transducers, the frequency of operation is related to the thickness of the elements. Thick elements are driven at their resonant frequency; thin ones can be made to operate over a wide range of frequencies. Beam shape depends on the frequency of the emitted ultrasound and the shape of the elements.

Ultrasonic beam shapes in CW techniques

It is the effective ultrasonic beam, which gives rise to detectable echoes, that is of interest in practice. This is particularly obvious in CW Doppler instruments in which the elements lie at an angle to one another such that the transmitted field and the zone of maximum receiving sensitivity overlap for a particular range (Fig. 19.2b). Any moving structure within this region of overlap contributes a component frequency to the total Doppler signal.

The receiving zone is usually assumed to have the same shape as the transmitting field for similarly shaped elements. The region of overlap clearly depends on the field and zone shapes and on their angle of orientation to each other. A type of crude focus can be considered to exist at the centre of the region of overlap. Because reception is the converse of transmission, Doppler beam shapes are often studied by making each element transmit and then measuring its intensity pattern in front of the transducer. Knowing the pattern from each element, one can deduce the shape of the region of overlap. In practice, the effective beam regions are rarely well known for CW Doppler transducers. For a fetal-heart detector operating at 2 MHz, the focal region is usually centred at about 10 cm from the transducer face. A 5 MHz blood-flow instrument might be focused at a distance of 2 or 3 cm from the transducer, and a 10 MHz device at a distance of 0.5 to 1 cm.

Basic CW Doppler instruments have ultrasonic output intensities (Isp) of from 5 to 500 mW/cm^2.

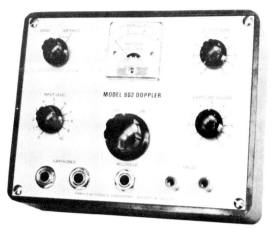

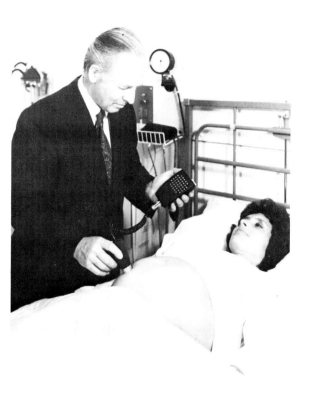

Fig. 19.3   A portable Doppler fetal-heart detector (courtesy of Sonicaid).

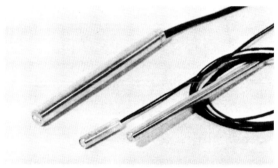

Fig. 19.4   A simple Doppler blood-flow detector (courtesy of Parks Electronics).

Well-designed fetal-heart detectors should have output intensities of less than 10 mW/cm^2. Further details of the output power, intensity, and pressure amplitude of Doppler units may be found in Chapter 8.

Examples of basic continuous-wave Doppler units are shown in Figures 19.3 and 19.4. It can be seen that they are usually small, simple instruments.

PULSED-WAVE DOPPLER INSTRUMENTS

A pulsed-wave Doppler instrument, sometimes called a range-gated Doppler, is illustrated in block form in Figure 19.5. The transmitter generates ultrasonic pulses, typically 5 cycles in length, at a high-repetition frequency. An instrument operating with 5 MHz ultrasonic pulses may have a PRF of 10 000 per second, i.e. 10 kHz. Because the highest velocity that the instrument can measure is directly proportional to its PRF, the

PRF is made as high as possible while still avoiding overlap among successive echo trains. Echo signals are produced as the transmitted pulse passes through reflecting interfaces and regions of scattering targets. This is exactly the same process as in A-scanning, so the echo train can be presented on a cathode-ray tube screen. After amplification, successive echo signals from a specific depth are selected by electronic gating, using a CRT display or a numeric depth indicator, and then mixed with a reference signal from the transmitter to produce the beats as described earlier. The beat frequency, that is, the Doppler-shift frequency, is again extracted in the demodulator. The quality of the output Doppler signal depends to a large extent on how well it is extracted without evidence of the original pulsed nature of the information or other electronic noise.

The Doppler shift signal is further amplified

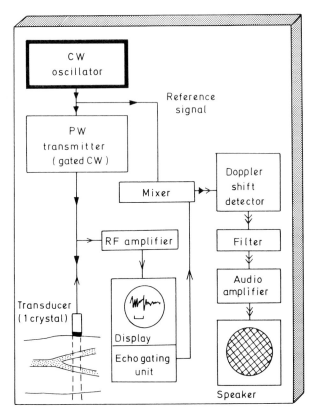

Fig. 19.5 Block diagram of a basic, pulsed-wave (PW) Doppler instrument.

and fed to an output device which, in a simple form, is a loudspeaker or earphones.

Pulsed Doppler devices can be used on their own by altering slowly the beam direction or the gated-range depth while listening to the output. Since the transducer is small, this is a flexible way of examining structures, especially the heart. Identification of vessels and chambers may be greatly assisted by combining the PW Doppler mode with an echo-imaging unit, a real-time B-scanner being most appropriate. The echo-imaging signals are usually generated separately from the Doppler-mode ones. It is possible, however, to use the echoes from the tissues received in the PW Doppler mode to make an echo image as well as to provide Doppler information. With the Doppler-beam direction fixed, the echo images are in the form of A-scan and M-scan recordings which can be related to the Doppler information. In Chapter 20, it will be seen that it is possible to sweep the beam from the Doppler transducer to produce both Doppler-flow and echo images. When the Doppler-probe echoes are used to make echo images, the axial resolution is slightly poorer than in conventional M-scan or real-time B-scan images, because the transmitted Doppler pulses are longer than ideal for imaging.

Transducers in PW instruments

Since the ultrasound is pulsed in this mode, a single-element transducer is employed for transmission and reception. The transducers are similar and sometimes identical to those used in ultrasonic echo imaging. The latter case is often convenient, but is not ideal since PW Doppler probes can be less heavily damped than imaging ones, with a resultant increase in sensitivity.

Ultrasonic beam shapes in PW techniques

Single-element probes generate more symmetrical and more directional beam distributions than do those from dual-element transducers in CW units. When the electronic gate is set to select a signal from a specific range, reflectors within a volume, known as the sample volume, contribute to the signal. The shape and size of the sample volume are determined by a number of factors: the transmitted pulse length, the beam width, the gated-range length, and the characteristics of the electronics and transducer. The sample volume is often described as a tear drop in shape (Fig. 19.6).

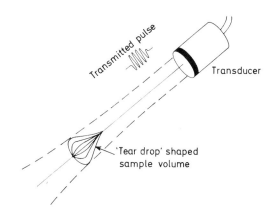

Fig. 19.6 A transducer for a PW-Doppler unit, and the sample volume shape from which signals are detected.

Studies of velocity profiles in blood vessels and quantitative blood-flow measurement require the shape of the sample volume to be taken into account. The length of the sample volume is given by

$$\text{Sample volume length} = c(tg + tp)/2$$

where tg is the gated-range length and tp is the ultrasonic pulse length. Sample volume lengths are usually altered by changing the gated-range length (tg). In a blood-flow unit for superficial vessels, the length may be as short as 1 mm, whereas in a transcranial device it can be 1 or 2 cm.

The ultrasonic output intensity of pulsed Doppler instruments varies considerably from unit to unit and should be checked at the time of purchase. For well designed units, the intensity (Ispta) should be less than 100 mW/cm^2. In a few instances, it may be justifiable to exceed this value (Ch. 8). There has been a tendency to increase the intensities of PW Doppler units for a number of reasons; for example, the use of a high PRF to measure high velocities or of increased power to compensate for the reduced sensitivity when echo-imaging transducers are employed.

DIRECTIONAL DOPPLER INSTRUMENTS

Additional circuitry in both CW and PW Doppler instruments results in the capacity to discriminate between flow toward and flow away from the transducer. Various techniques are exploited to achieve this end.

Filtering (single sideband detection)

From the basic physics of the Doppler effect, motion toward the transducer produces an increase in frequency while motion away gives a reduction. The Doppler shift is small, in the region of 1 part in 1000; for example, at 5 MHz, a velocity of 10 cm/s parallel to the beam produces a shift of 650 Hz. Specially selective filters can be designed to separate out the shifted frequencies from moving blood and the unshifted ones from static tissue. Such filters are difficult to make, so this technique for direction sensing is found in few Doppler units.

Heterodyne detection

In a simple, non-directional Doppler instrument, the beat frequency is obtained as the difference between the received signal frequency, f_1, and the reference signal frequency f_0; that is,

$$f_D = f_1 - f_0$$

If, however, the difference between the received signal frequency f_1 and a reference signal frequency such as $(f_0 - 5 \text{ kHz})$ is produced, then

$$f_D = f_1 - (f_0 - 5) = f_1 - f_0 + 5$$

So for $f_1 > f_0$ (flow toward transducer), f_D is above 5 kHz, and for $f_1 < f_0$ (flow away from transducer), f_D is below 5 kHz. In practice, when this type of signal mixing technique is used, the Doppler signal (f_D) is passed to a frequency-spectrum analyser in which forward flow signals are displayed in the range 5–15 kHz, and reverse flow in the range 5–0 kHz. The 5 kHz level is labelled the zero velocity baseline.

Phase quadrature detection

Circuits can be designed which can separate the forward and reverse flow signals through an electronic technique called phase quadrature processing (Ch. 6). Details of phase quadrature circuitry are appropriate in an electronics text, but not in this textbook. We should, however, be familiar with the types of output signals from this circuitry, since these are passed to spectrum analysers to generate sonograms. The term 'phase quadrature' arises from the fact that the received signal is passed along two parallel circuit paths; in one path, it is multiplied with a reference signal, while in the other it is multiplied with a second reference signal, which is 90° out of phase with that used in the other path. The two output signals after the mixing are called the 'phase-quadrature' signals (Fig. 19.7). After further electronic processing, the separated forward and reverse signals are obtained.

With this type of processing circuitry, we therefore get two pairs of signals, the quadrature pair and the forward-and reverse pair. Either pair or both may be supplied as outputs from a Doppler unit. Some spectrum analysers can accept either

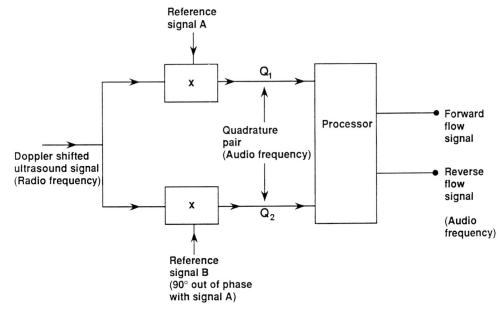

Fig. 19.7 The extraction of forward and reverse flow components from a Doppler signal.

pair for the generation of a sonogram, provided the appropriate switch is in the correct position: others may accept only one pair. Recently, the trend has been to simplify the situation by having only the forward-and-reverse pair from the Doppler units and designing the analysers accordingly. Reference to quadrature signals is still found in the literature.

From this brief discussion of direction-sensing techniques, it is apparent that the principle used in any instrument and also how well it performs the task should be ascertained. The phase-quadrature technique is the most commonly employed. The compatibility of the Doppler unit and a spectrum analyser should be checked. To avoid problems, one finds the best solution is to buy a combined Doppler and spectrum analyser. Even for this last course, the performance of the system in separating forward and reverse flow should be carefully checked, especially when they occur simultaneously.

OUTPUTS FOR BASIC DOPPLER INSTRUMENTS

Several output devices are used to present a signal to the investigator. Examples of these devices in their simplest form are loudspeakers and signal-level meters. Some processing circuitry may also be included, perhaps to produce a signal related to the average velocity of the blood cells at each instant. For more thorough analysis, the Doppler signal is passed to a spectrum analyser or computer. The properties of processing circuitry and more complex analytical techniques are discussed in Chapter 21.

Loudspeaker, stethoscope, earphones

The Doppler-shift frequencies produced by an ultrasonic instrument are in the audible range and can be dealt with directly by any of these listening devices. Although simple, these outputs make good use of the capacity of our hearing faculties to analyse sounds. Component frequencies can be related to moving reflectors, in order, for example, to separate the sounds of venous and arterial flow. With directional Doppler units, signals corresponding to forward flow can be fed to one side of a set of stereo earphones while those of reverse flow go to the other.

Plugging in the earphones or stethoscope usually cuts out the loudspeaker, permitting a searching procedure which does not alarm the patient.

Zero-crossing and average velocity outputs

These output signals are derived by circuits acting on the Doppler-shift signal and are used to obtain an indication of the average flow velocity. A zero-crossing circuit is so called because it generates its output by counting the number of times the Doppler signal crosses its own average value. The output may be in the form of a socket for passing signals to a chart recorder, a panel meter, an array of light-emitting diodes (LEDs), or a numerical display. These circuits are very prone to error, such as that caused by electronic noise.

Direction of flow indicator

Average velocity circuits may act on the forward- and reverse-flow signals to give an output signal for each. These signals are then presented on meters or on LED displays. An alternative is to add the forward and reverse flows to obtain the net flow and present that on one meter.

Maximum frequency follower

Of interest in blood-flow studies is the maximum velocity of flow of cells in a vessel at any instant. Circuitry has been designed to detect the instantaneous maximum Doppler-shift frequency. A related voltage is then fed to a chart recorder. This type of circuit is also prone to error.

Doppler signal outputs

Behind most instruments, sockets are provided where the forward-and-reverse pair of Doppler signals are available for passing to tape recorders, analysers, etc. A phase-quadrature pair may also be available.

Simple circuits providing outputs tend to require strong, clear Doppler signals to work well. They are best used as quick rough guides to the velocity of flow.

CONTROLS OF BASIC DOPPLER INSTRUMENTS

Basic Doppler units have few controls. Most controls are common to both PW and CW instruments. The controls include the following:

1. Volume

This merely controls the loudness of the output signal, but it is worth adjusting when weak flow is being searched for.

2. Low-frequency cut-off filter (Wall-thump filter)

Vessel wall sounds are loud and of low frequency. A filter is included in most instruments to remove them; that is, a high-pass filter is used to let through the blood signal. The frequency level above which signals are passed may be variable. If this is the case, its value should be carefully checked during use.

3. Noise reduction

Doppler units operate at high gain since blood is a weak scatterer of ultrasound. Electronic noise may therefore be evident when the gain is high to detect weak signals. Noise reduction techniques may be employed like Dolby techniques in tape recorders.

4. Gain

It may be possible to adjust the gain of the RF receiver to alter the sensitivity of the unit.

5. Automatic Gain Control (AGC)

It may be possible to switch to a mode where the unit senses the size of the Doppler signal and automatically adjusts the receiver gain to keep it within a specified range; strong signals are reduced and weak ones are amplified more. This technique is commonly employed in radios to reduce the need for constant manipulation of the gain as the signal level varies.

6. Time gain compensation (TGC)

With a pulsed-Doppler device, it is possible to relate the gain of the receiver to the time of the returned echo and, therefore, to compensate for the attenuation of tissue layers between the transducer and the blood vessel. The gated range may then be altered in position without manually altering the gain. This TGC technique is the same as in echo imaging. TGC controls such as initial attenuation and slope are not found on all pulsed units.

7. Gated-range width and position

In PW instruments, the gated range can usually be varied from a small value e.g. 2 mm, to a large one for straddling vessels, e.g. 2 cm. The position along the beam from which scattered sound from blood is to be accepted can also be adjusted, from close to the skin to the maximum working range of the equipment.

8. Calibration signals

The instrument may generate one or more internal signals of a well-defined frequency for superimposing on chart records or sonograms related to Doppler signals. It should be noted that these calibration signals normally do not allow for the beam-to-vessel angle, so frequency calibration is not easily converted to velocity.

These are the controls common to many Doppler instruments. Many variations are to be found among the products of different manufacturers. Additional controls usually have a secondary function, which should be clearly explained in the user's manual.

ACCESSORIES FOR BASIC DOPPLER INSTRUMENTS

A number of accessories may be linked to Doppler units to make them better suited to clinical application. The most common accessories, a spectrum analyser and a computer, are considered in Chapter 21, in which signal processing is examined. Other accessories include:

1. Circuitry for measuring fetal heart rate and plotting it on chart paper.

2. Telemetry equipment to allow the patient to move freely within a limited range. This has been developed for application in obstetrics.

3. Air-emboli detection circuitry for intra-operative or renal dialysis work.

4. Blood-pressure measurement equipment. A pressure cuff of a sphygmomanometer may be used with a Doppler unit to measure systolic and diastolic pressure.

5. A simple pulse-echo ultrasonic system which can detect the walls of the blood vessel may be linked with a Doppler device to measure blood flow quantitatively.

6. The Doppler transducer may be incorporated into a catheter or an endoscope for invasive work.

7. Recording devices, such as chart recorders, printers, memory scopes, audio-tape recorders, and digital discs, may be included in a total system.

8. A range of transducers of different size, shape, and frequency may be available for different studies. The frequency ranges from 2 to 10 MHz in some systems.

These variations and accessories emphasize the versatility of Doppler methods.

SUMMARY

The features of basic CW and PW Doppler instruments were described in detail, including for example, electronic systems, transducers, and beam shapes. Methods of detecting direction of flow were explained, in particular, heterodyne and phase-quadrature detection. Five outputs of Doppler devices were considered and also eight controls. Finally, it was noted that a variety of accessories exist for purposes such as heart-rate recording, telemetry, emboli detection, pressure measurement, and flow monitoring.

REFERENCES

Baker D W 1970 Pulsed ultrasonic Doppler blood-flow sensing. IEEE Trans Sonics Ultrasonics SU-17: 170–185
Coghlan B A, Taylor M G 1976 Directional Doppler techniques for detection of blood velocities. Ultrasound Med Biol 2: 181–188

Evans D H, Parton L 1981 The directional characteristics of some ultrasonic Doppler blood-flow probes. Ultrasound Med Biol 7: 51–62
Wells P N T 1969 A range-gated ultrasonic Doppler system. Med Biol Eng 7: 641–652

20. Doppler plus imaging

There are two ways in which Doppler and imaging techniques are combined. One employs a real-time B-scanner to locate the site at which blood flow is to be examined. A Doppler beam is then directed towards that site. This is known as a 'duplex' system. The second type of device creates an image from Doppler information; in other words, an image of regions of blood flow. This type of Doppler image is known as a 'colour-flow image' and is normally combined with a conventional real-time B-scan to display both structure and areas of flow.

Features of the instrumentation will be discussed in this chapter.

REAL-TIME B-SCAN PLUS DOPPLER (DUPLEX INSTRUMENTS)

A CW or PW Doppler mode can be combined with any real-time B-scanner in such a way that the Doppler beam may be directed to interrogate almost any location in the B-scan image (Fig. 20.1). The Doppler beam direction is indicated in the image by a line. In the PW case, a marker on the line shows the position of the sample volume. These systems are commonly known as duplex instruments since they incorporate two distinct modalities. The same transducer may be employed for both imaging and Doppler, or two separate ones may be linked together. Separate ones are probably better since Doppler transducers are less highly damped than those for imaging. In addition, blood vessels are imaged best when the ultrasound beam strikes the walls perpendicularly, whereas the prerequisite for a good blood-flow signal is that the beam should be directed at an angle to the vessel. These two conditions are most easily fulfilled with separate transducers. However, in some situations, limited access to the examination site may dictate the use of one transducer.

It would be very convenient if the imager and the Doppler instrument in a duplex system could be run simultaneously. In practice, it is then difficult to prevent ultrasonic pulses from one unit being picked up by the other. In theory, it is possible if the units operate at different frequencies. A satisfactory solution to this problem, employed by many manufacturers, is to spend most time in the Doppler mode and to refresh the image at, say, 1 second intervals. This allows the operator to check that the ultrasound beam is still intersecting the site of interest. Alternatively, the imaging mode is switched off completely once the Doppler beam direction has been fixed. It is often not clear what technique is utilized in a system when simultaneous imaging and Doppler is quoted in sales literature. Clarification is worthwhile, before a purchase is made, to ensure that the equipment will suit the proposed application.

The aliasing problem with pulsed Doppler at high velocity flow has resulted in many duplex systems being designed to cater for both PW and CW Doppler techniques. This requires that the Doppler transducer incorporate more than one element. The latter design feature is easily accomplished when array transducers are used for both real-time B-scanning and Doppler modes.

Another feature of duplex systems, resulting from the aliasing problem, is that the transmitted ultrasound frequency in the Doppler mode is lower than that for the imaging mode. The former is made low to reduce the likelihood of aliasing, while the latter is high to optimize the resolution

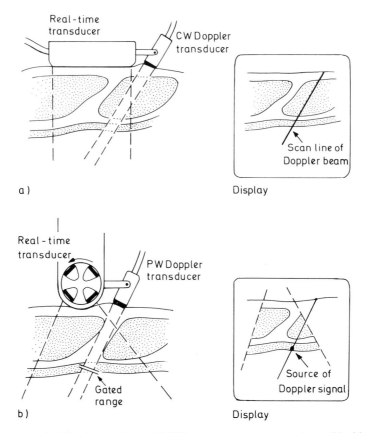

Fig. 20.1   Real-time B-scanner plus Doppler transducer: (**a**) With a continuous-wave transducer, (**b**) with a pulsed-wave transducer.

in the image. An example of different frequencies is 2 MHz for Doppler and 3.5 MHz for imaging in obstetric examinations.

Mechanical sector plus Doppler

A duplex system is easily made using a mechanical sector scanner and an independent Doppler unit (Fig. 20.2a). In addition to preventing the separate imaging transducer from transmitting ultrasound while the Doppler mode is in use, it is also necessary to stop it from moving, since the motion will be detected by off-axis ultrasound from the Doppler transducer.

An alternative approach is to use the same transducer for imaging and Doppler-flow detection (Fig. 20.2b). In cardiology, this type of system is advantageous since access to the heart is limited by lung and bone.

The attractions of this approach are the good quality results obtained with simple transducers at low cost. The disadvantages are the moving parts and the lower flexibility as compared to electronic arrays.

Linear and curved array plus Doppler

A duplex system may be based on a linear or curved array as illustrated in Figure 20.2c. With a linear or curved array, it is difficult to use the imaging transducer for Doppler measurement since many vessels are then interrogated at angles near 90°. To help overcome this problem, one can attach a Doppler probe to the end of the array at a fixed angle. A few systems have been constructed in which the angle of the Doppler beam is variable. In fact, the fixed-angle beam is less limiting than it looks for many purposes such as the study of blood flow in the fetus or superficial

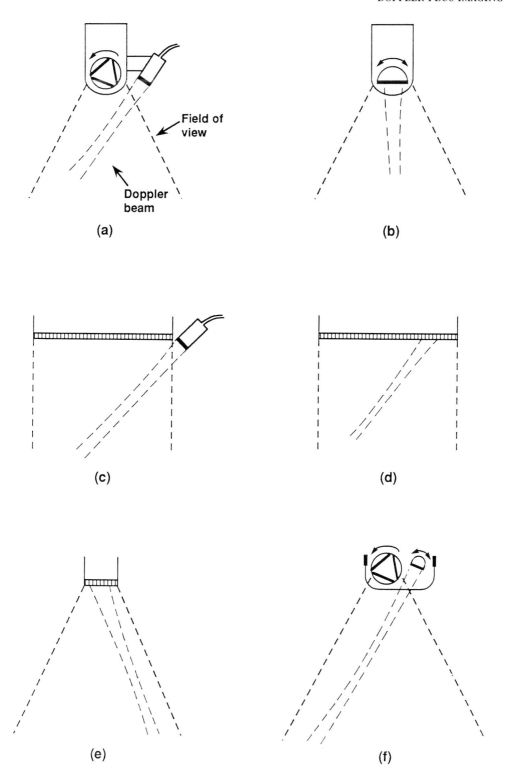

Fig. 20.2 Examples of duplex systems.

arteries. Another approach is to generate the Doppler beam from a few neighbouring elements in the array and to phase their excitation and reception such that the beam is at an angle to the imaging beams (Fig. 20.2d).

Phased array plus Doppler

Since most phased arrays with Doppler are aimed at cardiology, in which ultrasonic access to the heart is limited, it is rare for a separate Doppler transducer to be attached to the side of the array. The elements of the array are used to generate PW and CW Doppler beams which can be steered to the desired direction in the sector (Fig. 20.2e). The facility of switching easily between PW and CW is important in cardiac work where diseased states can give rise to high velocity jets of blood.

Small parts plus Doppler

A small-parts duplex system often takes the form of a mechanical scanner and a separate Doppler probe in a small oil-or water-bath which provides a stand-off layer between the ultrasonic units and the superficial structures being studied (Fig. 20.2f). Similar systems could be designed with linear, curved, or phased arrays. Typical ultrasonic frequencies are 5 MHz for Doppler and 7 or 10 MHz for imaging.

Water-bath plus Doppler

Duplex systems have been made comprising large water-baths and Doppler probes. An example of such a system is the Octoson plus PW Doppler (Ch. 17). The time taken to collect ultrasonic echoes from a blood vessel is longer with a water-bath scanner than with a contact scanner because of the increased path length through the water. The PRF of the pulsed Doppler is, therefore, usually reduced, resulting in aliasing at relatively low velocities.

M-SCAN PLUS DOPPLER

This combination is usually found as a feature of a real-time B-scan plus Doppler system for cardiology. When the pulsed-Doppler beam is aimed along a path through the tissues, signals are received from both moving blood and tissue boundaries such as heart walls. The Doppler instrument ignores the signals from the slow-moving walls and produces an output related to velocity of flow. However, it is possible to use the signals from the walls to make an M-scan in the normal way. The flow velocity sonogram and the M-scan are generated simultaneously. The axial resolution in the M-scan is poorer than normal since the pulses from the Doppler unit are longer than those from a conventional M-mode unit. Nonetheless, the quality is quite acceptable.

This combination of M-scan and Doppler is not particularly popular since the optimum beam direction for an M-scan is not often the same as that for a Doppler recording. For example, the optimum beam direction is between the ribs for an M-scan of the mitral valve, whereas flow through the valve is best examined from a subcostal view.

MANUAL COLOUR-FLOW IMAGING (MANUAL COLOUR-FLOW MAPPING)

Continuous- and pulsed-wave Doppler colour-flow imaging units, in which the transducer is moved by hand, have been available for a number of years. They are now being largely superseded by real-time colour-flow imaging instruments. The manual Doppler units have been designed primarily for peripheral vascular studies, whereas the real-time colour-flow instruments are applied throughout the body.

Another difference between these two approaches is that the transducer of a manual Doppler device is mounted on the arm of a gantry in a manner similar to a B-scanner, while the transducer assembly of a real-time Doppler unit is identical to that of a real-time imager. Indeed, mechanical scanners and all types of electronic arrays can be used to perform real-time Doppler and echo imaging simultaneously.

Manual CW Doppler flow-imaging instruments

Figure 20.3 illustrates the way in which CW instruments are used to produce images. The probe is mounted in a frame that permits it to move in

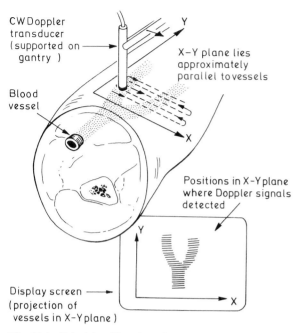

Fig. 20.3 Principle of imaging with a manual CW Doppler instrument.

we can locate the moving blood by measuring the echo-return time and the beam direction. This is the information required to produce an image of regions of tissue movement within the body.

One line of an image is created in the following manner. A pulsed beam of ultrasound is directed to intersect a blood vessel. Reflected and scattered ultrasound is detected at the transducer, as in A- and B-scanning. The pulse-repetition rate is high (e.g. 10 kHz), so signals are received from the structures at short, regular time intervals. By electronic gating, signals from a selected depth can be picked out and then tested for a Doppler shift which will tell if there is motion at that depth. This provides one spot in the image if motion is detected. To speed up the imaging process, the instrument examines simultaneously signals from several adjacent depth ranges (e.g. 32) for Doppler shifts. This gives a line of image information corresponding to the beam direction at that time. Points on this line are increased in brightness if they correspond to a depth range in which a Doppler signal is detected (Fig. 20.4). To produce a

a plane, and its position in this plane is measured by X and Y linear potentiometers. The plane of motion of the transducer is arranged to lie approximately parallel to the blood vessel, and the ultrasound beam intersects the vessel at an angle (e.g. around 45°) to obtain a distinct Doppler signal.

The transducer is moved manually to perform a raster-pattern scan in the X–Y plane. Its position is traced on the display by a dim spot. If no Doppler signal is received, the spot remains dim. When the beam intersects a vessel and picks up a Doppler signal, a related signal is stored in an electronic memory, and the spot brightness is increased. A directional Doppler unit eliminates some venous or collateral flow signals and helps to reduce noise caused by patient movement. Alternatively, colour-coding can be employed to present forward and reverse flow in different colours, commonly red and blue.

Manual PW Doppler flow-imaging instruments

We noted with pulsed-wave Doppler devices that, in addition to obtaining the Doppler shift signal,

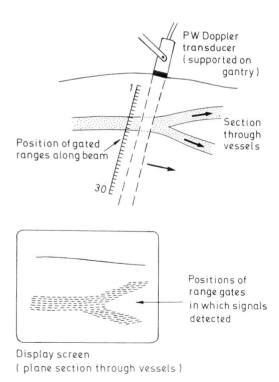

Fig. 20.4 Principle of imaging with a manual PW Doppler instrument.

picture, the operator sweeps the ultrasonic beam through a plane of scan, and related lines of bright spots are presented on the display at locations where blood flow is detected.

It is obvious that manual, pulsed-wave Doppler imaging is analogous to B-scanning. Sensitivity is governed by output power, gain, TGC, and frequency, as described in Chapter 7. A significant difference from echo imaging is that since a PW Doppler unit is being employed, the ultrasonic beam is required to interrogate each site until sufficient sample signals have been received to determine the beat frequencies, that is, the Doppler-shift frequencies (Ch. 18). In addition, if allowance is made for the variations in blood flow in the cardiac cycle, by ECG gating or by recording only the dominant systolic flow, it may take 2 or 3 minutes to complete an image.

REAL-TIME COLOUR-FLOW IMAGING (COLOUR-FLOW MAPPING)

We noted in the sections on PW Doppler that about 50 consecutive ultrasonic pulses are usually transmitted in each beam direction to determine the velocities of blood in sample volumes along that beam path. The beam cannot therefore be moved rapidly through the scan plane to generate real-time Doppler flow images. Before this rapid scanning could be achieved, means were required to extract at least an estimate of blood velocity at each site from a small number of ultrasonic echo pulses. The necessary breakthrough was made by manipulating the autocorrelation function of the

Doppler signals from blood to give an estimate of the mean velocity in each small sample volume along the beam (Ch. 18). Real-time colour-flow imaging is achieved in commercially available units by processing between 3 and 12 sets of echo signals from each sample volume. The direction of flow is also extracted by manipulating the autocorrelation function (Ch. 18). The direction is colour-coded in the image; for example, red for flow toward, and blue for flow away from the transducer (Plate 1).

All types of real-time scan transducer that can sweep the beam at the requisite speed are used for Doppler imaging; this includes mechanical scanners as well as phased and linear arrays. Invasive transducers, such as a 5 MHz transoesophageal phased array for heart studies, have also been made. The signals from the blood and tissues are passed along two paths through the electronic system (Fig. 20.5). In one path, the signals are used to generate a real-time B-scan image; in the other, they are subject to autocorrelation function processing to create a colour-flow image. An exclusion circuit in the autocorrelation path identifies large-amplitude signals as arising from tissue and prevents their processing as blood signals. The two images are then superimposed in the final display. In some machines the echo image signals are generated independently of the Doppler signal (Fig. 20.6).

The Doppler image is normally colour-coded, though other methods of presenting the velocity information as a two-dimensional image have been proposed. The latter types of image

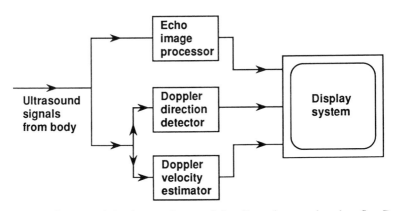

Fig. 20.5 Processing of ultrasound signals to produce a real-time B-scan image and a colour-flow Doppler image.

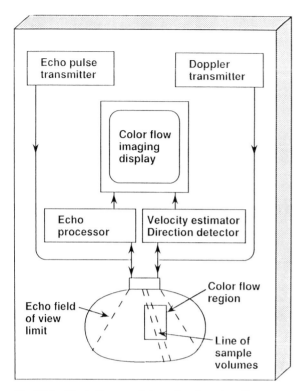

Fig. 20.6 Block diagram of the units of a colour-flow Doppler imaging system.

are in the form of a variety of computer graphics; for example, the rapid motion of dots may represent blood. In addition to basic colour-coding to show direction, colour hue or colour saturation can indicate the magnitude of the velocity approximately; for example, light red for high speed and dark red for low speed. Turbulence, assessed from the spread in detected velocities, may be presented as a different colour or as a mosaic of differently coloured dots (Plate 2).

Real-time Doppler images typically contain about 64 genuine lines of information and 128 gated sample volumes along each line. In practice, the frame rate varies from 5 to 40 frames per second, depending on the depth of penetration and the size of the field of view. The appearance of the image may be improved by inserting artificial lines or additional frames. If the field of view is reduced from, say, 90° to 30°, the line density in the Doppler image or the depth of penetration can be increased.

The image may be frozen at an arbitrary time or at a selected phase of the cardiac cycle, using an ECG signal to activate the freeze mode. Since alterations and events in the flow of blood occur rapidly, a most useful feature of a colour-flow system is the cine-loop store. Typically, in such a cine-loop, 64 consecutive colour-image frames are captured and may be replayed at various speeds to permit examination of the flow images.

M-mode scans and Doppler sonograms can be generated in correspondence to one or two beam directions in the real-time image and Doppler sample volume positions. PW and CW Doppler techniques provide more accurate information on blood velocities than do the estimates from autocorrelation processing; hence, the sonograms are still a valuable means of getting detailed information on velocities.

SUMMARY

Doppler techniques plus imaging are a very powerful combination for the study of blood flow. Such techiques are still developing rapidly.

1. Duplex systems, in which Doppler techniques were linked to all types of real-time B-scanner, were presented.

2. The M-mode can also be presented with a related sonogram.

3. Doppler colour-flow imaging was considered in detail. Both older manual and real-time Doppler imaging instruments were studied.

REFERENCES

Barber F E, Baker D W, Nation A W C, Strandness D E, Reid J M 1974 Ultrasonic duplex echo-Doppler scanner. IEEE Trans Biomed Eng BME-21: 109–113.
Fish P 1972 Visualizing blood flow vessels by ultrasound. In: Roberts V C (ed) Blood flow measurements. Sector Publishing, London
Kasai C, Namekawa K, Koyano A, Omoto R 1985 Real-time two-dimensional blood flow imaging using an autocorrelation technique. IEEE Trans Sonics Ultrasonics SU-32: 458–464
Omoto R (ed) 1987 Color atlas of real-time two-dimensional Doppler echocardiography, 2nd edn. Shindan-To-Chiryo, Tokyo
Reid J M, Spencer M P 1972 Ultrasonic Doppler technique for imaging blood vessels. Science 176: 1235–1236
Taylor K J W, Strandness D F (eds) 1990 Duplex Doppler ultrasound. Churchill Livingstone, New York

21. Processing of Doppler signals

Once a Doppler signal is being produced by an instrument, it is necessary to interpret it directly or to analyse it to obtain clinically relevant information. It is also often desirable to record the basic Doppler signal for future reference. This chapter describes analytic techniques employed for Doppler signals. As for analysis in most fields, it is not necessary to study all the details of the analyser, but it is important to interpret the final output accurately and to be aware of the limitations of the method. It is also essential to obtain good-quality signals prior to analysis in order to be able to detect the changes which occur when disease is present. The importance of this last point cannot be overemphasized.

PROCESSING CIRCUITRY

A Doppler blood-flow signal can be fed into electronic circuitry which produces an output suitable for a chart recorder. The trace on the chart paper is a feature of the Doppler signal, e.g. the maximum Doppler frequency. The circuitry used to produce this trace is usually called a maximum-frequency follower. Such a circuit should be able to follow the maximum frequency for forward and reverse flow. Another common circuit generates a trace of the average (mean) Doppler frequency.

A third circuit, the zero-crossing circuit, measures the number of times the oscillatory Doppler signal crosses its own mean amplitude level in a short time interval. The output of a zero-crossing circuit, the root mean square (RMS) frequency, has a value close to the mean frequency. RMS stands for the square root of the mean of the frequency components squared — if you meet this quantity you are safe to ignore it.

These circuits were developed mainly because they are a cheap way of drawing a trace related to blood flow. However, they are often very subject to error caused by factors such as noise in the Doppler signal, simultaneous forward and reverse flow, temporary loss of signal, and incorrect signal level. They have now largely been replaced by spectrum analysers, which provide a more accurate and detailed record of the velocities in the flowing blood.

The maximum, average, and RMS frequencies can be converted to the corresponding velocities of blood flow if the beam-to-vessel angle is known.

SPECTRUM ANALYSERS (FREQUENCY ANALYSERS)

When a Doppler sound is rapidly analysed into its frequency components, a pattern is produced, representing the velocities of the flowing red blood cells at each instant (Fig. 21.1). The Doppler signal is analysed in short time intervals, typically of 5 ms, and this produces an instantaneous frequency spectrum, i.e. an instantaneous velocity spectrum. When the consecutive velocity spectra are placed side by side, the sonogram is built up (Fig. 21.1). It is important to distinguish between the instantaneous velocity spectrum and the sonogram. The sonogram is of great importance in studies of blood flow since it shows how the velocities of the cells alter with time. Modern analysers are well-suited to medical application since they produce the sonogram in real-time during the clinical examination.

The spectrum analyser is an important part of most Doppler systems and performs the following functions:

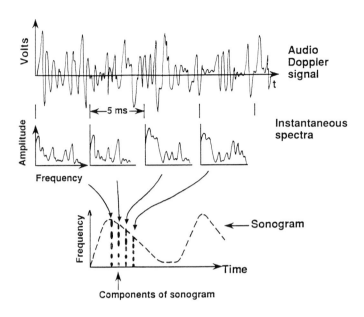

Fig. 21.1 The build-up of a sonogram by frequency-analysing successive portions of a Doppler signal.

1. Takes in the signal from the Doppler instrument. Analysers based on digital techniques digitize and store consecutive parts of the signal so that calculations can be performed on it.

2. Analyses the Doppler signal to form a sonogram.

3. Presents the sonogram on a display screen.

4. Performs calculations using the sonogram data.

5. Feeds the sonogram to a recording unit such as a multiformat imager or a fibre-optic recorder.

6. Outputs the sonogram data to a computer for further analysis.

These tasks are accomplished in different ways by different analysers, so it is important to identify clearly the features required of an analyser for the envisaged applications.

Filter bank analyser

With this type of analyser, the Doppler signal is fed simultaneously to a group of filters, typically around 20. Each filter is designed to pass a particular range of frequency (for example, 2400–2600 Hz) and the group of filters might be arranged to cover a total range of 0–4000 Hz (Fig. 6.5). When a frequency component passes

through one of the filters, a mark is made on chart paper at a position corresponding to the range of frequency passed by that filter. In this way, the components passing through the bank of filters create a sonogram.

A limitation of this approach to frequency analysis is the large number of filters required for the frequency ranges encountered in blood-flow studies. Resolution in frequency of 200 Hz for a range of 15 kHz (10 kHz for forward flow, 5 kHz for slower reverse flow) needs a bank of about 75 filters. This is expensive, and, as a result, this type of analyser has now largely been replaced by devices based on computer technology.

Digital spectrum analysers

Microcomputers, digital memory, and specialized circuitry for performing rapid calculations, as used in scan converters for storing images, are also components used in modern spectrum analysers. As for scan converters, it is not necessary for the user to know the details of their structure, but he or she should be familiar with their different modes of operation and the facilities they offer to get the most out of them. Names such as DFT (discrete Fourier transform) and FFT (fast Fourier transform) are given to digital analysers. As far as the user is concerned, they are all the same, and there is no need to be concerned with the different mathematical processing in these units.

With a digital spectrum analyser, the Doppler signal is fed in, and successive portions of it are digitized and analysed into frequency components by the computational circuitry (Fig. 6.6). The length of each portion is typically in the range 5–10 ms. Although the analysis is an ongoing process, the total duration of the signal analysed and stored at any time is usually around 3 seconds. Longer sonograms are either fed to a fibre-optic chart recorder or to a digital store of large capacity, perhaps a floppy or hard digital disc.

The sonogram generated by a digital spectrum analyser is similar in many ways to a grey-shade image from a scanner. It is presented in a two-dimensional array of pixels, and the shade of grey at each pixel is a measure of the power of the frequency component at that pixel (Fig. 21.2). Indeed, one of the most profitable ways of interpreting a sonogram is to regard it as a type of diagnostic image of the flow pattern in a blood vessel, rather than to try to relate it to the details of the haemodynamics. In a basic sonogram, the horizontal length of each pixel is equal to the duration of the portion of the signal analysed. The vertical length of each pixel is typically one-hundredth of the total frequency range selected. To make the sonogram appear smoother, the manufacturer ofter inserts additional pixels into the display, their shade of grey being an average derived from surrounding pixels. This is essentially a cosmetic operation.

From Figure 21.1, it can be seen that the temporal resolution in a sonogram, that is, the smallest discernible time interval, is equal to the lengths of the portions of the analysed signal, 5–10 ms. The frequency (velocity) axis of the sonogram is usually divided into about 100 parts, so, for a selected total frequency range of 10 kHz, each part represents a small range of 100 Hz, which is therefore the frequency resolution of the sonogram. The power or magnitude, of the frequency component at any point in the sonogram is related to the shade of grey at that pixel. Shades of grey are not always as well presented as they should be in sonograms, so it is not always possible to observe the strength of a frequency component at a point in a sonogram. In addition, averaging is necessary to reduce noise in the sonogram before power at a pixel can be estimated.

The term 'time compression is occasionally encountered in discussions of analysers. When a

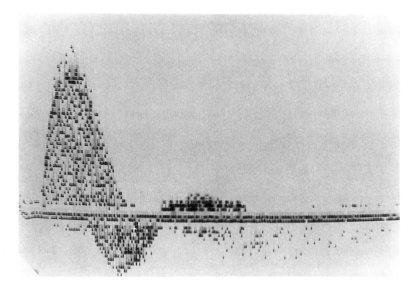

Fig. 21.2 A sonogram as a two-dimensional array of pixels, each with an allocated shade of grey.

portion of Doppler signal is digitized and stored in memory, it can be read out of the memory to the computer at a much faster rate than that at which it was stored. The signal is therefore compressed in time, and its component frequencies are increased, but it can still be analysed. The output display is labelled so that the original Doppler-shift frequencies can be noted. The advantage of this time-compression technique is that fast calculations can be carried out on the compressed signal. While these fast calculations are being carried out on one portion of the Doppler signal, the following portion of signal is being stored at the slow rate in a second memory store. This second portion is then analysed and the process is repeated for the whole duration of the Doppler signal.

Signal power versus frequency display

The analytic techniques described above generate sonograms, in other words, the instantaneous frequency components of the signal displayed versus time. Variation of a signal with time is a good way of presenting physiologic information. Occasionally, a second type of presentation of Doppler information is encountered. Here frequency is plotted along the horizontal axis, and the power of each frequency component is represented as a vertical line rising from the appropriate position on the horizontal axis (Fig. 21.3). If the Doppler signal is changing continually, this line pattern changes. A pattern at any particular moment of interest can be stored.

This sort of display of frequency components is

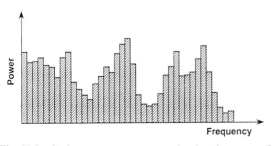

Fig. 21.3 An instantaneous spectrum showing the power of each frequency component.

not of much value in the study of blood flow. It has been used to show turbulence where the high-frequency content and spatial width of the spectrum are seen to be increased.

Desirable features of spectrum analysers

An analyser may be purchased as part of a complete system containing a Doppler unit, or as a separate device to be used with one or more independent Doppler instruments. In both cases, it is advisable to list the desired features prior to purchase.

1. Input Doppler signals

All spectrum analysers should be able to accept forward- and reverse-flow signals either from a Doppler unit or from a stereo tape recorder. It increases the analysers' flexibility if they can also handle two quadrature signals from a Doppler unit.

A third option of some value is the ability to accept two heterodyne signals. Since one heterodyne signal from a Doppler unit contains both forward- and reverse-flow information, the ability to accept two such signals means that flow signals from two independent Doppler units can be analysed and displayed simultaneously, and so two blood vessels can be examined at the same time. This third option is rarely available.

2. Frequency range

Since different ranges of Doppler-shift frequencies are obtained from different vessels, disease states, and input ultrasonic frequencies, it is important to be able to vary the displayed frequency range; for example, from 2 kHz for venous flow using a 2 MHz Doppler unit to 15 kHz for a stenosed artery with a 10 MHz Doppler unit.

Typically three quarters of the displayed frequency range will be used to show forward-flow spectra and the remaining quarter for reverse flow. It is most useful to be able to alter this allocation of frequency range to suit the flow velocities encountered in any particular problem. This is usually described as moving the baseline or offset frequency. It is also very desirable to be able to invert the displayed spectra at the flick of a switch. This flexibility is recommended since the range and direction of velocities in any particular case may not be known until the examination is underway.

The resolution along the vertical frequency axis should be about one-hundredth of the total range presented. A calibration scale should be clearly marked on the vertical axis of the sonogram.

3. Time range

The individual spectra in a sonogram should be produced rapidly so that changes in the flow pattern are accurately recorded. The time interval for analysis leading to each spectrum is around 5–10 ms, and this is therefore equal to the smallest time interval which can be resolved on the time axis.

The total length of a sonogram stored in a spectrum analyser is normally 3 or 4 seconds. The amount that is displayed at any one time is variable, and the operator can search, or scroll, through the whole sonogram presenting portions of it for detailed examination.

4. Display

A sonogram is best presented on a reasonably large TV screen. Black-and-white monitors appear to be very satisfactory for this purpose, the shade of grey at each point in the sonogram being related to the power of the frequency component at that point. However, colour monitors are sometimes used to emphasize the different powers of frequency components.

The display should contain at least 16 grey levels; this means that the sonogram should be stored in a memory of at least 4 bits' depth (Ch. 10). The duration of the displayed sonogram can be varied, usually to show one or more cardiac cycles.

Two independent stores are available in some analysers. This allows a stored sonogram from one site to be compared with that from another.

5. Measurement facilities

Having obtained a sonogram, one must often make measurements on it; for example, measurements of the start and stop times of a portion, or of the maximum velocity. Measurement is performed using cursors or a light pen as for images of anatomy. A light pen is generally considered to be the easiest to use, particularly if the envelope of the waveform is to be traced out by hand.

6. Calculation facilities

Since a modern analyser is, in effect, a digital computing device which stores the sonogram in memory, calculations can be made using data from the sonogram. For example, some calculations produce indices related to waveform shape or to the instantaneous mean and maximum velocity through the cardiac cycle. The computer programs to carry out these calculations are usually stored in separate memories (called PROMS and EPROMS) in the analyser. It may also be possible to display the normal and disease ranges of indices and to superimpose the newly calculated values on them.

It is important to check the types of calculation program offered with a spectrum analyser and to confirm that new ones can be inserted in the future.

7. Keyboard control

Analysers are best controlled by conventional computer keyboards. These allow entry of patient data, labelling of sonograms, and selection of calculation programs. They may also be the means of controlling the whole analyser. A helpful feature is the provision to call up instruction menus which aid the operator in setting up the unit. Keyboards with fewer keys are more easily incorporated into control panels and are therefore found in many instruments.

8. Signal outputs

It may be desired to perform calculations on the sonogram data in addition to those provided by the analyser. In this case, it is convenient to be able to transfer the data to an external computer. The ability to link the analyser easily to an external computer may prevent it from becoming obsolete.

To obtain hard copy of sonograms, one requires

outputs to a video multiformat camera, a fibreoptic recorder, a thermal printer, or a computer printer.

9. *Ease of use*

For the analysis to be carried out correctly, the signal fed to the internal circuitry should be neither too large nor too small. It should be possible to alter the Doppler signal size by adjusting one gain control on the analyser. Some analysers use automatic gain control to assist with this process, but it is likely that manual adjustment of the gain will also be necessary. If the signal is too large, a warning should be clearly shown to the operator.

A test signal containing some well-defined frequencies should be available for switching into the analyser to check that it is functioning properly.

ANALYSIS OF DOPPLER TRACES AND SONOGRAMS

The traces and sonograms derived from Doppler signals can be considered in two ways. The first approach is to regard them as types of images whose features are observed and related to disease states. The second is to make measurements on them to extract numeric indices related to their features.

Traces and sonograms as images

Treating the derived traces and sonograms as types of images may seem to be a simple-minded approach. In fact, it is probably our most powerful way of examining their content. This applies particularly to sonograms, and it emphasizes the need to present them on a large scale with good grey tones. The human brain and eye is particularly good at picking out characteristics from images. Studying the whole sonogram rather than extracted indices may also alert the user to artefacts in the recording. The main disadvantage of the 'image' approach, as opposed to the numeric index approach, is that it is more difficult to use statistical methods to relate the results to disease states. However, regarding a sonogram as an image makes more use of all of the available information. The sorts of features which have been found to be valuable are listed below. Examples of these features can be identified in the spectra presented in this text.

1. The shape, e.g. pulsatile or damped (Fig. 18.6)
2. Plug or parabolic flow pattern (Fig. 21.6 and Fig. 23.4, respectively)
3. Maximum velocity (frequency) at systole and diastole (Fig. 23.4).
4. Spectral broadening (Fig. 21.6).
5. Spikes caused by flow vortices in disturbed flow (Fig. 24.3).
6. Shoulder on the down slope of the systolic peak caused by a reflected pressure wave from a structure distal to the examination site (Fig. 18.6a).
7. Lack of diastolic flow (Fig. 18.6a).
8. Presence or lack of a reverse-flow component (Fig. 21.2)
9. Artefacts (Ch. 24).

Note that the vertical axis of a sonogram can be labelled in units of velocity only if the beam-to-vessel angle has been taken into account; otherwise the labelling is in units of frequency.

A distinct and easily heard Doppler signal results in a good quality sonogram image. Two sources of degradation are electronic and acoustic noise. These should be a problem only when the gain of the Doppler unit or analyser is very high for the detection of weak signals. If noise is present in a Doppler signal or sonogram, great care should be exercised in the interpretation of indices calculated automatically from such signals or sonograms. In this situation, it is very difficult to measure automatically waveform parameters such as the maximum velocity, and the indices are usually in error.

To acquire a good understanding of Doppler techniques, one should always attempt to relate the appearance of a sonogram to the flow pattern in the vessel.

Waveform indices

Waveform traces can be produced from the Doppler signal in a number of ways. It is most common to do this by first producing a sonogram and then performing computer manipulations on the sonogram data to obtain a waveform trace. Another approach, described above, is to feed the Doppler signal to circuitry which generates traces directly.

From these traces, indices can be calculated which characterize them. It is desirable that such calculations should be performed in real-time during the clinical examination. Flow waveform indices are not based on theory, but are merely derived from a combination of a few dominant features of the waveform. When an index is used, its definition should be carefully checked. Similarly, named indices in the literature are occasionally defined differently.

One example of a waveform trace is the variation of the maximum velocity with time (Fig. 21.4a). A light pen or a cursor is often employed to draw the maximum velocity trace on the displayed sonogram. This also stores maximum velocity values from points along the sonogram in the computer so that they are readily available for calculations. With some spectrum analysers, the internal microcomputer automatically detects and plots the maximum velocity at each instant.

It is not always easy to identify the maximum velocity in a sonogram, so waveforms and indices produced automatically should be checked. As a result of this difficulty, some analysers are designed to produce traces which are closely related to the maximum velocity trace; for example, a trace showing the upper velocity boundary below which the velocity components contain seven-eighths of the power of the Doppler signal. These difficulties highlight the ability of the human operator to trace patterns ignoring the noise and artefacts which seriously limit computers.

Another popular waveform to use is that of the mean velocity, i.e. the average velocity (Fig. 21.4b). This trace takes into account not only the values of velocity present, but also the number of blood cells moving with each velocity, so it is more representative of the flow rate of the blood at each instant. Indeed, the mean velocity is often used along with the vessel cross-sectional area to calculate blood flow rate. It should be noted that it is difficult to measure mean velocity accurately since it requires uniform insonation of the blood vessel to ensure that ultrasound is scattered from all cells.

Indices can be defined to try to characterize the shape of a waveform. Usually some measurements are made from the waveform and substituted into a formula to give the value of the index in a particular case. This value may contribute to the diagnosis of a disease state. To reduce errors from variations in different heart beats, one usually makes measurements over 5 to 10 cardiac cycles. The calculation of indices ignores most of the information in the sonogram, and the range of values for a disease state may overlap, to some extent, the values for the normal state. Efforts are still being made to define or identify the most suitable indices for each clinical problem.

In practice, the waveforms or sonograms we produce are often not of the blood velocity (u) versus time, but of the blood velocity component ($u\cos\theta$) along the ultrasound beam versus time.

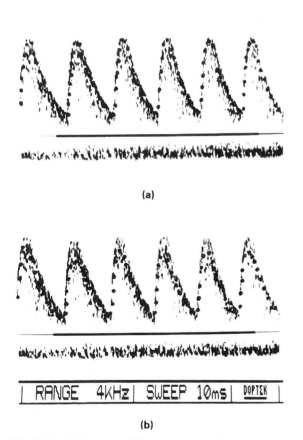

Fig. 21.4 (a) Sequence of dots superimposed on sonogram to show maximum velocity, (b) dots showing mean velocity.

In other words, they have not been corrected for beam angle. Therefore an index is often defined involving ratios of velocities. If we insert velocity components into such an index, the cosine factors appear on the top and bottom of the ratios and cancel out, so that the index is independent of beam angle.

The classification of disease by different indices is often very similar, since many of them give a measure of the oscillatory shape of the waveform. It is sometimes claimed that the measurement of indices or the more complex types of analysis described in the next section are a more sensitive way of classifying disease than looking at the sonogram, but this is debatable.

A number of the most commonly encountered indices will now be briefly discussed. These indices are usually calculated from measurements made on maximum-velocity waveforms since these are the easiest to obtain, but they can be used with data from any type of waveform, provided it is specified. It is particularly important to know the precise physiologic conditions under which each index can be expected to give reliable clinical results. For example, if possible, the normality of the cardiac output waveform should be checked, as should the dependence of the index on heart rate. Another important consideration is the minimum degree of disease which the index can be expected to detect. It is worth noting that the combined utilization of several indices will often improve the accuracy of the Doppler method.

1. A/B ratio

The A/B ratio is the ratio of the velocities at two specified times in the cardiac cycle (Fig. 21.5). The A/B ratio is commonly employed where there is no reverse flow, an example being carotid-artery flow. It has the disadvantage that as B gets smaller and approaches zero, the numeric value of A/B gets very large, rising to infinity.

2. (S−D)/S ratio

This index is known as the Pourcelot index or the resistance index (Fig. 21.5). If the resistance to flow is low in the vascular bed supplied by the artery, the index has a low value since there is high flow in diastole. Conversely, high resistance gives a high value (close to 1) for the index since the diastolic flow is low.

3. Pulsatility index

The pulsatility index (PI) is a measure of the oscillatory nature of the waveform; it is defined as follows:

$$PI = \frac{(\text{maximum velocity excursion})}{(\text{mean of the maximum velocity})}$$

PI is used in vessels where reverse flow may occur (Fig. 21.5). It has been widely employed to characterize waveforms from arteries in the lower limbs. For example, the value of PI at a site on the normal common femoral artery may be around 10, but it may drop to around 2 when proximal disease severely dampens the waveform.

It is important to note that if the heart rate is variable, the mean maximum velocity in each cycle will probably also vary. One way to avoid the resultant undesirable variation in PI is to calculate the mean velocity over a specified time from the start of systole, e.g. for the first 500 ms. The pulsatility index so calculated should be labelled accordingly, i.e. PI(500).

4. Damping Factor

The shape of a pulsed waveform is more damped in diseased vessels as the examination site is moved further downstream. The damping factor is the ratio of pulsatility indices measured at two sites, one on each side of a region of interest.

Damping factor = PI(proximal site) / PI(distal site)

For normal vessels, this index is less than 1 and increases to higher values with disease state. Values around 2 are observed for a large degree of damping. Some investigators prefer an index which decreases as disease increases, and they therefore use the inverse damping factor, which is the reciprocal of the above.

5. Spectral broadening

We have seen that a diagnostic CW field has one ultrasonic frequency, whereas a PW field has a

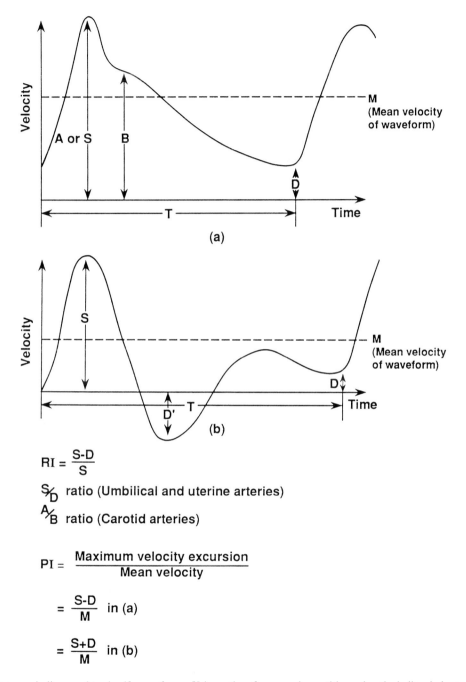

Fig. 21.5 Common indices used to classify waveforms. Using ratios of measured quantities makes the indices independent of beam-to-vessel angle.

range of frequencies called the bandwidth of the pulse (Ch. 5). If flowing blood is examined with a CW Doppler unit, the sonogram contains a range of frequencies at each instant, a range caused mainly by the spread of blood-cell velocities. If the same flowing blood is examined with a PW Doppler device, the sonogram will exhibit a broader range of frequencies. This arises since each frequency component of the pulse produces a range of Doppler frequencies just as the CW field did. Since the broadening of the sonogram at each instant is fundamentally related to the frequency range in the pulse, it is known as 'intrinsic spectral broadening'. The amount of broadening might typically be 10%, but it could be as high as 100% depending on the bandwidth of the pulse.

Another source of 'intrinsic spectral broadening' for both CW and PW beams results from blood cells crossing the beam and causing fluctuations in the received signal at the transducer. This is also known as 'transit-time broadening'. It can be seen from the above discussion that CW techniques suffer less from intrinsic spectral broadening than do PW techniques.

Disturbed flow and turbulence increase the range of velocities present in a vessel (Fig. 21.6). The value of the maximum velocity is then further

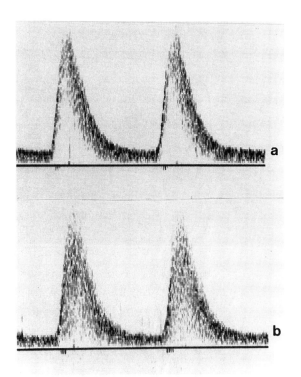

Fig. 21.6 (a) Plug-flow sonogram showing clear window under the depicted velocity components; (b) introduction of turbulence broadens the instantaneous spectra and therefore fills in the clear window. The maximum-velocity outline also becomes more spiked as a result of the presence of vortices.

removed from the mean velocity in the vessel than it would be for laminar flow. Several indices have been reported that characterize disturbed flow and turbulence based on this divergence of velocity values; for example:

Spectral broadening index (at systole) = maximum frequency/mean frequency

This divergence of maximum and mean velocity may be observed in the sonogram. However, the deduction of the presence of disturbed or turbulent flow should be made with caution, and only after one is familiar with the pattern for laminar flow for the particular instrument.

6. Transit time

The transit time of the pulse-pressure wave in travelling a length of artery can be measured by placing a Doppler probe at either end of it and recording the time at which pulsed flow occurs at each probe (Fig. 21.7a). If the length is also measured, the pulse-wave velocity (PWV) can be calculated.

Using the ECG and one Doppler unit, one can also measure the transit time. (Fig. 21.7b). The QRS complex of the ECG is taken to signify the time when the pulse pressure wave leaves the heart. Therefore, using the ECG and a Doppler unit, one can measure the time for the pulse to travel from the heart to the proximal artery site. A second time is then measured for the pulse to go from the heart to the distal site. Subtracting these two times gives the transit time, and, if the length of the artery is known, the PWV can be calculated.

For a normal aorta, the pulse-wave velocity (PWV) is typically around 5 m/s. The transit time along 0.5 m is then around 100 msec. The pulse-wave velocity is influenced by disease states of the artery wall and blood pressure.

Waveform analysis

More complex mathematical techniques can be employed to extract information from waveform traces. The underlying idea is still that the shape

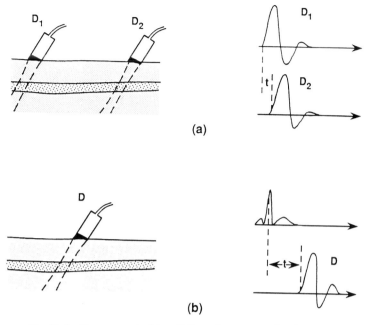

Fig. 21.7 Measurement of transit time of pressure pulse down artery.

of a waveform in a vessel is strongly influenced by the input waveform, the structure and elasticity of the vessel and related vascular bed, and the anatomy of the tissue supplied. It may therefore be possible to describe the waveform shape in terms of a few parameters which, in turn, may be related to a disease state. Much of this thinking is derived from electrical engineering, in which filters which influence voltage waveforms can be described in terms of a few parameters. It remains to be seen if these more complex ways of analysing waveforms will find widespread application. If a particular technique is found to be of value, it can be implemented on a computer for easy clinical use. The basic ideas will now be briefly described. (This section can be omitted in an initial study.)

1. Fourier analysis

We noted in Chapter 6 that Fourier analysis derives the frequency components of a waveform signal, and we have seen that this analysis is extensively applied to generate sonograms. Fourier analysis can also be applied to maximum- or mean-velocity waveforms. The more pulsatile a waveform, the more high-frequency components

are in its spectrum. This technique has not been extensively used to characterize waveforms.

2. Laplace transform analysis

In electrical engineering, a circuit may be used to shape a short pulsed signal. The mathematical expression which describes how the voltage of a signal varies with time is difficult to manipulate, so it is transformed into a related expression which is easier to use. The 'Laplace transform' is an example of such a transform.

Signal related to time, $V(t)$ is transformed to $H(S)$

where $H(S) = 1/(S^2 + 2\delta\omega_0 S + \omega_0^2)(S + \gamma)$

The details of the mathematics need not concern us. The important point to note is that the coefficients (ω_0, γ and δ, often called 'poles') are related to the features of the circuit, such as the resistance components, which determine the voltage waveform.

For a Doppler blood flow trace of maximum velocity versus time, $v(t)$, a Laplace transform can be derived similar to that above. The coefficients in the transform are now related to the features of the vascular bed which determine the shape of the velocity waveform, e.g. the resistance caused by stenosis.

Clinical studies have reported that ω_0, γ and δ, are related, respectively, to arterial stiffness, distal impedance, and proximal lumen size.

The computations involved in deriving the Laplace transform from the original waveform are fairly time-consuming and have not been performed in real-time.

3. Principal component analysis

In Chapter 6, we noted the converse of Fourier analysis, namely that any waveform can be constructed by adding sine and cosine waveforms in different proportions. This is a technique of very general application and is not particularly well-matched to constructing physiologic waveforms in an economic way. Most waveforms require several Fourier components to be known.

Blood-flow waveform traces, of maximum or mean velocity, corresponding to normal and disease states of a particular vessel usually have a limited range of shapes. It is possible to reconstruct these shapes using a few component waveforms, known as principal component waveforms, which have previously been determined as being suitable for that range of shapes. These components are pulsatile, but they are not sine and cosine waveforms. Principal components are added in different proportions to reconstruct a waveform of particular shape. The size of each principal component required is called the principal-component factor (PCF).

The use of principal-component analysis involves two stages:

1. The study of a representative population to determine the principal components. This stage may be avoided by getting results from another centre.

2. The determination of the size of each component (the PCF) required to produce a waveform which matches that from the patient. Since waveforms from healthy and disease states are different, they require different PCFs to describe them.

A good fit to a blood-velocity waveform can often be obtained using as few as two components. When only two components are required, the values of the two PCFs can be used as the coordinates of a point on an X–Y plot. If the technique is successful in separating normal and disease states, the points corresponding to them will be located in different regions of the X–Y plane.

This technique is more efficient and accurate than the Fourier method. It has been applied to fields such as carotid, aortic-iliac, and cerebral haemodynamics. The computation of PCFs for a waveform can be performed in real-time.

QUANTITATIVE FLOW MEASUREMENT

The blood supply by an artery to a region of the body is of fundamental importance, and, in theory, it is possible to measure it absolutely, say, in units of ml/s, by ultrasonic methods (Fig. 21.8). However, so far, it has been possible to do it with reasonable accuracy only for large arteries of simple structure, and even in this case the errors are usually around $\pm 20\%$.

Measurement of blood flow is based on the formula:

Instantaneous flow rate = cross-section × instantaneous average velocity

Averaging the flow rate over the cardiac cycle gives the average flow rate.

It is important to have a good appreciation of the sources of error, so that steps may be taken to minimize them. Although the list of errors presented later is rather daunting, it is worth remembering that Doppler techniques can measure pulsatile flow in test phantoms with an accuracy of 5–10%. Another point is that other non-invasive techniques which can measure blood flow usually have even poorer accuracy. We will now consider how to measure the quantities required for the above equation.

Measurement of average velocity from a sonogram

1. One way of measuring an instantaneous average velocity from a sonogram is to calculate

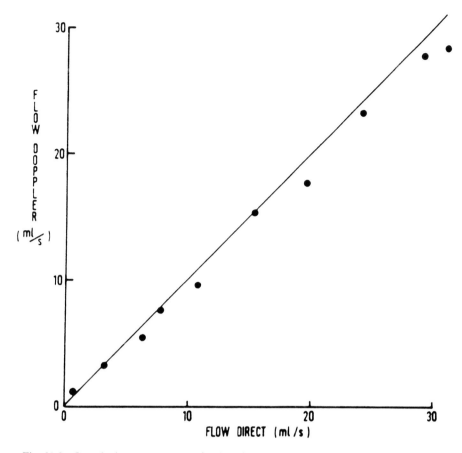

Fig. 21.8 Quantitative measurement of pulsed flow in a test-object using a Doppler unit.

the instantaneous average for the appropriate spectrum in the sonogram. The calculation of the average for a spectrum involves using both the power level of each velocity component in the spectrum as well as the velocity itself. The power level of each velocity component is a measure of the number of cells moving with that velocity, provided the blood vessel is uniformly irradiated. The latter is not easy to guarantee as a result of beam misalignment and distortion.

2. A second way to get a value for the instantaneous average velocity at any time is to measure the maximum velocity from a sonogram and assume a profile for the velocities across the vessel. It is usual to assume a simple profile corresponding to plug or parabolic flow. In the case of plug flow, all of the blood cells are travelling with the same velocity, so the instantaneous average velocity equals the maximum. For parabolic flow,

the instantaneous average velocity equals half of the maximum. Having obtained instantaneous average velocities at regular points along a sonogram, we calculate the average velocity over the cardiac cycle. Maximum velocity is fairly readily measured from a sonogram. Even if the ultrasound beam does not irradiate all of the blood cells, the maximum velocity may be measured if part of the beam passes through the centre of the vessel.

3. The third way of measuring the instantaneous average velocity is to use a multigated pulsed Doppler to measure the velocity profile across the vessel. Instantaneous average velocity is then calculated from the profile. A few systems have been marketed which perform these calculations.

The last two approaches assume that the flow pattern is symmetrical around the central axis of the vessel. This is reasonable if the vessel is not sharply curved or the measurement site is not just beyond a bifurcation. It has also been shown that the assumption of parabolic flow is good more often than might be expected, since variable and complex profiles are equivalent to parabolic flow when the average is taken over the cardiac cycle.

Measurement of beam-to-vessel angle

We have noted earlier that the velocities presented in a sonogram are, in fact, the component of the blood velocity along the ultrasound beam ($u \cos \theta$). To get the true velocity, we divide the sonogram values by $\cos \theta$. The angle θ therefore has to be measured from the ultrasonic image. If care is taken, this can be done with acceptable accuracy, provided the beam-to-vessel angle is less than 45°. Angle measurement can often be undertaken by manipulating an angle indicator line which is superimposed on an image of the blood vessel.

Measurement of vessel cross-section

The diameter of the vessel, d, at the measurement site is measured, and the cross section is given by the formula,

$$\text{Cross-sectional area} = \frac{\pi d^2}{4}$$

Error in the diameter measurement is particularly serious since the diameter is squared in the formula, doubling the error.

The cross-sectional area of a vessel can occasionally be measured directly from an image if a section perpendicular to the vessel axis is clearly depicted.

Sources of error in flow measurement

1. Average velocity

As was noted above, measurement of the true average velocity from a sonogram requires uniform insonation of the blood vessel. Tests with a flow phantom show that, provided the beam width is large enough to encompass the whole vessel and the vessel is clearly depicted, the average velocity can be measured with an error of less than ± 10%

for continuous flow. The error for pulsed flow is slightly larger and dependent on the pulse shape. A clearly imaged vessel indicates that the ultrasound beam has not been badly distorted. It is difficult to ensure uniform irradiation in practice, and the resultant error can be very large, perhaps greater than 50%.

The technique which relies on calculating the average velocity from the maximum velocity requires the ultrasound beam to be transmitted through the centre of the vessel. This can be arranged by observing the sonogram and listening to the pitch of the Doppler signal. The assumption of plug or parabolic flow is reasonable in some vessels; for example, plug flow in the ascending aorta and parabolic flow in the carotid. Texts on haemodynamics and the Doppler literature provide some guidance concerning the assumption of flow pattern in particular instances. Maximum velocity can often be measured with an error of less than ±5% from a sonogram. Flow phantom tests show that the average velocity can then be measured with an error of less than ±5% for continuous flow and ±10% for pulsed flow.

2. Beam-to-vessel angle

If a blood vessel is reasonably straight the beam-to-vessel angle can be determined to within 2 or 3°. Examples of such vessels are the common carotid and fetal aorta. Table 21.1 shows how a 3° error in angle at different beam-to-vessel angles affects the calculation of velocity. It is obvious that it is necessary to make a careful measurement of angle.

Table 21.1 Error in velocity at different beam angles for 3° error in angle measurement

Angle θ	$\cos \theta$	Velocity error (%)
0°	1.000	0.1
10°	0.985	1.1
20°	0.984	2.0
30°	0.866	3.1
40°	0.766	4.6
50°	0.602	6.4
60°	0.500	9.2
70°	0.342	14.3
80°	0.174	29.9

If a blood vessel is curved, it is difficult to measure the beam-to-vessel angle. An added complication is that the blood cells in the vessel cannot be guaranteed to be moving parallel to the vessel walls.

3. Cross-sectional area of vessel

Table 21.2 presents data showing the errors in cross section arising from errors in diameter measurement. It can be seen that these errors are always quite large and render the technique of doubtful value for small vessels. The importance of minimizing the error in diameter is evident.

Table 21.2 Error in area and, hence, flow for a 1 mm error in the measurement of the diameter for a range of vessel sizes.

Diameter (mm)	Area (mm^2)	Error in area (%)
2	3.14	75
5	19.60	36
10	78.50	19
15	176.50	13
20	314.00	10
25	490.00	10

A second source of error is the variation in cross section of pulsatile arteries. A change in area of 10% is typical of larger arteries. Allowance can be made for this error by noting the correct diameter for each point in the cardiac cycle from an M-mode trace. This makes the calculation of average flow rather laborious. A compromise solution is to use the cross section measured during systole when most of the flow occurs.

The assumption that a vessel is circular in cross section appears to be reasonable for arteries and introduces little error. The situation for veins should be checked with the ultrasonic scanner.

Another point to note is that the cross section and the velocity should be measured at exactly the same site.

4. Wall-thump filter

To reduce the effect of the very large echo signals from the artery wall relative to blood, one cus-tomarily filters out Doppler signals corresponding to low velocity. A contribution to the flow signal from slowly moving blood is also removed by this filter. Since the blood is moving slowly, this contribution should not be large. The need for the wall-thump filter is reduced if the incident beam is at an angle well removed from 90° to the wall due to a reduction in both the echo size and the component of the wall velocity along the ultrasound beam. The cut-off value of the filter can therefore be reduced in some instances.

5. Vessel motion

Overall vessel motion from respiration or fetal movement may cause the Doppler signal to be altered or lost altogether. The real-time scan image should permit this source of error to be avoided to a great extent.

6. Turbulence

We saw earlier that turbulence can be present in normal vessels and becomes very marked in diseased ones where the structure is altered. The effect of turbulence on a sonogram complicates the process of finding the average velocity of flow down the vessel. The seriousness of the problem ranges from negligible to completely inhibiting. Any sign of turbulence in a sonogram casts doubts on the validity of flow measurement.

7. Spectral broadening

Intrinsic spectral broadening effects do not appear to degrade flow measurement to any great extent if CW or long PW techniques are used. This may be concluded from the accuracy of measurements in test phantoms.

8. Spectral noise

The speckle noise in a sonogram introduces an error to the determination of the average velocity, but, again, the effect does not appear to be of major significance.

Development continues to reduce the error in the quantitative measurement of blood flow (Ch. 28).

PRESSURE-GRADIENT MEASUREMENT

The flow of blood through an orifice such as a diseased heart valve or a shunt between chambers takes the form of a jet in the receiving chamber. It turns out, somewhat surprisingly, that the maximum velocity of flow in the jet at any time gives a useful measure of the pressure drop (gradient) through the orifice at that time (Fig. 21.9). The pressure drop is calculated by inserting the maximum velocity into a simple equation (Ch. 18).

$$\text{Pressure drop} = p_1 - p_2 = 4v^2 \text{ (for } v \text{ in m/s,}$$
$$\text{and pressure drop in mmHg)}$$

where p_1 and p_2 are the pressures on either side of the orifice, and v is the maximum velocity in the jet. This is a simplified version of the Bernoulli equation. The above equation ignores the effect of viscosity and the acceleration and deceleration at the opening and closing of a valve. These exclu-

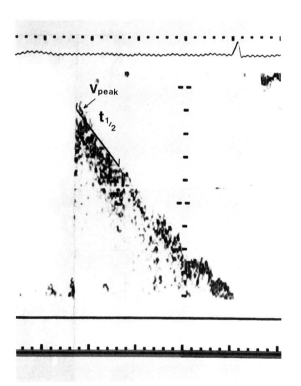

Fig. 21.9 Measurement of the peak velocity to permit calculation of the peak pressure gradient across a heart valve. The time needed for the maximum velocity to drop to $\frac{1}{\sqrt{2}}$ of the peak velocity is the pressure half-time (courtesy of Bloomfield P).

sions have been shown to be reasonable approximations. The pressure gradient obtained from the Doppler method is close to that from catheter measurements. On average, the Doppler result is lower than the catheter result by about 20%, but it still provides clinically useful information.

The time for the pressure gradient to drop from its peak value to half of it, the pressure half time, is of clinical interest. The pressure half time is the same as that taken for the maximum velocity to drop by a quarter from its peak value (Fig. 21.9).

The above equation is based on the simple model of flow through an orifice, as illustrated in Figure 18.7. Blood is considered to flow along well-defined streamlines through the orifice. In the chamber on the input side, the blood is moving slowly towards the orifice. As the streamlines converge through the orifice, the blood velocity is greatly increased to form a fast jet. The increased kinetic energy of the blood cells is a result of the high input pressure pushing them to the region of lower pressure beyond the orifice. The velocity of the blood on the input side is taken to be much lower than that in the jet and is ignored.

The above formula has been found to be valid for orifices down to a diameter of 8 mm, below which viscosity cannot be ignored. Valid use also requires that the maximum velocity not be measured in the sonogram near the start and finish of the flow. Considerable care should be taken to ensure that the angle between the direction of the jet and the ultrasound beam is accurately known, to provide the true maximum velocity. Remember that it is a three-dimensional problem. In practice, this is best done by directing the beam along the jet while listening for the highest pitched signal. When the beam-to-jet angle is 0 or 180°, the cosine has a magnitude of 1 and changes slowly with the angle, so reducing the error in velocity attributable to error in angle.

Pressure measurement is carried out by using both hand-held Doppler probes and combinations of real-time imagers and Doppler transducers. Since the velocities in jets are usually high, PW Doppler signals suffer from aliasing. This problem is overcome by switching to a CW or a high-PRF Doppler mode. The increased use of real-time colour-flow Doppler imaging should ease the problems of detecting and ascertaining the direction of blood-flow jets.

The approach described here for pressure measurement has been shown to be valid in many situations related to the heart. It may also be applicable in other areas.

SUMMARY

Considerable efforts are made to extract haemodynamic information from Doppler signals.

1. Spectrum analysers which produce instantaneous spectra and songrams are the main tools. Six functions of analysers were listed.

2. The desirable features of a spectrum analyser were considered to be acceptance of different types of signal, appropriate frequency and time ranges, large area display, measurement and calculation facilities, keyboard control, outputs to recorders and computers, and ease of use.

3. Sonograms can be regarded as images. Nine features of such images were listed.

4. Indices are often calculated from sonograms; in particular, from the maximum-velocity envelope. These indices are used to characterize the waveforms and to relate them to disease states. As examples, six indices were studied — A/B ratio, $(S–D)/S$ ratio (resistance index), PI index, damping factor, spectral broadening index, and transit time.

5. A few examples of more complex types of waveform analysis were given — Fourier analysis, Laplace transform, and principal component analysis. These types of analysis have still to be fully evaluated in clinical practice.

6. Quantitative blood flow was stated to be difficult, but possible. Most approaches require the measurement of average velocity, beam-to-vessel angle, and vessel cross-section. Eight sources of error were listed.

7. Pressure-gradient measurement was described.

REFERENCES

Evans D H, McDicken W N, Skidmore R, Woodcock J P 1989 Doppler ultrasound: Physics, instrumentation and clinical applications. Wiley, Chichester

Hoskins P R, Haddad N G, Johnstone F D, Chambers S E, McDicken W N 1989 The choice of index for umbilical artery Doppler waveforms. Ultrasound Med. Biol. 15: 107–111

Hoskins P R 1990 Measurement of arterial blood flow by Doppler ultrasound. Clin. Phys. Physiol. Meas. 11: 1–26

Hottinger C F, Meindl J D 1979 Blood flow measurement using the attenuation-compensated volume flowmeter. Ultrasonic Imaging 1: 1–15

Taylor K J W, Burns P N, Wells P N T 1988 Clinical applications of Doppler ultrasound. Raven Press, New York

22. Performance of Doppler instruments

In the previous four chapters the operation of Doppler instruments has been considered under idealized conditions. The question immediately arises, 'How well do the instruments perform in clinical use?' An understanding of the performance achieved by each type of instrument is important, since errors and limitations can be difficult to identify. Artefacts and techniques of usage will be discussed in subsequent chapters.

As with pulse-echo imaging instruments, the performance of Doppler units is closely related to the factors which contribute to their resolving power, that is, their ability to resolve values in space, time, velocity, and signal power.

CONTINUOUS-WAVE DOPPLER

CW Doppler resolution

The definitions of resolution for CW techniques also apply to PW techniques

1. Axial resolution

The axial resolution of a Doppler unit is the minimum separation of two moving reflectors lying one behind the other along the beam for which separate signals can be identified.

Since a CW Doppler unit emits an ultrasound beam and receives echoes continuously, any moving structure in the region of overlap of the transmit field and the reception zone will be detected. We cannot resolve the signals from structures at different positions on the transducer axis. The concept of axial resolution is not applicable to CW Doppler units.

2. Lateral resolution (azimuthal resolution, beam-width resolution)

The lateral resolution of a Doppler unit is the minimum separation of two moving reflectors lying in the direction across the beam for which separate signals can be identified.

As for echo-imaging techniques (Ch. 12), lateral resolution with a Doppler device is a measure of the ability of the instrument to separate the signals from structures that are placed side by side in a direction perpendicular to the beam axis (Fig. 22.1). Lateral resolution at each depth is obviously related to the width of the sensitive zone

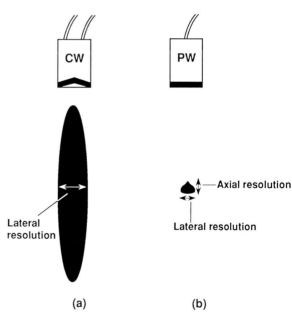

Fig. 22.1 Spatial resolution in CW and PW Doppler systems.

249

Table 22.1 Examples of resolution in Doppler technique

	Frequency (MHz)	Lateral resolution (mm)	Axial resolution (mm)
CW Doppler			
	2	10	——
	3	7	——
	5	4	——
	7	3	——
	10	2	——
PW and Colour-Flow Imaging			
	2	5	2.5
	3	3	1.5
	5	2	1.0
	7	1.5	0.7
	10	1	0.5

at each depth. There have been few detailed studies of the shapes of the sensitive zones of CW units. Table 22.1 provides a rough indication of values for Doppler units operating in the frequency range 2–10 MHz. It should be noted that, as for echo imaging, the lateral resolution is not a fixed quantity, but it is dependent on machine settings such as gain and transmitted power.

3. Velocity resolution

The velocity resolution of a Doppler unit is the minimum difference in velocity which it can detect.

Electronic equipment can measure very accurately the frequency of a signal and, hence, the velocity of motion. Very high accuracy is rather academic, in practice, since, as we noted in Chapter 21, a number of factors broaden the spectrum of frequencies generated for each time interval in the sonogram.

With a high-resolution spectrum analyser, it is possible to measure speed with an error of 2%.

4. Temporal resolution

The temporal resolution of a Doppler unit is the mimimum time interval between events which it can detect.

Timing measurements from Doppler signals can be made on a sonogram or signal trace with an error which is typically ±5 ms. In the case of measurement from a sonogram, the temporal resolution usually depends on the time interval over which the Doppler signal is analysed to produce each spectrum (Ch. 21). Typically this time interval is between 5 and 10 ms, but it can be as low as 1 ms or as high as 40 ms.

5. Power resolution (sonogram contrast resolution)

The power resolution of a Doppler unit is the minimum change in the power of the Doppler signal which it can detect.

It was noted in Chapter 21 that the grey-shade level in a sonogram is greatly affected by a noise speckle. It is therefore difficult to measure the power of a frequency component at any point in a sonogram with good accuracy. Indeed, sonograms are often presented in a simple two-tone display or recording. A number of sonograms are displayed in colour which helps to show the different power levels of the components.

At present, with a good grey tone or colour display, the power level of a component can be measured with an error of less than ±20%. In the future, this may be improved by averaging over several heart cycles.

CW Doppler advantages

1. The instrumentation is simple and inexpensive. Although it suffers from a number of limitations, CW Doppler has been shown to be valuable in several applications; for example, in the study of high-velocity flow, the assessment of carotid arteries, and in the study of umbilical artery flow where the signal can be readily detected in isolation.

2. The units are small and portable.

3. Good-quality, low-noise signals are produced.

4. Adequate performance can be achieved with low output power.

5. There is no practical limit of the speed which can be measured.

CW Doppler limitations

1. The signal generated by a CW Doppler unit comes from any structure in the sample volume which reflects sufficient ultrasound and is moving at an adequate velocity. This lack of localization may make it difficult to obtain a signal from only one vessel.

2. The lack of localization may also make it difficult to identify the vessel in which blood flow is giving rise to the signal.

3. It can be difficult to interpret Doppler signals from basic instruments except in simple situations; even then, most of the information in the signal is ignored.

4. The lowest velocity which can be measured is determined by the wall-thump filter, which is designed to cut out the large signal from slow-moving tissue. The lowest value of such a filter is typically 80 Hz for a 2 MHz Doppler unit, and 200 Hz for a 10 MHz device. Using the basic Doppler shift formula, one can calculate the corresponding velocities for any beam-to-vessel angle.

5. From a sonogram, it is usually fairly easy to trace out the maximum frequency and, hence, calculate the maximum velocity. Likewise, the mean velocity may be calculated, but this calculation is dependent on uniform irradiation of the vessel and can be subject to large error. It is difficult, but not impossible, to quantify the results from CW Doppler units.

6. Doppler-shift information is obtained from structures lying along only one line through the body. As with M-scanning, an initial search is performed before the final direction of the ultrasonic beam is fixed.

7. With CW instruments, attenuation of the ultrasound beam in tissue cannot be compensated for; that is, there is no TGC. Superficial moving structures are therefore more readily detected than deep ones.

8. Difficulty in detection of the direction of flow is exhibited by some instruments. The most common cause is the simultaneous occurrence of forward and reverse flow. Other factors which upset these techniques are a weak, rapidly changing, or variable strength signal. This limitation usually arises with circuits designed to provide a trace for a chart recorder. It should not arise with modern spectrum analysers.

9. Not all blood vessels are accessible by ultrasound. Bone and gas cause considerable problems in some parts of the body.

10. When interrogating a vessel, one does not usually know the beam-to-vessel angle accurately.

11. The diameter of a blood vessel cannot be ascertained with a CW Doppler instrument.

PULSED-WAVE DOPPLER

PW Doppler resolution

The definitions of resolution for CW techniques also apply to PW techniques.

1. Axial resolution

If two small moving reflectors on the beam axis of a pulsed-Doppler unit are within the same sample volume, located at a particular range, they will both contribute to the output signal (Fig. 22.1). Since they are not identified separately, they are not considered to be resolved. To be resolved for all sample-volume positions, the reflectors must be separated by more than the sample-volume length. The axial resolution of a PW Doppler is therefore equal to the length of the sample volume.

We noted in Chapter 19 that the sample-volume length can be altered by changing the length of the transmitted pulse or the duration of the electronic gate. It is quite common to alter it by using the gate duration. The axial resolution is therefore not a constant; it depends on the machine settings. Table 22.1 gives an indication of values of axial resolution for Doppler units of different ultrasonic frequency.

2. Lateral resolution

Once again, lateral resolution is determined by the width of the ultrasonic beam at the range of interest and is therefore dependent on machine settings such as gain and transmitted power. We noted earlier that the width of the sample volume is determined by the width of the beam. An instrument operating at 10 MHz might have a lateral resolution of 1 mm while that of a 5 MHz unit could be 2 mm (Table 22.1).

3. Velocity resolution

The velocity resolution of a PW instrument is similar to that of a CW instrument.

4. Temporal resolution

The temporal resolution of a PW instrument is similar to the resolution of a continuous-wave device. As for the CW unit, it is the spectrum analyser which determines the temporal resolution in practice.

5. Power resolution (sonogram contrast resolution)

As in the CW case, a sonogram derived from the output of a PW instrument suffers from speckle, making it difficult to measure the power of a component with an error of less than ±20%.

PW Doppler advantages

1. The equipment is reasonably simple and inexpensive when compared to the price of imaging machines.

2. PW Doppler units are portable. A typical instrument plus a spectrum analyser can be accommodated on a small trolley.

3. A small, single-crystal transducer is convenient for examining the patient from a number of entry points. This is of particular value in cardiology.

4. The sample volume can be located precisely at any selected depth. Identification of the source of the signal is therefore quite feasible.

5. The ultrasound beam shape is narrower than that from a CW unit since it is generated from a single crystal.

6. Blood-flow signals can be obtained from more than one gated range. For example, 32 adjacent ranges may be selected along the beam to give information on the velocity profile across a vessel.

PW Doppler limitations

1. Although the flowing blood producing the Doppler-shifted signal is much better localized than in the CW case, difficulties can arise in the identification of the vessel or site.

2. Interpretation of the Doppler signal is difficult, but valuable clinical data can be obtained.

3. The lowest measurable velocity is determined by the wall-thump filter, which is usually set at around 100 Hz. The highest velocity is determined by the PRF of the unit. Velocities above this upper limit give rise to lower-than-expected Doppler-shift signals as a result of aliasing (Ch. 18).

4. As in the CW case, the maximum velocity can be fairly readily calculated from a sonogram, but the mean velocity depends on uniform irradiation of the vessel.

5. At any particular time, flow information is obtained for only one beam direction through the body.

6. The performance of direction-sensing circuitry in the instrumentation needs to be carefully checked. The problem of the simultaneous detection of forward and reverse flow in neighbouring vessels is much less than with CW-Doppler techniques.

7. Not all blood vessels are accessible with ultrasound.

8. The quality of a PW Doppler signal may suffer from background noise caused by the switching circuitry in the electronics. PW units are often inferior to CW units in this respect.

9. With a stand-alone PW instrument, the beam-to-vessel angle is usually not known accurately. Hence, it is difficult to convert from Doppler frequency to velocity.

10. The diameter of the blood vessel is not known, although, in theory, it is possible to move a small sample volume across the vessel and measure it by noting the appearance and disappearance of the signal.

11. The output power of a PW unit is usually greater than that of a CW unit of similar ultrasonic frequency (Ch. 8).

DUPLEX DOPPLER

We have seen in earlier chapters that both continuous- and pulsed-wave Doppler devices can be linked to echo-imaging machines.

Duplex resolution

The different resolutions of a Doppler instrument (axial, lateral, speed, temporal, and power) should not be affected by incorporation into a duplex system. This is true, provided some compromise design has not been adopted. There may be good, practical reasons for a compromise such as the use of the same transducer for both Doppler and echo imaging in order to enable good access to the heart at a rib space.

The performance of the echo imager should also be little affected during use in a duplex mode. If the image is refreshed only once or twice per second, then it is obviously no longer true real-time imaging.

Duplex advantages

1. The site of the Doppler examination can be identified on the ultrasonic image. In particular, this allows deep vessels to be studied.
2. The beam-to-vessel angle can be measured to within 2 or 3 degrees.
3. The vessel diameter can often be measured. However, the error is typically 10% or more, with a resultant large error in the calculation of flow.
4. The size of the sample volume can be chosen to suit the examination site and technique; small for location within the vessel or large to straddle it.
5. The sample volume can be placed to avoid undesirable contributions from neighbouring vessels or moving tissue.
6. Patient motion may be noted.

Duplex limitations

1. The beam-to-vessel angle is restricted if the imaging transducer also acts as the Doppler transducer. If the scanning direction is optimum for imaging the vessel walls, it is not usually well

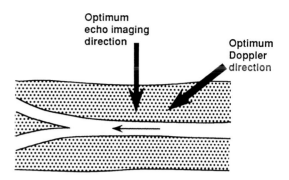

Fig. 22.2 Optimum scanning directions for examining blood vessels with echo-imaging and Doppler instruments.

suited to produce a good Doppler signal (Fig. 22.2).
2. Blood flow information is obtained from one site in the image. A velocity profile can be produced by examining several sites across a vessel. For this to be practical, a multigate unit which can examine several sites simultaneously is required.
3. With a separate Doppler transducer, it is not always certain that the Doppler beam has reached the blood vessel without degradation or deviation.
4. In many duplex systems, the sonogram is presented on too small a display scale for detailed study of the velocity patterns.

COLOUR-FLOW IMAGING

Colour-flow-imaging instruments are all based on pulsed-wave principles. The number of lines in a real-time Doppler image (e.g. 64) and the number of sampled gated ranges along each line (e.g. 128) result in the spatial resolutions being less than that of a real-time echo image. Resolution of velocity in the image depends on brightness differences of the colour presentation. Velocity resolution is therefore poorer than that in a sonogram. However, the quality of Doppler images is such that very useful images of regions of flowing blood are obtained.

Colour-flow Doppler resolution

1. *Axial resolution*
Consider the case of a 3 MHz PW-Doppler unit

being used to image to a depth of 18 cm into the body. If there are 128 gated ranges along each line, the length of each gated range is approximately 1.5 mm. The sample-volume length for this size of gated range and, say, a 5 cycle pulse is around 3 mm. The axial resolution is therefore also 3 mm. The axial resolution in an imaging Doppler unit is therefore similar to that of a basic PW Doppler unit.

2. Lateral resolution

The number of lines in a typical real-time Doppler image is 64. At a range of 10 cm in a 60° sector shaped image, these lines are typically 1.5 mm apart. This is less than the width of the ultrasonic beam, so the line density should not severely affect the lateral resolution, which will be largely determined by the beam width. We noted that the effective beam width is not a fixed quantity, but is dependent on factors such as the sensitivity settings. In practice, the beam widths, and, hence, lateral resolutions, of a 3 MHz and 5 MHz Doppler imager are around 3 mm and 2 mm, respectively.

3. Velocity resolution

Even though the velocity is displayed as 8 different brightness levels in an image, the resolution is unlikely to be better than ±20%, that is, ±10 cm/s for a velocity of 50 cm/s. By reducing the size of the field, e.g. from 90 to 30°, we can collect more samples from each beam direction. This improves the accuracy with which the Doppler-shift frequency from each gated range is measured and, hence, improves the velocity resolution. However, the effect on the colour brightness is not significant, so the improvement in velocity resolution is also limited. To measure velocity accurately, we produce a sonogram, using the Doppler signal from the region of interest.

4. Temporal resolution

Normally, about 25 images are presented per second. Events separated in time by less than 1/25 of a second will not be resolved in the image. In practice, the temporal resolution is more likely to

be nearer 1/10 of a second, since it is difficult clearly to appreciate rapidly occurring events. To obtain good temporal resolution in the study of flow, one generates a sonogram for the point of interest.

5. Power resolution

Since the brightness at each point in the image has been employed to denote a velocity magnitude, it is not possible to display the power of the signal received from each point. Instruments can be designed in which brightness in the display represents the power of the Doppler signal rather than velocity. In practice, the power of the Doppler signal from each point in an image is not of much interest. This is because, within a vessel, the power from different regions of blood should be the same since it depends on the number of blood cells in the region. An exception to this is the study of vascular structures such as tumours.

Colour-flow imaging advantages

Many of the attractions of colour-flow imaging are similar to those of pulsed-wave duplex systems: flow can be studied at a well-defined site; the beam-to-vessel angle and the vessel diameter can be measured. However, there are a number of advantages which make flow imaging more compatible with clinical use.

1. The two-dimensional colour-flow map makes it easier to find specific regions of flow such as a regurgitant jet in the heart, or disturbed flow at a bifurcation of a vessel. In general, it is easier to search through the heart or a complex vascular structure. Blood vessels are more easily identified in organs like the liver and kidneys.

2. Direction of flow is quickly ascertained from the colour coding.

3. The flow can be related to the associated structures presented in the real-time echo image. For example, the degree of stenosis of a vessel can be measured.

4. The true lines of flow through a region can be observed. It is no longer necessary to assume that the flow is always parallel to the walls of a vessel or outflow tract.

5. The extent of a jet into a cardiac chamber from a diseased valve can be measured and used to assess stenosis roughly.

6. The effect of more than one cardiac defect can be imaged at the same time.

7. Patient or heart movement can be allowed for.

Colour-flow imaging limitations

1. The velocity depicted is the component of the actual velocity along the ultrasonic beam axis. The velocity components perpendicular to the beam axis, both in the scan plane and out of it, are not presented. In other words, we are looking at a limited two-dimensional image of three-dimensional flow.

2. The ultrasound beam-to-flow angle is variable throughout the image. Interpretation of the colour-flow image can therefore be complex. For example, where the beam-to-flow angle is around 90°, the presence of flow may not be depicted, since the Doppler-shift frequencies are low.

3. High velocities which cause aliasing errors are depicted in the wrong colour; in other words, as flowing in the opposite direction to that actually occurring. This can be helpful in the identification of high-velocity jets.

4. The axial, lateral, velocity, temporal, and power resolutions of colour-flow imagers are poorer than desired.

5. Although a colour-flow image can be superimposed on a real-time echo image, the ideal viewing direcction for the one does not always correspond to that for the other. This is essentially the same limitation, as depicted in Figure 22.2, for duplex systems.

6. The equipment is expensive.

MANUAL DOPPLER IMAGING

Manual Doppler imaging instruments are based on both continuous- and pulsed-wave principles. Pulsed-wave manual units have not been purchased on a large scale and are likely to be completely replaced by real-time colour-flow units. Manual instruments have resolution factors similar to those discussed above for colour-flow imaging. The image quality is slightly better with

manual devices as a result of a higher line density. PW manual instruments are probably best regarded as stepping stones on the way to real-time colour-flow machines.

We noted in Chapter 20 that CW Doppler images are intrinsically different from PW images since they give an image of regions of flow projected on to a plane approximately parallel to the skin surface. CW devices are unlikely to appear in a real-time form since, for each beam direction, only one point of data is obtained for the flow image, rather than a complete line of data as in the PW case.

Manual CW Doppler resolution

1. Axial resolution

Since continuous-wave ultrasound is employed, there is no resolution of structure along the beam axis. Any vessel falling within the sensitive zone can contribute to the image.

2. Lateral resolution

A CW Doppler beam can be focused, to some extent, and this focal region can be placed at the expected depth of the vessel. However, CW Doppler beams resulting from the action of two crystals cannot be as sharply focused as a single-crystal transducer. As is the case with echo imaging, lateral resolution is not fixed and depends on the sensitivity settings of the instrument. With a 5 MHz unit imaging the carotid, a lateral resolution of 4 mm can be achieved.

3. Velocity resolution

Velocity resolution in the image depends on the brightness of the colour (e.g. dark red for low velocity) or on a different colour being allocated to each velocity. The velocity is unlikely to be resolved to better than 10% accuracy from the image. The velocity at selected points in the image is measured in detail by generating a sonogram.

4. Temporal resolution

Since the image is not presented in real-time, events cannot be distinguished as occurring at different times. Sonograms are again used to study the temporal dependence of events.

5. *Power resolution*

As in colour-flow imaging, when the brightness of the display is used to indicate velocity, the power of the signal at each point cannot be depicted. If different velocities are shown as different colours, brightness could be used to present the power level of the signal. On a display, the power resolution is unlikely to be better than ±20%.

Manual Doppler advantages

1. The higher line density in the image results in slightly higher spatial resolution than is common with colour-flow devices.

2. Manual CW Doppler images represent the flow in vessels in a three-dimensional volume of tissue, whereas both manual PW and colour-flow images are of slices through the tissue.

3. The equipment could be made relatively inexpensively, though, since it has not been manufactured on a large scale, low cost has not always been achieved.

Manual Doppler limitations

1. Blood flow is not displayed as a dynamic process.

2. The duration of the scan is long, typically several minutes.

3. Unless an ECG signal is used to gate the flow signal at a particular time in the cardiac cycle, the image of arterial flow is likely to be dominated by flow occurring during systole.

4. The image is degraded by patient movement.

5. An uneven scanning action impairs the image quality.

6. The CW manual technique is really suitable only for superficial vessels where there is no confusion caused by signals from neighbouring vessels.

7. Manual Doppler imaging techniques are not conveniently linked to real-time echo-imaging systems.

It is obvious that the restrictions of manual Doppler are quite severe.

SUMMARY

In this chapter, five components of resolution have been considered for each Doppler modality. They are axial, lateral, velocity, temporal, and power resolution. The Doppler modes discussed are CW, PW, duplex, colour-flow imaging, and manual imaging. The advantages and limitations of these techniques were also listed.

23. Using Doppler instruments

It is obvious that the more complex Doppler devices must be used in a scientific fashion, and the same is true of the basic units. Even when a simple fetal heart detector is used, the narrowness of the beam and the phenomena which could degrade it should be considered, as a systematic search is made for heart sounds. We will see later that a number of factors need to be taken into account when examining blood flow in vessels.

In Chapter 4, the physical processes which influence ultrasound passing through tissue were discussed. The effects of processes, such as absorption or reflection, are evident when images are produced. These processes are equally significant, but less evident, in most Doppler applications. The operator is therefore required to be more vigilant when using Doppler equipment.

Many basic Doppler units are designed to be powered by replaceable or rechargeable batteries. Batteries in need of recharge or replacement degrade the performance of the instrument.

FETAL HEART DETECTION

Features of fetal-heart detector

Fetal-heart detectors based on the CW Doppler principle are small, inexpensive, and highly sensitive. Their high sensitivity makes them suitable for detecting the weakly reflected ultrasound from a fetal heart in early pregnancy. The directional nature of the ultrasonic beam allows the heart to be located roughly. These instruments usually operate at a fixed ultrasonic frequency of 2 MHz, although some use frequencies up to 5 MHz. An ultrasonic frequency of 2 MHz gives adequate penetration for detecting fetal hearts at depths up to 15 cm from the surface of the abdomen.

In our discussion of pulsed imaging techniques, frequency was seen to be an important parameter in determining sensitivity. Frequency, ultrasonic intensity, and suppression level are not normally variable in simple Doppler instruments. The sensitivity is usually variable only by means of the amplifier gain. The control knob governing sensitivity is often labelled 'volume' or 'sensitivity'. It is meaningless to talk of compensation for attenuation with depth (TGC) in relation to continuous wave units since there is no way of measuring depth. A CW Doppler device merely indicates that a moving structure is in its beam. Filters are often used on the output Doppler-shift signal, and so influence sensitivity. They are almost always used to remove very low-frequency components (below about 100 Hz) that correspond to slow movements within the body. With a 2 MHz instrument, the most significant fetal-heart sounds are considered to be in the range 500 Hz to 1 kHz, so some instruments also allow Doppler-shift components of frequency greater than 1 kHz to be removed by filtering.

The control panel of a Doppler fetal-heart detector contains four or five features whose functions are almost self-explanatory; for example battery meter, and filter and volume control. There are also one or two sockets for taking the output signal to earphones (a plug-in 'stethoscope') or a tape recorder. The earphones usually cut out the signal to the loudspeaker, thus preventing the patient from being alarmed by artefact sounds during searching.

Use of fetal-heart detector

Because detection of the fetal heart is fairly easy,

the part played by processes such as absorption or refraction is rarely considered in detail. Nevertheless, some care has to be taken in the use of these instruments. Good acoustic coupling is required between the transducer face and the skin surface. As the beam is only 1 or 2 cm in effective width, it is necessary to search thoroughly for the fetal heart. If detection proves difficult, a check should be made to see that the sensitivity is at a maximum and that the beam is not being swept too quickly through the tissues. In such a situation, careful listening and a fairly slow rate of change of beam direction by the operator, e.g. 30° of arc per second, may result in success.

Fetal-heart sounds are distinguished from other sounds by their crispness and repetition rate, e.g. 150/s. Manufacturers provide tape recordings of typical Doppler sounds as a useful guide. The placenta, for example, gives rise to a low-pitched audible output as a result of the low speed of blood flow in it. Simple Doppler techniques have been unsuccessful in locating the placenta, since the moving red cells can lie at any depth along the beam.

Note that Doppler signals are produced by moving structures and are not the same as heart sounds heard with stethoscopes; the latter result from impacting structures or turbulent blood flow.

FETAL HEART-RATE MONITOR

Several systems incorporate a continuous-wave Doppler unit as one means of monitoring a fetus (Fig. 23.1). The role of the Doppler instrument is to provide a simple means of measuring fetal-heart rate. The heart rate is obtained by filtering dominant and regular sounds from the Doppler signal and feeding them to a counting device.

The ultrasonic transducers are designed to produce a wide beam so that the heart signal is not lost when the fetus moves. Wide beams are usually generated, using several piezoelectric elements for transmission and reception; for example, two or three performing each function. Basic Doppler fetal-heart detectors can be converted to simple monitors by using a wide-beam transducer. When assessing a monitoring system, operate it over a period of time to gauge how consistently the heart signal is recorded.

BLOOD-FLOW DETECTION

Valuable information can be obtained in a number of fields by using a basic CW or PW Doppler instrument, particularly when it is linked to a spectrum analyser. Examples of this are flow in umbilical arteries, through heart valves, and in peripheral or cerebral arteries.

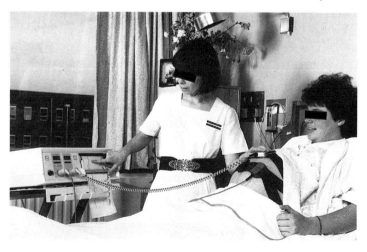

Fig. 23.1 A fetal monitoring system in which the ultrasonic transducer is strapped to the abdomen (courtesy of Sonicaid).

Ultrasonic frequency selection

The frequency of ultrasound used to detect blood flow depends on the application. Detection of flow in deep vessels such as deep veins or the abdominal aorta, is usually accomplished with an instrument transmitting 2 MHz ultrasound. The umbilical arteries and vein, though often deep in the body, can be studied with frequencies in the range 2–4 MHz. The higher frequency is permissible since amniotic fluid has low attenuation. Fetal-heart detectors can be used to study flow in deep vessels. Flow in less deeply located vessels may be recorded with 5 MHz ultrasound, and, for superficial vessels, 8 to 10 MHz is suitable. Table 23.1 gives the working ranges of Doppler instruments of different frequencies. This table should be used only as a rough guide, because the tissues to be penetrated vary for different applications, and the sensitivities of instruments are also not identical.

Table 23.1 Guide to useful depth of penetration of Doppler instruments at different frequencies

Freqency (MHz)	Depth (cm)
1	15
2	10
5	5
8	3
10	2

For several reasons, it is advisable to work with the highest input ultrasonic frequency that will give the necessary penetration:

1. The higher the input frequency f_0, the greater is the Doppler shift for a particular velocity.
2. A higher frequency f_0 results in a greater magnitude of scattered wave at small point targets, i.e. at blood cells.
3. Beams more sharply defined can be generated at high frequencies. This may be helpful in excluding contributions from neighbouring blood vessels.

It should be remembered, however, that the prime factor in determining the ultrasonic frequency is the need to overcome attenuation in tissue. It should also be remembered that with pulsed-Doppler units the aliasing artefact is encountered at lower velocities when high-frequency ultrasound is used.

Features of CW blood-flow detector

The main features of blood-flow detectors are the same as those mentioned above for fetal-heart detectors. Blood-flow instruments normally operate at one frequency in the range 2–10 MHz. Occasionally, a few frequencies and some transducers of different design are offered. A gain control and filters are also found on these instruments. A number of instruments contain outputs from circuits such as zero-crossing ratemeters to provide a signal related to velocity of flow. The Doppler-shift signal is available at the rear of most units. In many modern directional Doppler devices, the forward and reverse signals are presented separately and can be recorded on the two channels of a stereo tape recorder. A few instruments provide a pair of phase-quadrature signals which may be fed to a spectrum analyser, but which cannot be recorded on a tape recorder (Ch. 21).

When slow flow is to be detected, for example, at the end of diastole, there is often interest in having a wall-thump filter which is as low as possible. Typically, filters are set to pass frequencies above 80 Hz, though reports have been made of lower values such as 25 Hz. Automatic filters are feasible where the instrument senses the frequencies from very strong tissue signals and sets a high-pass filter just above them. These devices have not been thoroughly evaluated in clinical practice. The difficulty associated with the use of very low wall-thump filters is that if strong tissue signals of low frequency are passed, the amplifier of the Doppler instrument becomes saturated.

Use of CW blood-flow detector

CW blood-flow instruments can be employed to study flow through arteries, veins, and orifices in the heart. Stenosed and blocked vessels are examined by listening to the Doppler signal produced at a number of sites. Though a diagnosis may be obtained by listening alone, it is also highly desirable to obtain a sonogram. Flow is detected by applying the transducer to the skin of the patient and directing the beam to intersect the vessel. In some applications, the transducer is placed on the vessel wall during surgery. The literature contains descriptions of many applications, such as the assessment of the degree of stenosis of arteries or the resistance to flow in the fetal circulation. To some extent, many of these applications are still in a research phase of development. The object of this section is to point out technical factors which are relevant to most fields.

The Doppler-shift equation is useful when considering the application of an instrument, since this equation clearly indicates which factors influence the output Doppler-shift frequency.

$$f_D = f_o \, (2\mu \cos \theta / c)$$

This equation gives the Doppler-shift frequency for an ultrasonic wave reflected from one moving surface.

From this formula, several important points can be noted:

1. The Doppler-shift frequency depends on the speed, u, of the moving surface. A higher speed results in a greater shift frequency, f_D, which is heard as a higher pitch of output Doppler signal.

2. The size of the Doppler-shift frequency, f_D, is related to the angle θ between the direction of the ultrasonic beam and the direction of reflector movement. It is easy, in practice, to observe the changing pitch of an output signal, as the angle between the ultrasonic beam and the direction of blood flow is varied (Fig. 23.2).

3. The output frequency, f_D, is also determined by the magnitude of the transmitted ultrasonic frequency, f_o. Occasionally, flow in limbs is compared by using two blood-flow detectors simultaneously at corresponding points on each limb. These Doppler units should operate at the same frequency and, if possible, be of the same design. When noting a frequency value in a sonogram, say, at peak systole, the input ultrasonic frequency should be taken in account.

During detection of blood flow, the beam should be moved slowly in the neighbourhood of the vessel until the desired signal is heard. This will normally occur when the beam has been

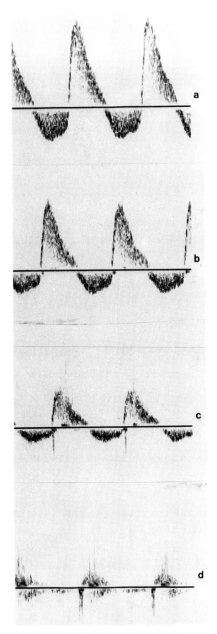

Fig. 23.2   The changes in a sonogram as a result of changing the beam-to-vessel angle: (**a**) 30° (**b**) 45° (**c**) 70° (**d**) 90°.

directed at a specified angle to the vessel, and the audible output is at a maximum. The formula shows that the highest-pitched Doppler signal is obtained, when the angle, θ, has a value of zero degrees, that is, the beam is parallel to the direction of flow. This is usually impractical with a non-invasive technique. Angles from 30° to 60° are a good compromise between obtaining a large Doppler shift in the reflected ultrasound and readily directing the beam into the blood vessel. Use of a gel coupling medium helps to eliminate air between the transducer face and the skin when the transducer is manipulated to optimize the angle of contact. With a basic non-directional unit, only the value of the angle, θ, matters. Whether the beam is pointing with or against the flow is immaterial, because the magnitude of the component of the velocity along the beam, $u\cos\theta$, is the same in each case.

Simple theory predicts that no Doppler shift should be heard when the ultrasonic beam is held at right angles to a blood vessel. However, cells passing in and out of the beam also cause fluctuations in the scattered ultrasound signal which result in an output from the Doppler device. Finally, the problem of determining the angle of the beam to the direction of flow should not be underestimated, particularly if the vessel is curved in any way. In the section in this chapter on duplex Doppler systems, it can be seen that imaging of the vessel is one way of determining the orientation of the beam to the vessel.

The frequencies in a Doppler-shift signal that occur in practice depend on the factors mentioned: f_0, u, and $\cos\theta$. They depend therefore on the design of the instrument and the application. For example, when using an instrument transmitting 10 MHz ultrasound at an angle of 45° to a normal femoral artery, we find Doppler frequencies up to 6 or 7 kHz. Femoral-vein Doppler frequencies for the same instrument and angle of beam propagation have values up to 2 or 3 kHz. Instruments operating at other ultrasonic frequencies have correspondingly altered Doppler-shift fre-

quencies. Tapes are often supplied with instruments to illustrate the sounds heard in particular studies; for example, the high-pitch sounds at stenosed segments of arteries; or the low-pitch venous sounds being influenced by respiration or limb compression.

Features of PW Doppler instruments

Pulsed Doppler devices are commonly used in conjunction with imaging instruments which are employed to identify the sites for blood-flow study. However, they can be successfully used on their own, provided the sample volume can be located at the examination site with reasonable confidence. This technique has been most widely applied in the heart and in the brain; for example, to measure the maximum velocity of flow through the mitral valve, or record the velocity waveform in the mid-cerebral artery. Superficial vessels can also be examined with a stand-alone PW unit. A few instruments of the multigate type have been designed to provide a velocity profile across a superficial vessel.

In addition to the ability to obtain flow information from specific sites within the body, an attraction of PW instruments is the well-defined beam shape produced by the single-crystal transducer. Once again the frequency of the transducer best suited to an application is determined by the penetration required. PW instruments are found with ultrasonic frequencies in the range of 1–10 MHz.

A variable PRF is a feature of pulsed-wave instruments. For superficial vessels, a high PRF can be employed. Unfortunately, to interrogate deeper vessels, one must reduce the PRF to allow more time for the echoes to be collected. This reduces the upper velocity that can be measured. Data for

Table 23.2 The relationship between the maximum measurable velocities and range for PW Doppler units operating at ultrasonic frequencies of 2, 5 and 10 MHz. Beam to vessel angle equal to 45°.

Range (cm)	Maximum PRF (kHz)	2 MHz Maximum velocity (cm/s)	5 MHz Maximum velocity (cm/s)	10 MHz Maximum velocity (cm/s)
5	12	328	131	62
10	6	164	65	33
15	4	109	43	22
20	3	82	33	17

2, 5, and 10 MHz instruments are shown in Table 23.2. These upper-velocity limits were calculated using the formula quoted in Chapter 18. As the range gate is altered, the PW instrument may automatically select the maximum PRF, with the maximum velocity being shown on a numeric display.

The sensitivity of a PW unit is normally controlled by varying the gain of the receiving amplifier (Fig. 23.3). Another possibility is to alter the transmitted power. Since pulsed ultrasound is being used, it is feasible to compensate for increasing attenuation with increasing depth by using TGC circuitry and controls. TGC is found with multigate instruments, but it is not necessary with single-gate units since the gain can be altered manually to suit the depth selected.

A wall-thump filter is included in all machines. It may be fixed to reject frequencies below about 100 Hz or variable, for example from 100 to 1000 Hz (Fig. 23.4).

A meter displaying mean or maximum velocity is found on some instruments. In addition, outputs for a chart recorder may be available to allow mean or maximum velocity to be recorded. As noted earlier, the validity of such records should be carefully checked since the performance of processing circuitry is usually dependent on the quality of the blood-flow signal.

The option of altering the sample volume is a fairly common feature; for instance, it may alter in steps from 1 to 20 mm. This enables the operator to match the sample volume to the technique; to cover the whole vessel or to make measurements at a specific internal point. We noted in Chapter 19 that the sample volume is tear-drop shaped, so the labelling of the control in millimetres should be regarded as a rough guide to size.

Several instruments have a noise-reduction switch which acts to remove some high-frequency sounds in a manner similar to the noise-reduction control on a tape recorder. Since Doppler signals contain high frequencies and resemble noise signals, this control should be used with caution.

Use of PW-Doppler instruments

The dependence of the Doppler frequency f_D on velocity u, angle θ and transmitted frequency f_o is the same for PW and CW instruments. In other words, the Doppler-shift formula still applies. Many of the points described for the CW method are also relevant for the PW one. Particular attention should be paid to the following:

1. When high velocities are expected, check that the PRF is sufficiently high to avoid aliasing errors. This may not always be possible; if not, then the aliasing artefact should be noted in the sonogram (Ch. 24). The PRF limitation can be compensated for, to some extent, by directing the beam at a large angle to the vessel to reduce the velocity component along the beam. For example,

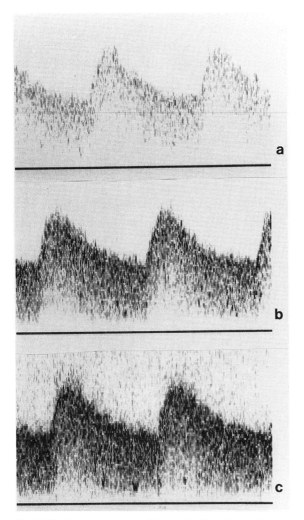

Fig. 23.3 Increasing the sensitivity of a Doppler unit by increasing the receiver-amplifier gain. (**a**) Gain to low, (**b**) correct gain, (**c**) gain too high.

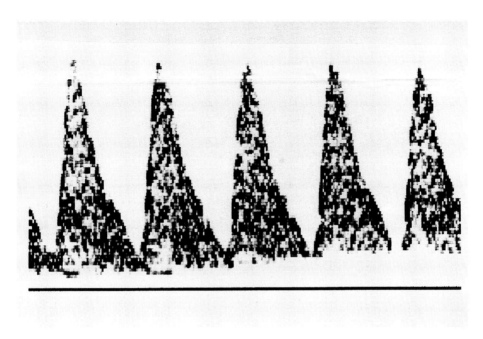

Fig. 23.4 Increasing the level of a wall-thump filter from 100 to 400 Hz. Low frequencies are removed from left to right in sonogram corresponding to shift of filter level.

with a 5 MHz unit and a velocity of flow of 100 cm/s along the vessel, viewing at 45° requires a PRF of 9180 Hz, whereas at 75° the requisite PRF is 3360 Hz. However, the quality of the signal is degraded at the larger angle.

2. Confirm that the sample is optimally located on the vessel by making slight adjustments to the selected range.

3. It is worth bearing the range-ambiguity artefact in mind, especially when high PRFs are being employed (Ch. 24).

4. As in CW techniques, estimate the beam-to-vessel angle as well as possible in order to give an accurate conversion to velocity. Recall that making measurements close to 0° minimizes the angle error in this conversion.

5. If the option is available of switching easily to the CW mode, this mode may serve to overcome any aliasing problem and possibly provide a better-quality signal. Bear in mind that the sample volume of a CW and PW mode of operation are normally very different.

6. When a sonogram obtained with a pulsed-Doppler unit is examined for broadening caused by disturbed or turbulent flow, two points should be recalled. The first is that a small sample volume

may result in broadening caused by cells passing in and out of the volume — transit-time broadening. The second is that a large sample volume may result in broadening caused by a range of cell velocities in the volume — profile broadening. It is apparent that clinical experience must be acquired in normal subjects before a diagnosis of disease is attempted on the basis of the detection of spectral broadening.

DUPLEX SCANNING

The combination of real-time echo imaging and Doppler instrumentation has led to a large increase in ultrasonic blood-flow examinations. The linking of the two ultrasonic methods involves the learning of no new physical principles, but merely careful consideration of how to use the combined system. The controls of the Doppler units are similar to those described above for stand-alone instruments.

Features of duplex systems

The echo-imaging unit of a duplex system can be any type of ultrasonic scanner. It is usually a hand-held real-time B-scanner.

The Doppler transducer may be that used for the imaging, or a completely independent one attached to the imaging-transducer assembly. Where access to the examination site is limited, as it is to the heart or the neonatal brain, a common imaging and Doppler transducer is preferred. Examples of this are a duplex phased array or duplex mechanical oscillator. In obstetrics, where access is not a problem, the Doppler transducer may be attached to a larger imaging transducer, such as a linear array or rotating-transducer scanner.

The Doppler device may be PW, CW, or both. For the CW mode, the transducer requires two or more crystals. Array transducers, linear or annular, are obviously well suited to operating in the PW or CW mode. If it is anticipated that the CW mode will be required to record high velocities accurately, the ease with which the PW can be switched to the CW mode should be checked.

The theoretical path of the Doppler beam across the ultrasonic image is usually depicted by a line. In the pulsed mode, the sample-volume position is indicated by a marker on the line. The shape of the marker is usually related only very roughly to the shape of the sample volume; indeed, often the two shapes are not related at all.

A lower frequency is often used for the Doppler mode than for the imaging one. This is related to the fact that the higher the ultrasonic frequency of a PW Doppler unit, the lower the velocity which gives rise to aliasing problems. Another feature of present-day duplex systems is that the frequencies of the transducer assemblies are fixed and cannot be changed, say, by altering one transducer.

A stand-off water-bath or oil-bath is often a feature of duplex systems designed for the examination of superficial vessels. In the case of a Doppler transducer attached to the imaging one, a stand-off layer is usually essential to enable the Doppler beam to interrogate the superficial vessels. The Doppler beam also has a better shape at an increased distance from the transducer.

An essential feature of a duplex system is the simultaneous viewing of the ultrasonic image while receiving the Doppler signal. This allows a check on the position of the sample volume relative to the vascular anatomy. Since the ultrasonic pulses from the Doppler and the imaging units would interfere with each other if they were run truly simultaneously, the image is usually only refreshed at regular intervals, e.g. 1 second intervals. Some manufacturers run the real-time imager at a reduced frame rate and spend the rest of the time operating the PW Doppler unit. This gives an appearance of truly simultaneous operation, but reduces the PRF of the Doppler unit.

Use of duplex systems

The points noted for the use of CW and PW blood-flow detectors obviously still apply when the detectors are used in a duplex system. A number of additional points related to their use in a duplex mode will now be listed:

1. Check regularly to see that there is ample coupling gel between the Doppler transducer and the skin. If an adequate image is displayed, it is easy to assume, wrongly, that the Doppler beam is also passing into the tissues.

2. A preliminary scan is useful to see if the proposed Doppler beam path will be obstructed by gas or bone.

3. Bear in mind that the line indicating the Doppler beam path across the field of view may not correspond to the actual path. Refraction may cause deviation of the beam. This problem should not be frequently encountered, but it can give rise to an unexpected lack of flow signal.

4. Study the echo image to see if any other vessel or structure could give rise to a Doppler signal which might be wrongly attributed to the vessel of interest. This is particularly relevant to the use of CW instruments, but it also applies to the PW case, in which the range-ambiguity artefact may come into play (Ch. 24).

5. The beam-to-vessel angle should always be measured as accurately as possible since it is central to the conversion of frequency to velocity (Fig. 23.5). Techniques which attempt to make the beam-to-vessel angle take a value near zero have much to commend them since errors in angle size become less significant below 30° (Table 21.1). Changing the viewing point into the heart can often minimize the angle. If the direction of

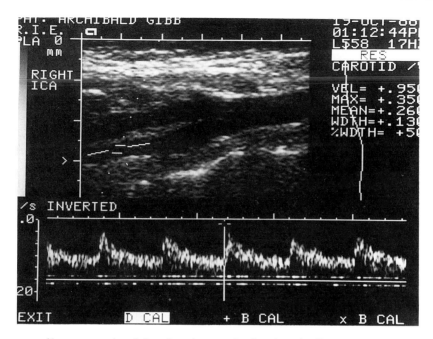

Fig. 23.5 Measurement of beam-to-vessel angle by orientating a marker line along the direction of the vessel. This is necessary to convert the vertical axis of a sonogram from frequency to velocity (courtesy of Allan P).

flow cannot be made to lie in the scan plane of the imager, the beam-to-vessel angle cannot be determined. The difficulty of determining this angle led to the development of flow-waveform indices which are not angle dependent (Ch. 21).

6. In attempts to quantify blood flow, one should measure the diameter of the vessel as accurately as possible at the site where the sample volume is located.

7. Bear in mind that flow occurs in three dimensions and not just in the plane shown in the image. This point is particularly relevant in the estimation of velocities of flow in the heart.

8. Note that the best access point for imaging a structure, where the beam intercepts the surfaces perpendicularly, may not be the best for obtaining a good Doppler signal where it is desirable to have the beam at an angle of 45° or less to the flow.

9. Although it is very useful to refresh the image during a Doppler study, the best-quality Doppler signal is obtained when the image is not being refreshed, and the PRF of the Doppler unit is not being restricted by the need to switch to the echo-imaging mode.

10. Valuable flow signals can be obtained from locations at which the vessel is not clearly depicted, e.g. renal or cerebral arteries.

11. Although it is desirable to record several cycles of flow, this may not be achievable if there is significant patient movement. Nonetheless, useful information can be gleaned from short recordings.

COLOUR-FLOW IMAGING (REAL-TIME DOPPLER IMAGING, COLOUR-FLOW MAPPING)

Colour-flow imaging equipment, as described in Chapter 20, is an example of technology well-suited to clinical use, since it not only provides more information, but also makes it easier to obtain with fewer errors. Flow imaging can be added to real-time, echo-imaging equipment without an excessive increase in the number of controls or procedures to be mastered. Indeed, the number of additional controls may be as few as four, and their function is fairly evident. Other machines offer greater flexibility, but are more demanding of the user. All of the clinical benefits of presenting data as real-time images apply to this technique.

Features of colour-flow imaging systems

On the colour-TV display of a flow-image system, the conventional real-time echo image is shown in grey tones, while the flow of blood is presented in colour (Plates 3, 4, 5 and 9). The colour-flow image may cover the whole field of view of the real-time image or a selected part of it.

As for real-time echo imaging, a finite amount of time is required to collect data at each beam position. The parameters related to the field are therefore linked: frame rate, depth of penetration, and field width are interdependent. In a typical phased-array system, the frame rate varies from 8 to 40 Hz, the field angle varies from 30 to 90°, and the depth of penetration ranges from 6 to 24 cm. Most flow-map systems are based on phased-array transducers; however, other types of scanner may be more suited to non-cardiac applications; for example, a linear array for small-parts scanning. The ultrasonic frequencies employed in flow mapping are similar to those for simple PW Doppler units, typically, 2.5, 3.5, and 5 MHz are employed.

Restricting the field-of-view size is not as limiting as it first appears, because it is difficult to interpret rapidly occurring events over a large image. Some machines outline a box of variable size within which colour flow is depicted. This box can be moved to any part of the pulse-echo image and can also be magnified by a zoom control.

The cine-loop facility is invaluable for unravelling complex flow patterns. It may be possible to replay it with different machine-control settings or colour-coding to clarify the image. For example, the echo level below which the machine treats the signal as coming from blood rather than tissue may be altered. This may help to present the blood flowing within a clearly defined vessel. An ECG signal displayed along with the flow image is also very helpful in the identification of events.

Since the Doppler beam takes a finite time to sweep across the field of view — for example, 50 ms — events in one region do not coincide exactly with those depicted in a neighbouring region. This is a limitation which needs to be borne in mind, particularly when the heart is being examined. If it is only desired to show the regions where blood flow occurs, several image frames can be added together, and then systolic flow will be presented in all regions.

With a linear array, pulse-echo images are produced by beams which emerge perpendicular to the face of the transducer. This often gives good images of blood-vessel walls which run parallel to the skin surface. To generate colour Doppler images of flow in such vessels, the instrument often generates the Doppler beams at an angle to the face of the transducer, e.g 30° to the perpendicular. The Doppler beams then avoid insonating the vessel at 90°. An alternative approach is to use a small prism on the transducer face to deflect the beams from the perpendicular.

The few electronic controls associated with flow imaging are similar to those described for PW instruments, that is, a wall-thump filter and gain control. A gated range may also be positioned anywhere in the image to generate a sonogram related to flow at that site.

An option to aid the detection of low-velocity flow, the slow-flow mode, may be offered. This is of interest for the study of small vessels and veins. The slow-flow mode involves gathering more signals from each beam direction so that low frequencies may be measured and greater sensitivity is achieved by averaging the velocity estimates from more signals. Since the beam dwells longer in each direction, the frame rate is reduced.

A particular feature of flow-imaging systems is that several types of display can be produced simultaneously; for example, flow and echo images with an M-scan containing colour-coded flow information, as described in the next section. It is also possible to present flow and echo images simultaneously with a sonogram from a specific site (Plate 4). The presentation of the colour-flow image and a sonogram is not truly simultaneous; the image is refreshed at selected time intervals. Colour-flow systems are usually sophisticated and expensive. Since colour-flow imaging is still a developing modality, it is probably wise to purchase a machine which is versatile and allows the operator to alter the method of use to suit new applications.

Use of colour-flow imaging systems

The frame rates offered by colour-flow systems

permit the plane of scan to be moved freely around to identify the views of interest. The following are points to note in practice:

1. Controls which affect the sensitivity of the system should be carefully adjusted for each study. Examples of these controls are the wall-thump filter, transmitted power, receiver gain, and TGC. Doppler detectors and analysers produce erroneous results when they are supplied with signals which are too large, and they produce noisy results when the input signals are too small. It is particularly important to know the effect of each control which influences the level of the received signal, since several machines separate the signals from blood and tissue, using signal-magnitude discrimination. Too low a gain or transmitted intensity results in moving tissue being colour-coded as blood, with an apparent 'leakage' of blood in the image (Plate 6). Too high a gain or intensity results in the tissue echo signals spreading out and reducing the areas of blood flow (Plate 7).

2. It is is also true for colour-flow imaging that the optimum view for echo imaging is not normally the best view for flow detection. For example, valve leaflets and vessel walls are best imaged by a beam scanning them perpendicularly, but flow through them is best detected by a beam parallel to the containing structures.

3. Note that the colour identifies the direction of flow with respect to the transducer, that is, toward or away from the transducer. The colour of flow at a particular site may therefore change when the transducer is moved to a different viewing point.

4. It is common practice to depict flow toward the transducer as red and flow away as blue. Different manufacturers use different conventions to represent velocity. Increasing velocity may be represented by changing the shade (saturation) or by altering the hue of the colour; for example, by making the red become more orange. It may be possible for the operator to choose which technique is used to indicate increasing velocity. A colour bar pattern on the screen is a helpful reminder of the relationship of colour to velocity.

5. The method employed by the manufacturer to present turbulent flow should be ascertained. It is fairly common to present it as a mosaic of colours related to the range of velocities in that region, that is, to the statistical spread (variance) of the velocities (Plate 2).

6. The PRF of a flow-imaging instrument which images along the full range of each beam direction is usually lower than that of a simple PW unit looking at a site of intermediate depth. The aliasing artefact therefore sets in for lower velocities. The aliasing artefact, while not desirable, has been found to be of some use in the identification of high-velocity jets whose centre appears in the wrong colour.

7. Short-duration events such as systolic-ejection flow can be difficult to study in detail in a flow-map presentation since they are over so quickly. One solution is to play back a video recording or a digital storage cine-loop at a slow rate or even frame by frame. A sonogram relating to a relevant location is also useful. It is a good practice to keep the cine-loop running so as continuously to record several seconds' worth of images. This prevents the loss of the best images before the operator can act to record them on a video recorder.

M-SCAN PLUS DOPPLER

The value of the M-scan is that it shows the variation of the position of structures with time. Similarly, one valuable aspect of a sonogram is that it also shows the variation of blood velocity with time (Plate 4). A third technique showing variations with time is colour-coded flow recording, in which the flow velocities at points along a fixed ultrasonic beam are recorded, at the appropriate points on the display line, as coloured dots (Plate 4). This display line sweeps across the screen at a uniform speed. An M-mode can be combined with both of these Doppler techniques with advantage to study physiologic variations with time.

Features and use of M-scan plus sonogram systems

Familiarity with M-scan and spectral-analysis equipment makes their combined use straightforward (Chs 16 and 21). As mentioned earlier, this combination is not as ideal as it first appears since the optimum beam direction for each mode is different. However, it is a good tool for the exact timing of cardiac events and associated blood flow since the temporal resolution of both M-scans and sonograms is around 10 ms. It is worth remembering that to see the full detail of both an M-scan and a sonogram, one must present them on a large display.

Features and use of M-scan plus colour-coded flow recording

This combination has not proven to be popular as a stand-alone system, but it is a useful adjunct to a colour-flow imaging system for timing events. Both M-scan and colour-coded flow recording, which measure motion along the ultrasound beam, are very much one-dimensional techniques applied to three-dimensional problems.

BLOOD-PRESSURE MEASUREMENT

Ultrasonic Doppler instruments can be incorporated into devices for measuring blood pressure. These are used when the pressures are low; for example, in neonates or in shock patients when the standard Korotkoff sounds cannot be heard with a stethoscope.

In most instruments, the Doppler transducer is placed under a cuff and coupled to the skin with gel. The cuff is then inflated above systolic pressure, as is normal in measuring blood pressure. Next, the cuff is slowly deflated. When the cuff pressure falls below that of systole, the artery opens and closes. The start of this movement of the artery walls is detected by the Doppler instrument. The pressure in the cuff is then equal to the systolic pressure. Moving blood cells also probably contribute to the Doppler-shift signal. On further deflation of the cuff, diastolic pressure is noted when the artery ceases opening and closing during the cardiac cycle. At diastole, no signals are detected from the artery walls. The Doppler signals can either be listened to directly in the usual manner or recorded on a chart recorder along with the cuff pressure.

A less common method of measuring blood pressure with a Doppler instrument is to place the transducer over an artery distal to the cuff. As the cuff is deflated, the start of intermittent flow allows the systolic pressure to be noted, while the onset of continuous flow gives the diastolic pressure.

Doppler instruments for measuring blood pressure have been operated with frequencies in the range 2–10 MHz. An accuracy of about ± 2 mmHg is usually quoted for the measurements.

Commercial instruments have been designed to detect arterial wall movements. Some of these can perform individual measurements; others are used as monitoring systems. A standard Doppler blood-flow device can be used to measure pressure if a slim transducer is inserted under the cuff. In this situation, the transducer design will probably not be the best to ensure that the ultrasonic beam intercepts the artery.

OPTIMIZATION OF A DOPPLER SIGNAL

During an examination it is difficult to be sure that the signal that has been obtained is the best possible for that particular patient in the time available. A few checks can reassure the operator:

1. Consider the Doppler beam path briefly from the point of view of beam degradation. Are there any tissues or materials, such as calcification, fat, bone, or gas, in the selected path which will affect the beam? A good test for a suitable beam path is to see if the blood vessel can be imaged from the entry point of the Doppler beam.

2. Ensure that the acoustic coupling between the Doppler transducer and the patient remains good.

3. Check that the ultrasonic frequency selected is low enough to give adequate penetration (Table 23.1).

4. Consider whether the examination is best carried out with a CW or PW instrument or both.

5. Choose a transducer which can produce a beam wide enough to encompass the whole width of the blood vessel. It is not easy to be sure of this, since the effective beam width is dependent on

several factors such as the sensitivity setting of the instrument.

6. Adjust the sensitivity controls to ensure that the strong velocity components are not saturated on the grey-tone or colour display of the sonogram, or that overload warning indicators are not operating. Weak signals should not be lost as a result of the sensitivity controls being set too low. Finally, it should be remembered that the position of any wall-thump filter is crucial to the detection of low velocities.

7. Try to make the beam-to-vessel angle as close as possible to $0°$ and below $45°$, if at all possible.

8. Background noise in a Doppler signal which is to be further processed is not desirable as it will confuse the computer. Reduce the noise in a sonogram by lowering the gain of the system, if this can be done without losing velocity information from the weaker signals.

9. The signal level may be improved by a slight sideways movement of the Doppler beam and, in the case of a PW unit, by moving the sample volume along the beam axis. These small manoeuvres may compensate for the sample volume's not being exactly in the position shown on the display.

10. Compare the audible Doppler sounds with the sonogram or chart trace to see if all of the features which can be heard are presented in these outputs.

11. Optimize the velocity and time scales on the sonogram to show fine detail in the velocity data.

12. Arrange the sensitivity settings to present the sonogram as a good-quality grey-tone (or colour) pattern in which the speckle is seen. That is to say, do not compress the spectrum to a simple black-and-white image.

13. Record and process the Doppler signal over several heart and respiration cycles.

14. Identify artefacts and features of sonograms associated with each application.

15. Check to ensure that forward and reverse flow are being properly handled by the system.

16. Check the recording levels on the indicators of the tape recorder.

17. Dub all recordings thoroughly with details of the patient and the examination.

This list is rather long but much of it soon becomes automatic. The perfect signal is probably never obtained.

SPECIFICATION OF A DOPPLER TECHNIQUE

As with echo imaging, a written account of an application of Doppler instruments is much more meaningful if the technique is clearly specified. Points of relevance in the technical specification are as follows:

1. Type of Doppler instrument: directional or non-directional, pulsed or continuous wave, duplex or colour-flow imaging

2. Trade name of instrument

3. Ultrasonic frequency of the Doppler unit and that of the imager in a duplex system

4. Shape, size and angle of crystals

5. Approximate shape of the Doppler beam, e.g. the location of the focus

6. Output intensity or power

7. Type of echo-imager transducer used in a duplex system and the relationship of Doppler beam to it

8. Pulse-repetition frequency (PRF) of pulsed Doppler or colour-flow image equipment

9. Site of application of the transducer to the skin

10. Angle of ultrasonic Doppler beam to the blood vessel

11. Size and shape of sample volume

12. Plane of scan associated with any image

13. Maximum velocity encountered in the application

15. Filters used to exclude low- or high-velocity signals

16. Details of the methods used to record or analyse the signals; in particular, the frequency and time resolution of the spectrum analyser

17. Details of the colour-flow system: frame rate, number of lines in image, and number of samples along each beam direction (The colour-coding should also be explained.)

18. Number of gated intervals in a velocity profile across a vessel and their physical length

It is unlikely that a complete specification will be

possible, but this type of information adds considerably to a publication.

SELECTION OF A DOPPLER INSTRUMENT

We have seen that Doppler instruments vary a great deal in complexity and cost. In some applications, it is desirable to have a complete flow-imaging system; however, it has been shown that results can be obtained in other situations with simpler equipment. The most important feature in the selection of a Doppler unit is the ultrasonic frequency, which can readily be related to depth of penetration (Table 23.1). An important test to carry out is the ability of the device to detect weak signals without their being lost in instrument noise. This test can be performed by examining flow in a small artery or vein situated at a depth similar to those in the proposed applications; for example, digital arteries for high-frequency instruments, or hepatic and umbilical veins for low-frequency units. Spectral analysis is mandatory in any serious study of blood flow with the Doppler technique. Before one purchases an instrument, it is essential to check that it can produce high-quality Doppler signals in the envisaged applications. Diagnoses cannot be made on the basis of signals which are merely average. The four common approaches to the study of blood flow are summarized below:

1. A basic CW unit is of value where a signal can be obtained from the site of interest without confusing sounds being picked up from other regions.
2. A stand-alone PW unit is useful when it is desired to examine a site which is easily interrogated by the Doppler beam and which is highly localized; for example, the orifice of a mitral valve or mid-cerebral artery.
3. A duplex system is used where an image is necessary to locate the examination site. This type of system is also essential if the diameter of a blood vessel is to be measured. Particular care should be paid to the selection of the echo imager in the duplex system, as this governs the coupling to the patient and the method by which the imaging and Doppler modes are actually linked.
4. A Doppler colour-flow imaging instrument is useful in the study of complex flow patterns which occur in many situations, in addition to those encountered in the heart, and to locate vessels which cannot be clearly seen using echo imaging alone. The simultaneous presentation of an echo image allows vessel dimensions to be measured and the flow to be related to anatomical structures.

Other techniques such as M-scan plus Doppler can be regarded as additional features of a principal technique and do not usually enter into the selection process.

SUMMARY

In this chapter, practical points related to the use of Doppler units were discussed. It was noted that it is usually advisable to work with the highest ultrasonic frequency possible, provided aliasing problems are not encountered. For each type of device, the features were first identified, and then guidance for use was provided. The basic Doppler equation was again seen to be helpful as a guide to obtaining and interpreting results. The controls associated with each type of Doppler are similar, and the lessons learned with one instrument can be applied to another. Just as in echo imaging, knowledge of the use of Doppler systems can be gradually accumulated. To make a diagnosis from a Doppler examination, the operator requires high-quality signals. Seventeen points were raised for the optimization of a Doppler signal. Eighteen points were noted for the specification of a Doppler technique. Finally, some guidance for the selection of a Doppler instrument was presented.

24. Artefacts in Doppler techniques

As with echo imaging, Doppler information is subject to artefacts. However, in the case of Doppler information, more of the artefacts arise from operator technique than from intrinsic aspects of the instrumentation. It is therefore important to build up knowledge of the sources of artefacts.

PROPAGATION ARTEFACTS

The phenomena which affect the ultrasound beam as it passes through tissue have a direct bearing on the scattered ultrasound picked up by the transducer. These phenomena have been discussed in Chapter 4. While scattering from blood cells provides us with the basic signal, the other phenomena can give rise to artefacts.

Attenuation

The reduction in amplitude of ultrasound as it passes through tissue results in stronger signals being detected from superficial vessels than from deep ones. With CW Doppler units, there is no way of compensating for this imbalance. With PW Doppler devices, signals are often accepted from a sample volume at a selected depth, and the gain can be adjusted to amplify suitably the received signal. If signals are accepted from a number of sample volumes along the beam, time-gain compensation (TGC) can be used to allow for attenuation. This is done in colour-flow imaging.

Refraction

Refraction may result in the Doppler beam's being deviated from the direction of the transducer axis so that it misses or only partially intercepts the vessel. Deviation at soft-tissue interfaces is usually only 1° or 2°, but situations can arise where it is more significant, such as those at wedge-shaped muscle or fat layers. With duplex systems, it is not uncommon to detect a weaker than expected signal from a well-imaged vessel, probably because the tissues in the Doppler beam path have refracted the beam.

Shadowing and enhancement

In some cases, the attenuation of the Doppler beam at a particular structure may be so large that it is difficult to detect blood flow behind it. The most common example of this is attenuation by calcium on a vessel wall. The fetal spine can also make the detection of flow in the fetal aorta difficult.

The converse of shadowing is enhancement, in which the Doppler signal is larger than might be expected from a vessel at a particular depth, because the beam passes through low-attenuating tissue to reach the vessel. A common example of this is the detection of blood flow in the umbilical artery, which is immersed in amniotic fluid. Blood flow in the heart is made easier to study by the relatively low attenuation of blood.

Multiple reflection

It is worth bearing in mind that the Doppler beam could reach a vessel by an indirect route; for example, it could do so after reflection at a strong reflector such as the diaphragm or a bone surface. This type of artefact is common in echo imaging, but is less often identified in Doppler techniques, possibly because Doppler signals from blood are intrinsically weak and become even weaker after multiple reflections. However smooth tissue/gas interfaces can act as mirrors and produce duplicate colour flow images of vessels, as noted for tissue structures in Chapter 15.

Beam width, side-lobes, and grating-lobes

Strong moving reflectors such as heart muscle may give rise to Doppler signals even though they appear to be quite far from the central axis of the Doppler beam. Strong reflectors can give rise to detectable signals when they lie in a low-intensity beam side-lobe. It is often quite difficult to get a Doppler signal from the fetal aorta without picking up a fetal cardiac component.

On the other hand, use of a narrow beam can be responsible for partial insonation of a vessel and, hence, for a Doppler signal related to only a portion of the moving cells. An example of this artefact is the enhancement of the contribution from the high-velocity flow at the centre of a vessel when a narrow beam passes through the centre but does not encompass some of the slower-moving blood at the side.

Sonogram speckle

It was noted in Chapter 21 that the power levels of the velocity components in a sonogram fluctuate from pixel to pixel and give it a speckled appearance. These amplitude fluctuations are a result of fluctuations in the magnitude of the ultrasonic signal received from the random distribution of blood cells. The way in which the frequency analysis is carried out also makes a contribution to the fluctuations. It is therefore not possible to interpret the power level in a pixel as an accurate measure of the number of cells moving with a particular velocity. Averaging or smoothing the power levels in neighbouring pixels gives a more accurate measure of the number of cells moving with each velocity (Fig. 24.1).

Transducer ring-down zone (transducer dead zone)

With a PW transducer, there is a zone close to the front face within which blood flow cannot be

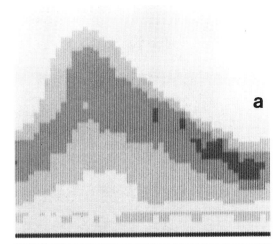

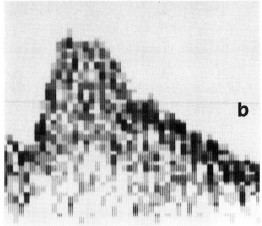

Fig. 24.1 Smoothing of the speckle noise in a sonogram (courtesy of Hoskins P).

detected. This is due to the fact that the transducer cannot detect echoes while it is still transmitting. The length of the ring-down zone is dependent on the length of the transmitted pulse, e.g. 5 mm for a 3 MHz pulse and 2 mm for a 7 MHz pulse. It is emphasized that these are only examples, since the length of the transmitted pulse varies quite substantially from machine to machine.

The dead zone for a CW instrument is due to the overlap of the transmit field and the receive zone occurring at a distance from the transducer (Ch. 19). The region of overlap of these zones in a CW beam is quite large, and the dead zone may be restricted to within a few millimetres of the transducer face.

Lack of coupling

Just as in imaging, weak signals may result from poor acoustic coupling between the transducer and the skin. The artefact is not as immediately obvious in Doppler applications as in imaging, where poor penetration is readily seen. This problem seems to arise most often with Doppler transducers attached to the side of imaging ones.

ELECTRONIC ARTEFACTS

Noise and pick-up

When weak Doppler signals are to be studied, say, from a small, deep vessel, it is necessary to turn up the gain of the receiving amplifier in the Doppler instrument. With high gain, other signals may become significant; for example, noise signals generated in the electronics of the instrument, or electromagnetic signals radiated from neighbouring equipment. Such signals add random noise to the sonogram, or even more definite signals at well-defined frequencies (Fig. 24.2c). Noise and pick-up can often be ignored by the operator, but they can upset automatic signal processing; for instance, where the average velocity trace is drawn on the sonogram. The possibility of spurious signals affecting the sonogram or associated processing should be checked. Some spectrum analysers allow the operator to attempt to clean up the sonogram by deleting spurious signals.

Compression of sonogram

If a sonogram is presented with few or no grey tones, a considerable amount of information is lost (Fig. 24.3). For example, it is extremely difficult to ascertain the degree of spectral broadening, since the window below the maximum velocity components may be filled with weak components which have been presented at too high a level.

A small scale of presentation is also undesirable, since it may make difficult the observation of details in the sonogram, such as small notches in the waveform pattern or spikes of high velocity caused by turbulence (Fig. 24.3). The accuracy of measurements from the sonogram will also be affected.

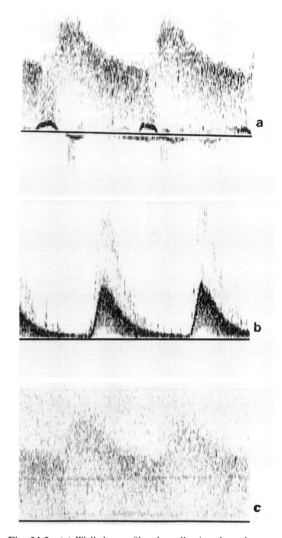

Fig. 24.2 (**a**) Wall-thump filter low allowing through strong signals from moving structure. (**b**) Additional high-frequency version of sonogram caused by large signal distortion which generates harmonics. (**c**) Random noise and pick-up in a sonogram when sensitivity is high to try to detect weak signals.

The frequency scale should be optimized for the preservation of detail (Fig. 24.4).

Poor direction sensing

Direction-sensing circuitry needs to be set up accurately since it has to measure small phase changes in the received signal. It is not uncommon for poor or badly set up circuits to indicate some

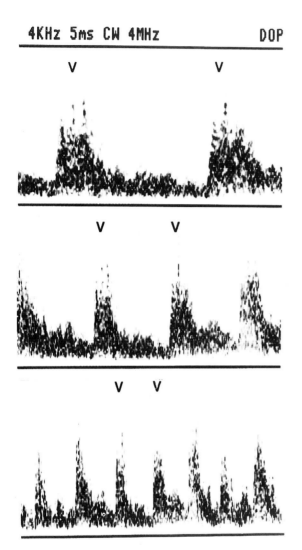

Fig. 24.3 Compression of the time axis of a sonogram illustrating how detail in the sonogram is lost. The arrows indicate the same time span in each sonogram. The spikes in the sonogram are due to vortices in the flow (courtesy of Pye S D).

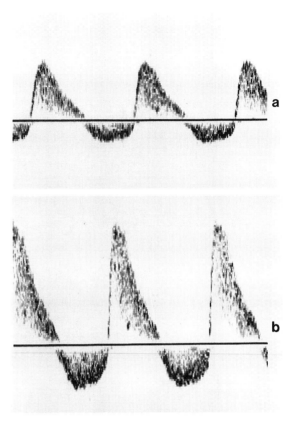

Fig. 24.4 Compression of the frequency axis in a sonogram illustrating how detail is lost. (a) Frequency range compressed, (b) frequency range more suitable.

flow in the wrong direction. Large signals, possibly caused by too high a gain, tend to become distorted and saturated, hence losing the phase information. In this case, the sonogram may even look completely symmetrical in the forward and reverse directions. The direction-sensing performance of a Doppler unit or colour-flow system should be tested in a flow phantom or in some normal arteries where the flow pattern is known.

Filtering

Filters are incorporated into instruments, usually in order to remove the low-frequency signals from moving soft tissue (Fig. 24.2a). In doing this, the system also removes information on slow-moving blood, as is evident on most sonograms or images of cardiac chambers (Fig. 23.4, Plate 7). It is also worth remembering that filters do not cut out signals completely, but do reduce their size very significantly. The size of the reduction and how well it is achieved depend on the design of the filters; typically, the reduction is around 40 dB. The signal from a strongly reflecting structure may still be significant after filtering.

Harmonic generation by large signals

It was seen in Chapter 5 that the harmonics of a frequency are multiples of it: the harmonics of 100 Hz are 200 Hz, 300 Hz, etc. When a signal of, say, 100 Hz becomes distorted, possibly by overamplification, the resultant signal contains frequency components at harmonic values. If this distorted signal is analysed, the harmonics appear at regular frequency intervals in the sonogram. When a large signal from a moving structure, such as a mitral valve, is analysed, regular bands of frequency components can be seen in the sonogram. The effect can also be seen in large blood-flow signals, in which a higher-frequency version of the sonogram may appear faintly above the true one (Fig. 24.2b).

We normally consider harmonics in a sound as part of its musical content.

High or low sensitivity

In a sonogram, it is usually fairly obvious when, as a result of inappropriate amplification or transmitted intensity, the sensitivity of the system is too low or too high. Too low a sensitivity may account for a weak signal; too high a sensitivity compresses the grey tone presentation and may introduce higher harmonic frequencies as a result of signal distortion. A feature of too high an amplification is a general background electronic noise (Fig. 24.5).

In colour-flow imaging, too low a sensitivity results in the blood flow not being detected and may also cause a weak signal from moving tissue to be colour-coded as blood. Too high a sensitivity causes saturation and, hence, spread of the echoes in the pulse-echo image, with a resultant decrease in the areas where blood flow can be detected (Plate 7).

Aliasing

We saw in Chapter 18 that pulsed Doppler and colour-flow units essentially examine a regular sequence of samples of the Doppler-shift signal. To generate the Doppler signal accurately, one must have a sampling rate of at least twice the highest frequency component in the Doppler signal (Fig.

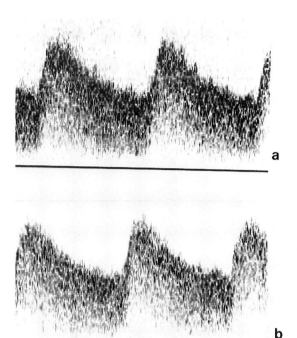

Fig. 24.5 High sensitivity compressing grey-shade range and introducing background noise. (a) Sensitivity (gain) too high, (b) sensitivity more suitable.

18.13). This is a fundamental theorem relating to the reconstruction of signals from samples. If the sampling rate is too low, the frequency of the reconstructed Doppler signal is also too low, and the phase information in it corresponds to flow in the wrong direction. In a sonogram or flow image, this low-sampling artefact, known as an aliasing artefact, appears as flow in the wrong direction at a velocity lower than the true value (Fig. 24.6, Plate 8).

The aliasing artefact is a problem when high-frequency Doppler-shift signals are produced. This occurs usually when there is high-velocity flow. It is worth bearing in mind that the Doppler-shift frequency also increases with the frequency of the transmitted ultrasound, so high-frequency units are more prone to aliasing than are low-frequency ones with the same sampling rate.

When deep structures are to be examined for blood flow, it is necessary to reduce the PRF of the Doppler unit (the sampling rate) to allow time to collect echoes from the blood before the next

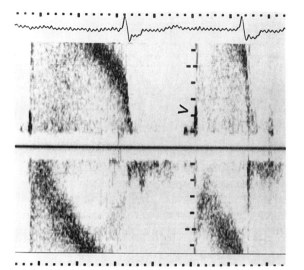

Fig. 24.6 During diastole, the high frequencies in the sonogram are presented as reverse flow caused by aliasing. The true sonogram in diastole is obtained by adding the lower part of the sonogram on to the top part. The low-velocity reverse flow in systole is correctly shown. The arrow indicates the signal from the opening flick of the mitral valve (courtesy of Bloomfield P).

pulse is sent out. Aliasing can, therefore, readily arise in such applications.

The sonogram in Figure 24.6 illustrates the aliasing artefact; the high-velocity forward-flow components appear as reverse flow. The computer can rearrange the display to add the reverse flow

on to the top of the forward flow components, by moving the zero-velocity baseline down the screen and relocating the reverse components at the top of the screen. This is useful in some situations. If aliasing is very marked, the artefactual signal may occupy all of the reverse-flow region in the sonogram, so this procedure is not profitable. In the case of severe aliasing, it can be difficult to distinguish the artefact from genuine reverse flow.

Aliasing is often considered to be of assistance in colour-flow imaging, since it allows high-velocity jets to be identified.

An indicator in the machine which draws the operator's attention to the presence of aliasing is a useful feature. A technique which allows the accurate measurement of high velocity at a particular site is to locate the flow with a duplex or colour-flow system, and then to switch to the CW mode to generate a sonogram.

Range ambiguity

It is a quite common practice in the design of PW Doppler units to arrange that the time between transmission pulses is just sufficient to collect echoes from the selected depth of the sample volume (Fig. 24.7). So after one cycle of transmit and receive, a second cycle is immediately started (the high PRF mode). However, during this second cycle, some echoes from a blood vessel at

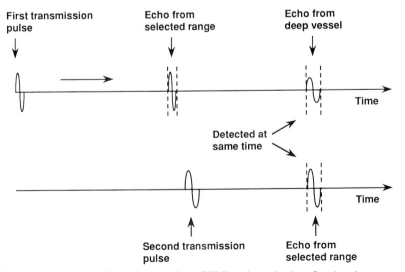

Fig. 24.7 Explanation of range ambiguity in PW Doppler and colour-flow imaging systems.

twice the depth of the sample volume may be received by the instrument as a result of the first transmission pulse, which is still travelling on into the tissue. The instrument cannot discriminate between these late echoes from the first pulse and the echoes from the second pulse. The late echoes from the deeper vessel are therefore added to the echoes from the sample volume and contribute to the Doppler signal. This range-ambiguity artefact occurs when the deeper vessel gives rise to a large signal which is detectable; for example, a maternal vessel reflecting at twice the range of a fetal one.

In flow imaging, deep vessels beyond the displayed range may also contribute to the image if they are detected, since the machine will attribute them to more superficial sites.

The high PRF mode is employed to reduce aliasing from high velocity flow at a known depth while bearing in mind the possibility of range ambiguity.

The 90° signal

When the axis of an ultrasound beam intercepts flowing blood at 90°, no Doppler signal is expected since, in the Doppler equation, $\cos 90° = 0$ (Fig. 23.2). However, a very distinct sound is usually heard. There are a number of sources which can contribute to this signal. Firstly, there may be some turbulence in the flow; in which case, the blood cells are not all travelling in parallel paths at 90° to the beam. Secondly, spectral broadening occurs as cells enter and leave the beam.

In colour-flow imaging, a vessel interrogated at 90° may appear to be dark, corresponding to zero or slow flow. For example, in a curved vessel in which the direction of flow alters with respect to the ultrasound beam, different regions of the same vessel may be coloured red and blue with a dark portion in between (Plate 1).

Beam-to-vessel angle changes

In colour-flow imaging, many colour changes are not due to flow reversal, but, rather, to changes in the beam-to-vessel angle. One source of this angle change is the curvature of vessels (Plate 1). Another is a result of the changing beam direction in a sector scanner.

Transducer movement

If the Doppler transducer operates next to a moving transducer of a real-time scanner, some ultrasound may well be reflected from the moving transducer and give rise to a Doppler signal. This artefact is avoided by stopping the moving transducer, but this may impair the ability of the duplex system to refresh its image at regular intervals. Another solution is to improve the acoustic insulation between the transducers.

We have noted that the same transducer is often used in a duplex scanner to produce real-time images with a mechanical scanning action and for PW-Doppler operation when it is stopped in a selected direction. Vibrations from the mechanical drive may cause the transducer to move slightly while in the stopped position. This gives rise to spurious Doppler signals.

Recording artefacts

Mistakes and artefacts can easily occur when one records Doppler signals on a tape recorder. Electrical pick-up can degrade the signal, for example, as a result of poor earth connections. It should be reasonably easy to eliminate this problem. Acoustic pick-up via the tape-recorder microphone could be superimposed on the Doppler sounds, but in most recorders the microphone input is disabled when the Doppler signal is being recorded, and vice versa.

As noted in Chapter 21, the phase information of quadrature signals may not be well preserved in a tape recording and, hence, direction of flow information is lost.

TECHNIQUE ARTEFACTS

Interference from neighbouring vessels

If, in addition to the vessel being studied, part or all of a neighbouring vessel is within the sample volume of a CW or PW instrument, the Doppler signal contains a contribution from the extra vessel (Fig. 24.8). This artefact can sometimes be removed by reducing or moving the sample volume or by redirecting the ultrasound beam to interrogate only the vessel of interest. The additional contribution from a neighbouring vessel can

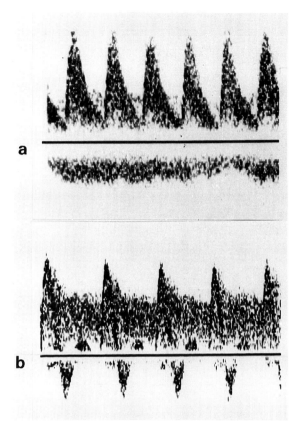

Fig. 24.8 Detection of flow from neighbouring vessels (courtesy of Hoskins P).

occasionally be of help in identifying the signal of interest. An example of this is the composite signal from the umbilical artery and vein. An advantage of colour-flow imaging is that neighbouring vessels are not confused.

Vessel compression

Superficial vessels may be inadvertently compressed by heavy-handed application of the transducer. As the vessel lumen is decreased, increased velocity of flow through the restriction results in a higher-pitched Doppler sound or a colour change in an image. Manipulation of a transducer on a superficial vessel does much to emphasize the dependence of the Doppler signal on velocity, angle, and position.

Factors affecting the patient

A complication of blood-flow investigations is the response of the cardiovascular system to many factors. Examples of these factors are exercise, temperature, anxiety, posture, food, smoking, and drugs. Strict protocols must be observed in investigative methods if the results are to be meaningful.

Patient or vessel movement

Obviously, if movement causes the sample volume of a CW or PW beam to interrogate a different region, the blood-flow signal will be altered. It can be difficult to eliminate this factor, and it is not always clear whether respiration has actually affected the flow or just moved the vessel. Particular care must be taken in the identification of reduced diastolic flow.

Beam position in vessel

The Doppler signal varies markedly when a beam insonates different regions across the vessel. This may be avoided if the beam is uniform and wider than the vessel. In practice, it is quite difficult to make wide uniform beams. Usually a beam through the centre of a vessel will overemphasize the high velocities, while at the side of the vessel the velocities detected will be lower.

Operator variability

We have noted that many factors, both physical and physiologic, influence the final outcome of a Doppler examination. It cannot be assumed, therefore, that different operators or the same operator on different occasions will produce the same result. A somewhat neglected aspect of Doppler techniques is the inter- and intra-operator variability. Even once a sonogram has been obtained, it cannot be assumed that different operators will apply the same criteria in coming to a diagnosis.

One-dimensional scan

If blood flow occurs in an unknown direction in

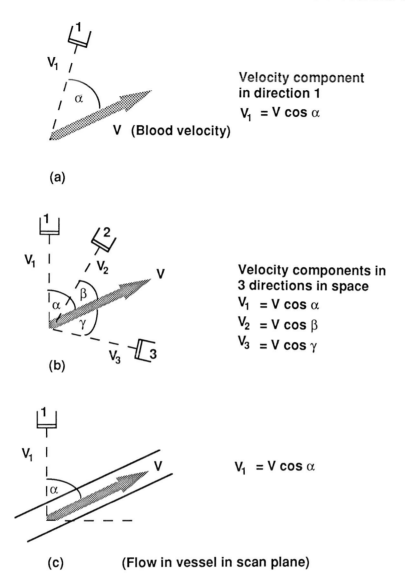

Velocity component in direction 1

$$V_1 = V \cos \alpha$$

V (Blood velocity)

(a)

Velocity components in 3 directions in space

$$V_1 = V \cos \alpha$$
$$V_2 = V \cos \beta$$
$$V_3 = V \cos \gamma$$

(b)

$$V_1 = V \cos \alpha$$

(c)   (Flow in vessel in scan plane)

Fig. 24.9   Difficulty of determination of true velocity of flow in three-dimensional space: (a) only component along beam direction is measured; (b) three components are required to measure true velocity, e.g. in heart chamber; (c) if the direction of a straight vessel in a plane is measured, then one velocity component is sufficient to determine the true velocity.

3-D space — for example, in the heart — detecting it from one direction only measures the velocity component along that beam direction (Fig. 24.9a). To measure the actual velocity requires components to be measured in three directions which are not in the same plane (Fig. 24.9b). If the flow occurs in a vessel lying in a scan plane, measurement of one velocity component and the angle between the beam and the vessel is sufficient to determine the actual velocity along the vessel (Fig. 24.9c).

Moving tissue

Moving tissue may appear in a sonogram as well as blood. Normally, the speed of motion will be low compared to that of blood, so the two can be distinguished. Heart valves travel at high speed, but such motion is of short duration, a fact which permits their identification (Fig. 24.6). Occasionally part of the heart valve structure is made

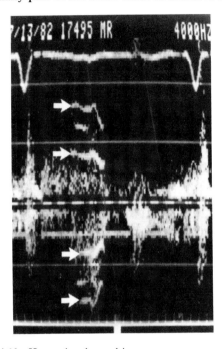

Fig. 24.10 Harmonics observed in a sonogram as a result of an oscillating structure modulating the Doppler beam. Frequency of oscillation equals the separation of the harmonic bands, approximately 1700 Hz. (Courtesy of Holen J, Waag R C and Gramiak R (1985) Ultrasound Med Biol 11: 267–272).

to oscillate by passing blood at a frequency of a few hundred Hz — the valve acts as a whistle. Ultrasound reflected from such a structure is frequency modulated. Harmonic bands are clearly seen in the sonogram (Fig. 24.10).

In colour flow imaging, tissue movement can give rise to large patches of colour which may obliterate all or part of the image. With mechanical scanners, the beam continually moves so tissue crosses it. The velocity component of the tissue along the beam is usually small and does not create a problem. However the slow-flow performance of mechanical colour flow instruments should be checked.

SUMMARY

The operator must be aware of possible sources of artefacts. They can be grouped into three classes.

1. Nine artefacts were listed as propagation artefacts.

2. Eleven examples of electronic artefacts were provided.

3. Eight technique artefacts were noted.

REFERENCE

Reading C C, Charboneau J W, Allison J W, Cooperberg P L 1990 Color and spectral Doppler mirror-image artifact of the subclavian artery. Radiology 174: 41–42

25. Invasive techniques

That ultrasonic techniques are non-invasive is commonly emphasized. However, they are, in fact, extremely well suited to invasive procedures, so we should not get too attached to the non-invasive dogma. A number of devices for invasive techniques are commercially available, and there is great potential for further development. The advent of small, portable scanners to which specialized transducers and biopsy needle systems can be added should help the spread of invasive ultrasonic methods. Probably the main barrier to advances in this area is the total time required, much of which is used for procedures not related to the actual ultrasonics. This is a problem of logistics and staff training, a problem which will, no doubt, be resolved if the demand for the techniques is sufficiently high. Ultrasonic techniques are well suited to invasive procedures since they operate in real-time and the transducers and associated devices can be made small and flexible.

It is interesting to note that with invasive transducers the four main problem factors of ultrasonics, gas, bone, fat, and muscle, are virtually eliminated. In addition, the utilization of high frequencies leads to high-resolution images. All of the imaging and Doppler technologies discussed so far are employed in invasive scanning.

INTERNAL SCANNERS

Internal scanners are used when the structures of interest cannot be imaged adequately from outside the body, usually as a result of bone or gas obstructing the beam. Internal transducers can often be placed close to the structures to be visualized, so frequencies in the range 5–20 MHz can be used. A disadvantage of internal scanning is that the scope for manipulating the scan plane is limited, although some transducers are now being produced in which the angle of the scan plane can be altered. The restricted manipulation means that careful thought has to be given to the selection or purchase of each transducer.

360° scanners — plan position indicator (PPI) scanning

In this technique, a transducer is inserted into the body, and the ultrasonic beam is swept in a plane through an angular range of 360°. A typical scanning rate is 6 revolutions per second; a frame rate of 6/s. Insertion is usually via an orifice such as the vagina or rectum, but, occasionally, the method is employed during surgery. A specially constructed transducer is required for 360° scanning. As shown in Figure 25.1, a small piezoelectric element is mounted on the side of a tube so that the ultrasonic beam is emitted perpendicularly to the tube axis. Electronic connections and backing material for the element are the same as in normal pulsed transducers. The necessity of keeping the element diameter small (typically 5 mm) makes the generation of a narrow beam difficult (see Ch. 27). Likewise, the limited space for backing material behind the element may hinder the generation of short pulses. The last two difficulties are of less significance in high-frequency scanners. It is advantageous to have elements of different operating frequency and focal range mounted on the tube.

During the scan, the direction of the beam is measured by an angular measuring device, and tissue interfaces are located by detecting echoes in the usual manner. As the beam sweeps round the

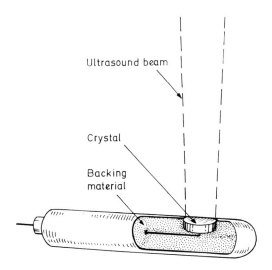

Ultrasound beam

Crystal

Backing material

Fig. 25.1 Transducer for 360° radial invasive scanning.

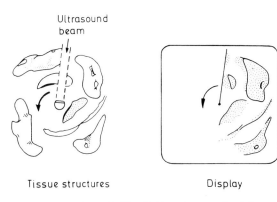

Ultrasound beam

Tissue structures   Display

Fig. 25.2 Principle of 360° radial invasive scanning (plan position indicator scanning).

scan plane, echoes are depicted as bright spots on a line that rotates about one end, positioned at the centre of the display screen (Fig. 25.2). A two-dimensional image is built up on the screen. As with all modern scanners, the echo information is, in fact, fed to the screen via a scan-converter memory store which enables additional frames to be inserted and, hence, image flicker to be eliminated. This type of scanning action is familiar as a means of displaying radar signals.

A commercially manufactured, 360° transducer is shown in Figure 25.3, and an image of a rectal tumour in Figure 25.4. Often two transducers are incorporated in the scanning head, which can therefore be switched to operate, typically, at 5 or 10 MHz. At 5 MHz, a penetration range of around 10 cm is possible, while at 10 MHz, ranges around 3 cm are accommodated. The probe is covered with a thin rubber sheath that is filled with water to ensure good acoustic coupling between the transducer and the tissues. It is not always necessary to employ a water-filled sheath. Multiple reflections in the water layer may create difficulties in imaging tissues close to the transducer. The amount of water in the sheath can be varied to avoid compressing structures, or to push them into the focal zone of the transducer. Some 360° scanners have been mounted on a motorized support which enables the scan plane to be changed in a controlled fashion.

Internal linear arrays

A linear array which operates at a frequency of 5 MHz or higher can be mounted on a tube of a diameter of approximately 1 cm (Fig. 25.5a). Such an array is typically 6 cm in length and has an imaging performance similar to a normal 5 MHz device designed for external use. The rectangular field of view is in a plane parallel to the axis of the tube. An internal linear array can be used with or without a water-filled sheath to assist acoustic coupling with the surrounding tissues. Alternative forms of small linear arrays can be mounted on the finger or held between two fingers.

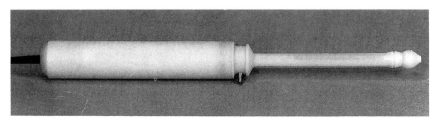

Fig. 25.3 Transducer assembly for invasive scanning (courtesy of Kretz).

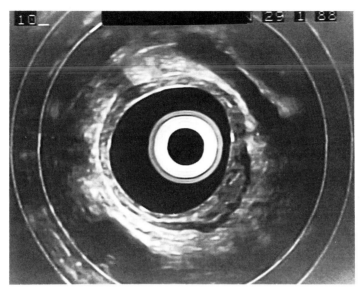

Fig. 25.4   360° radial scan at 10 MHz, showing tumour of rectal wall (courtesy of Wild S R and Pye S D).

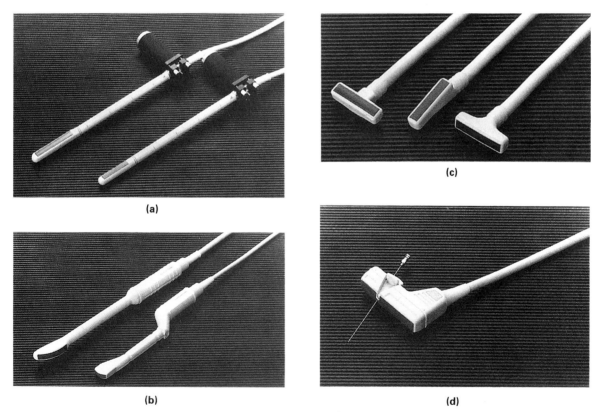

Fig. 25.5   (a) Linear arrays for invasive scanning, (b) curved forward- and side-viewing arrays for transvaginal scanning, (c) linear arrays for intra-operative scanning, (d) biopsy-guidance linear array (courtesy of Aloka).

Whereas a 360° scanner produces transverse sections of structures such as the prostate gland, a linear scanner provides longitudinal ones.

Internal sector scanners

Sector scanners can be reduced in size for internal applications. Both mechanical and phased-array techniques find application. Two phased arrays have been mounted on the same probe to permit scanning in two perpendicular planes. Curved linear arrays are also common (Fig. 25.5b). When a sector scanner is inserted into the body, the field of view normally encompasses tissues which lie ahead of the transducer. For example, the pregnant uterus can be examined with a sector scanner inserted into the vagina. This approach has been advocated as a means of using high-frequency ultrasound to get high-resolution images in early pregnancy (Fig. 25.6). Transoesophageal scanners are proving particularly popular in cardiology (Fig. 25.7).

Mechanical sector scanners have been developed in which the field-of-view direction is variable (Fig. 25.8).

Catheter scanners

It is possible to miniaturize scanners, both mechanical and electronic, so that they are only a few millimetres in diameter and can therefore be

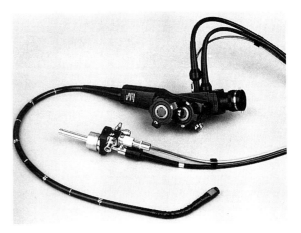

Fig. 25.7 Transoesophageal phased array for cardiology (courtesy of Toshiba).

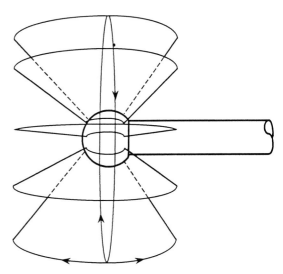

Fig. 25.8 Example of plane-of-scan variation in an invasive scanner.

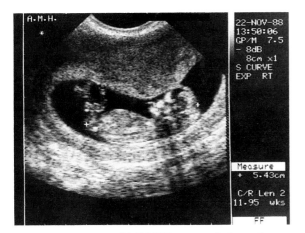

Fig. 25.6 Fetal scan with 7.5 MHz transvaginal transducer (courtesy of Smith A P M).

incorporated into catheters. Such scanners use high frequencies, 10 MHz or more, and are employed experimentally to study arteries.

INTRA-OPERATIVE SCANNERS

Intra-operative scanners are identical in principle to scanners for use external to the patient. The main differences are the smaller overall dimensions of the transducers and the fact that they usually function at frequencies of 5 MHz and above.

However, it is worth checking in each application that a high-frequency probe gives adequate penetration and that the transducer, plus cable arrangement, is suitable. Transducers for surgery take the form of sector scanners and linear arrays (Fig. 25.5c). Small dimensions and convenient shapes are prime attributes in surgical scanners. For instance, a small transducer is required for imaging via a burr hole in the skull, and a slim linear array is convenient for moving over the surface of an organ.

High-quality images can be obtained when superficial fat and muscle layers are removed, since these layers contribute greatly to distortion of the beam by processes such as refraction and absorption (Fig. 25.9).

NEEDLE GUIDANCE SYSTEMS

A real-time ultrasonic scanner is an excellent instrument for observing a needle as it penetrates soft tissue. When the comparison is made with

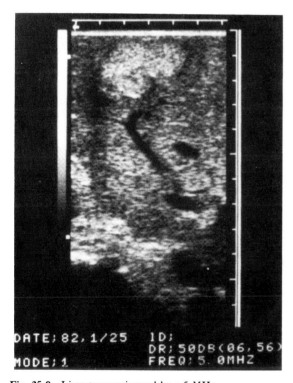

Fig. 25.9 Liver tumour imaged by a 5 MHz intra-operative linear array (courtesy of Aloka).

other medical imaging techniques such as X-ray CT or MRI, the value of ultrasonic guidance is even more evident.

The value of the technique is also made apparent by the diverse range of procedures which can be carried out when the needle is in place: soft-tissue and liquid sampling, injection of drugs and contrast agent, blood transfusion, surgical procedures, and radiotherapy implantations.

Guidance techniques

Four common approaches to ultrasonic guidance are illustrated in Figure 25.10:

1. In Figure 25.10a, a method is shown in which the region of interest is located by a scan, and the optimum needle path is determined from the image. The scanner is then removed, and the needle is inserted without further guidance. This approach is widely used for sampling large masses or liquid pools. Its main weakness is the possibility of patient movement after the scan, especially fetal movement.

2. Figure 25.10b represents a technique in which the imaging continues while the needle is inserted. However, the needle and the transducer are completely separate from one another, so the operator is required to keep the needle tip in the scan plane. This technique demands a high level of manipulative skill on the part of the operator, but it is popular since it minimizes sterility problems and allows considerable freedom of action during the procedure. The path of the needle across the ultrasonic image should be carefully worked out prior to insertion. Patient movements, large and small, may be allowed for with this method. Masses having a diameter of 1 or 2 cm can be sampled with this technique.

3. An easy, if somewhat imprecise, way of fixing the path of the needle across the field of view of the scanner is to hold the needle against the transducer as it is pushed into the tissues (Fig. 25.10c). This technique is not widely used, since, if it is important to define accurately the path of the needle, it is relatively easy to obtain a proper guidance device. However, this technique is a low-cost approach and allows freedom of action during the procedure.

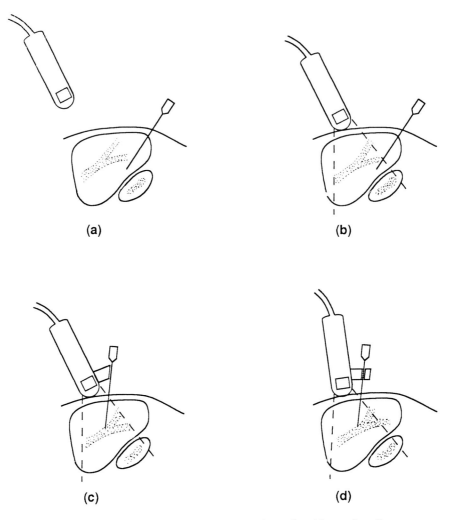

Fig. 25.10 Four conventional approaches to ultrasonic guidance of needles.

4. Most manufacturers supply either a special transducer or a transducer attachment containing a narrow guidance channel (Fig. 25.10d). As the orientation of the channel is known relative to the transducer, the needle path can be electronically marked as a line of bright dots in the image. Figure 25.5d shows a linear-array transducer with a guidance channel built into it, a few crystal elements being omitted from the array to give space for the channel. This creates a shadow across the image corresponding to the needle path. Transducer attachments are employed with all types of real-time scanner. Instruments with fixed channels vary considerably in size, design, and

ease of use. Some allow the needle orientation to be altered prior to use, while others are completely fixed. A thorough assessment of their ease of use and acceptability to the user should be carried out before purchase. The range of needle gauge accommodated by each device should also be noted, as should the feasibility of maintaining a sterile environment. Guidance channels can also be attached to invasive probes; for example, for follicle aspiration (Fig. 25.11).

A fifth method, which is less commonly employed, is one in which the needle path is not in the scan plane, but the tip of the needle is iden-

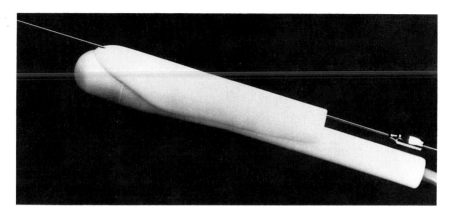

Fig. 25.11 Transvaginal transducer with needle-guidance channel (courtesy of Phillips).

tified as soon as it enters the plane. The needle is inserted along a predetermined path, and the appearance of the tip signal in the image confirms whether or not it is in a region of interest. This method is of some value where fine needles are prone to bend and cannot be relied upon to stay in the scan plane. In a few instances, this approach is the method of choice; for example, for inserting needles into the prostate gland.

Needle-tip identification

In practice, some difficulty can be experienced in detecting the echo from the needle tip. Tip-detection difficulties are usually encountered with fine needles, e.g. 20 or 22 gauge (0.92 or 0.71 mm). The degree of difficulty depends on which of the above guidance techniques is used and the echogenicity of the tissues.

Uncertainty as to the part of the needle producing the echo can arise with all gauges of needle. If the angle of the needle to the ultrasound beam is close to 90°, strong echoes may be obtained from the body of a smooth needle, as well as the tip. This difficulty can be overcome by additional scanning to establish the full extent of the needle in the field of view.

The difficulty in detecting the tip of a fine needle is probably the result of several factors. If the tip echo is of a size similar to that from surrounding tissues, it may appear momentarily as the scan plane is altered and not be recognized. In another situation, the tip echo may interfere with the echoes from organ parenchyma and become part of the speckle pattern. The echo signal may also be missed if the needle bends in such a way that the tip is not in the expected place. Attempts have been made to solve this problem by shaping the needle tip with the aim of increasing the level of ultrasound scattered back to the transducer. The smooth surface of a needle, inside or outside, is sometimes roughened to increase its scattering properties. These modifications are partially successful.

It is also worth noting that the size of the echo from the body of a smooth needle varies rapidly with the angle of orientation of the needle to the ultrasound beam. For example, if the beam-to-needle angle changes from 90 to 70°, the echo size drops by 100 to 1, a 40 dB drop. This explains why the echo along a needle may vary from very strong and saturated to extremely weak in the same image.

Given the suitability of ultrasonics for needle guidance, further sophistication of the equipment is justified to make the technique more precise and easy to use. One approach has been to attach a crystal to the needle or its stylet. Then a signal is generated when the scanning beam strikes the needle. This signal can be used to indicate the position of the tip in the image. Sonically sensitive needles have been fairly fully developed, but have not yet found widespread clinical application.

CATHETER GUIDANCE

Although not widely used, ultrasonic imaging can be employed to observe catheters directly and to manipulate them. Sonically sensitive catheters can also be made, based on the same principles as sonically sensitive needles. Since catheters or their stylets are typically a few millimetres in diameter, it is relatively easy to mount piezoelectric elements on their ends. Even though the catheter bends, the registration of the marker spot is still accurate.

LITHOTRIPSY GUIDANCE

Ultrasonic real-time B-scanners are often employed as the imaging devices for the localization of the focal region of a shock-wave lithotripter on the kidney stone or other matter to be destroyed. The transmission of the ultrasonic beam and the shock wave to the patient can be conveniently achieved by using a water-bath.

ULTRASONIC ENDOSCOPES

Both linear-array and rotating-transducer scanners have been built into the ends of flexible optical endoscopes. Figure 25.12 shows an ultrasonic endoscope with a rotating transducer on its end. The ability to position, optically, the ultrasonic probe on the inside wall of a body cavity for the examination of adjacent structures is proving valuable; e.g., to image the pancreas through the stomach wall (Fig. 25.13). At present, the highest-frequency device available functions at 10 MHz,

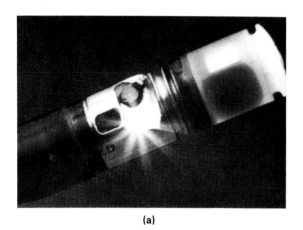

(a)

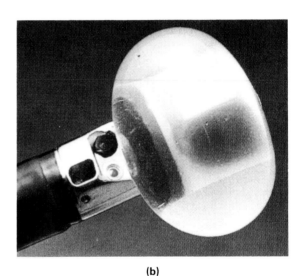

(b)

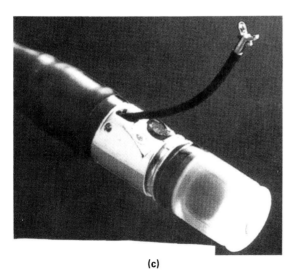

(c)

Fig. 25.12 Endoscopic rotating-transducer scanner showing (a) side-view fibre optics, with tranducer in plastic cylinder, (b) liquid-filled balloon to improve contact, and (c) biopsy channel (courtesy of Olympus).

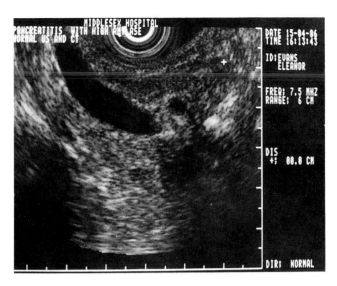

Fig. 25.13 Pancreatic image obtained with the 7.5 MHz endoscopic scanner in the stomach (courtesy of Lees W R).

but one hopes this will be increased in the future. Apart from giving better resolution, higher-frequency transducers can be made of smaller dimensions.

There is a conflict in the optimization of the design of the ultrasonic and optical parts of an endoscope. For example, in the instrument shown in Figure 25.12, the mounting of the ultrasound transducer on the end means that the optical view is at an angle to the forward direction. The pressure on space is further increased when it is desired to include a biopsy channel in the unit. A biopsy channel is not always available.

Considerable expertise is required to coordinate the optical and ultrasonic functions. Since the ultrasonic transducer cannot be directly observed, less positional information is supplied to aid the interpretation of the ultrasonic images. Familiar structures are also imaged from unusual angles. A water-filled balloon is often used to provide acoustic coupling between the transducer and the tissues. In addition, the balloon moves the scanned structures 1 or 2 cm from the transducer face to where the beam shape is improved, and reverberation echoes from the transducer head are not a problem.

INVASIVE DOPPLER METHODS

Simple continuous-wave Doppler units, duplex systems, and colour-flow imaging techniques can all be applied invasively (Plate 9). Only a few imaging techniques have been developed such as cardiac flow imaging by a phased-array transducer in the oesophagus, or the use of a CW device during peripheral vascular surgery. Such phased-array transducers typically contain 32 elements and the dimensions of their face are 10 by 10 mm (Fig. 25.7). Such instruments produce real-time pulse-echo and colour-flow images at frame rates up to 40/s.

STERILIZATION AND SAFETY

Unless it has been specifically stated that a transducer, needle, or catheter can be sterilized by high temperature in an autoclave unit, this method should be avoided since some plastics and bonding cements may be damaged. Ethylene oxide sterilization is often recommended, but it is slow and not always available. Advice on sterilization is readily available, but guarantees are not.

Scanning is most easily made sterile by covering

the probe with a sterile polythene or latex-rubber membrane and using a sterile coupling liquid.

Invasive devices should be carefully examined from the point of view of mechanical and electrical safety. With reference to electrical safety, suitability for use in the presence of anaesthetic gases should be checked.

SUMMARY

We saw that all of the imaging and Doppler technology that had been developed for transcutaneous applications could be modified for internal use. Ultrasonic methods are particularly well suited to the guidance of biopsy needles. Using invasive techniques greatly reduces the four main sources of degradation of ultrasonic images, namely bone, gas, fat, and muscle, and allows high frequencies to be employed.

26. Display and recording

CATHODE-RAY-TUBE (CRT) DISPLAYS

The basic operating principle of a CRT was described in Chapter 1. Here we will consider the display aspects of tubes. Under typical conditions of use, the echo-spot brilliance levels have a maximum ratio of 10 to 1, that is, 20 dB. With care, this can be extended, but the above figures are typical of viewing ultrasonic images.

A feature of a CRT display is the small spot that can be moved extremely quickly around the screen. The achievable spot size varies with the size of the tube; for example, a 0.3 mm diameter size for a screen of side length 10 cm; 0.4 mm for 20 cm; and 0.5 mm for 30 cm. The spot size is therefore larger relative to the screen size for small screens, and it can be comparable to the image resolution resulting from ultrasonic factors. For example, in a quarter-life-size image on a 10 cm screen, the spot size of 0.3 mm corresponds to 1.2 mm of tissue.

The persistence of both white and green, phosphor screens is short, the brightness decaying to 1% of the spot brilliance in about 0.5 ms after the removal of the echo signal.

Television CRTs

Tubes used in black-and-white television monitors are similar to the basic CRT units described. We noted earlier that the image is presented on them by moving the display spot in a raster (Ch. 1). The presence of raster lines has implications for the resolution of an image. Consider a television-raster display consisting of 500 horizontal lines. Observing test images, one finds that, in the vertical direction, detail down to 1/250 of the vertical dimension can just be resolved, that is, detail which straddles at least two lines. Resolution of adjacent spots along a television line is designed to be similar to the vertical resolution by constructing video amplifiers with adequate response. Thus, for an image of tissue area 250 × 250 mm filling the screen, the vertical and horizontal resolution owing to the television performance is 1 mm in either direction. If the image is magnified to, say, 50 × 50 mm of tissue area, the television factors put a limit on resolution of 0.2 mm in each direction. Nonstandard television displays with 1000 or more raster lines have not yet been employed in ultrasonic imaging, though they have been used in other medical imaging techniques which have higher resolution.

Distortion of an image on a television display can be quite marked and can introduce errors in distances measured from the screen. Distortion is checked by imaging a test piece consisting of a regular array of reflectors or by using a test-pattern generator (Fig. 15.15).

Television images are generated by reading echo data from a scan-converter memory.

Colour-television display

Colour displays are now being used more in medical ultrasound. A few experimental units have been produced in which echo amplitude is colour-coded. In Doppler imaging, blood velocity and direction are related to colour. The limited use of colour is somewhat surprising, considering the increased information content of domestic colour television compared to black-and-white. It may be that ultrasonic images are only acceptable when the echo data is greatly compressed, as in a grey-tone display, or that the best way of utilizing a colour display has still to be discovered.

Colour-television tubes differ from a standard CRT in three ways.

1. The screen usually consists of a regular array of extremely small dots of red, green, and blue phosphor material (Fig. 26.1a). There are over one million phosphor dots in a colour-television tube.

2. Three electron guns are built into the tube to provide three beams.

3. A metal shadow mask, with many holes, accurately aligned with the phosphor dots, allows each beam to strike only one type of phosphor (Fig. 26.1b).

There are, effectively, three CRT displays in the one vacuum vessel. Each beam scans in the normal raster fashion and generates bright spots of its allocated colour. The phosphor dots are very close together and are not resolved by the eye at a normal viewing distance. At any point in the screen, the eye sees a combination of red, blue, and green light, and the relative amounts of these primary colours determine the actual colour perceived.

Relating a physical quantity, such as speed or echo amplitude, to colour is rather arbitrary and usually determined by what the instrument designer thinks the user will find most useful. The most popular colour-coding is to relate the size of the quantity to a 'temperature' colour scale in which low values are coded as shades of blue while increasing values are presented as red through orange to white. This is considered to be a natural scale familiar to users. Alternative colour-coding has been tried, but has rarely been found to be popular; for example, the sequence of colours in the rainbow has been related to signal size.

Liquid-crystal displays

Liquid crystals alter their transparency when a voltage is applied to them. Compact panels of liquid crystals are constructed which are convenient for the display of diagrams and data. Portable personal computers make use of these display panels. Liquid-crystal displays do not exhibit grey tones, so their use in ultrasonics is limited as a means of presenting information. Crystal displays for colour images are available. Slim display devices which can be hung on the wall have long been the dream of designers in this field.

FILM RECORDING OF IMAGES

Transparency film

Film has some obvious attractions as a means of recording grey tones: high resolution, convenience, and reasonable cost. Its main deficiency is that it is not reusable. Comparison of films is undertaken by studying their characteristic curves of optical density versus exposure, where exposure is the intensity of the incident light multiplied by the duration of the recording (Fig. 26.2). Two important parameters can be identified from comparison of these curves. The first is the speed of the film. It can be seen that some films require a larger exposure than others before they begin to exhibit blackening. The second parameter is the gradient of the curve, referred to as the film contrast, or film gamma. High-gamma films are said to have high-contrast properties; that is, for a relatively small increase in exposure, they quickly change from clear to dark. In medical imaging, the

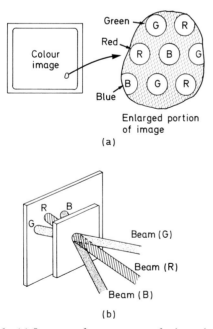

Fig. 26.1 (a) Structure of common type of colour-television screen, (b) three electron beams that strike the screen, producing a range of colours.

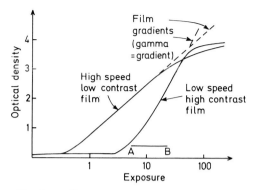

Fig. 26.2 Characteristic response curves of film.

speed and contrast of a film are rarely quoted absolutely; rather, the film is compared qualitatively with other films, and the display and camera settings for its use are established by trial and error.

The idea of film latitude, that is, margin for error in exposure, is important in practice. Consider the situation in which a certain range of brightness levels has to be recorded, for example, in correspondence to the brilliance levels of echo dots. The exposure range to be accommodated is shown by the length of the bar AB in Figure 26.2. By careful setting up of the exposure, one can record the brightness levels in both the high-and low-gamma films. On the other hand, if the exposure level is set, for example, slightly high, as the brightness levels drift, the high brightness levels will be recorded almost equally black on the high-gamma film, but their differences will be preserved in the lower-gamma film. The lower-gamma film is said to have a better latitude. Note that if the film gamma is very high, it will probably never be possible to accommodate the exposure range. With a very low-gamma film, the high-density levels of blackness are never produced on the film, and the image lacks contrast.

Commercially available films have been developed especially for grey-tone imaging from CRT screens. Because their gamma values cover a small range, the final selection of a film boils down to personal preference. These films are available in a variety of forms; for example, 10 × 8 inch sheet or 100 mm sheet for cassette cameras, and 35 or 70 mm roll film. The availability of daylight rapid-processing facilities makes film recording a popular technique. In particular, multiformat

cameras are a convenient way of recording several images on sheet film (Fig. 26.3). These cameras record a variable number of exposures per sheet, for example, 1, 4, 6, 9, and 16.

Laser imagers

In this type of device, the image signal varies with the intensity of a laser beam as it is scanned systematically across a film. Very high-resolution recording is possible; for example, 4000 × 5000 pixels and 256 exposure levels on a 35 × 43 cm film. The image information is fed to the unit in digital or video form and stored in an internal memory. Laser imagers are very expensive and are designed to serve many imaging modalities at the same time.

Polaroid film

The attractions of Polaroid film are the speed and convenience with which the final image is obtained. On the debit side, although the capital costs are low, the running costs are high. Greytone Polaroid films have been developed for medical imaging (Type 611, 8.3 × 10.8 cm prints). As with normal film, the resolution of Polaroid film is high compared to that of ultrasonic images.

Some points are worth noting regarding the handling of Polaroid film:

1. The camera rollers should be cleaned regularly; otherwise, solidified developing-liquid produces regularly spaced white marks on the print.

2. The film should be extracted from the camera-back by a straight, steady pull. Deviations from this technique can cause the resultant image to have a corner missing, or to have a variation in the grey-shade pattern. Too rapid a pull produces bubbles in the developing-liquid, resulting in fine white dots in the image.

3. During the developing time, the print and the negative should not be pressed or bent, as this influences the uniformity of the developer layer between them.

4. The developing time for the particular room temperature should be ascertained from the chart

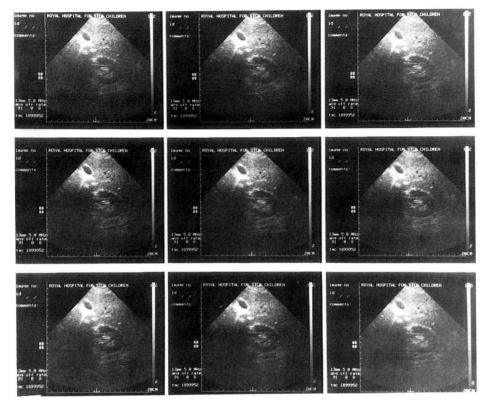

Fig. 26.3 Example of the versatility of multiformat image recording — one large image per sheet or groups of images.

supplied with each packet, and it should be adhered to for best grey-tone results.

Cameras which produce a finished print automatically avoid these problems.

Matching display to film gamma (gamma correction)

Consider a display system in which the light intensity of the displayed spots is directly related to the echo-signal amplitude in a linear fashion (Fig. 26.4a). When the echoes are recorded on film, the response characteristic of the film will probably result in their optical film densities not being linearly related to their amplitudes (Fig. 26.4b). This distortion in grey tones can be corrected by an amplifier in the display module that alters the echo amplitudes to produce a linear increase in optical density (Fig. 26.4c). The display is then said

to have a gamma-correction feature to match it to the film.

Just as a display system can be designed to suit a film, it can also be designed to suit the response of the eye. In some equipment, the display is optimized for direct observation, and, when a camera is placed in position, a switch is activated automatically to alter the gamma correction from that for viewing to that for photography with a specified film.

Colour film

For convenience, large- and small-area Polaroid film packs are used (20 × 25 cm and 8.3 × 10.8 cm), but they are rather expensive; 35 mm colour film is also employed to make slides and subsequent prints, although it has slow speed and little latitude. Colour Polaroid has an acceptable quality for many applications.

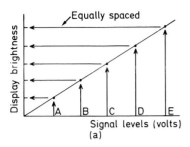

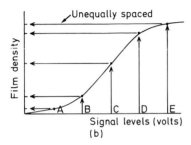

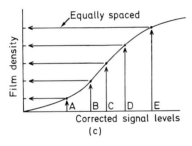

Fig. 26.4 Gamma correction to relate echo-signal level linearly to film density by allowing for the characteristics of the film.

PAPER RECORDING OF IMAGES

Direct print photography

Optical transfer of an image from a display screen to photographic paper results in high-quality prints. The bromide paper is supplied as a large roll and is advanced in steps into a cassette after each exposure. After processing in a rapid X-ray film processor, large glossy prints are obtained. This approach is economical and ergonomically suited to routine scanning sessions. A character generator for immediate labelling of the displayed image is useful. Since the final image is a print, some sacrifice of the number of presented grey shades is involved, as noted in Chapter 10. Recording paper is supplied by several manufac-

turers, including those who make photographic film. The development of photographic roll paper for recorders is a field in which new products are continually appearing.

Fibre-optic chart recording

Normal ultraviolet recording paper in a fibre-optic chart recorder stores images, but the range of grey tones is limited to 4 or 5. The image is usually transferred, line by line, to slowly moving paper. A thermal processor added to a fibre-optic chart recorder offers a wider grey-tone range on thermographic paper.

Video thermal imagers (black-and-white)

Reasonably small and inexpensive video image recorders have been manufactured in which a previously stored image is transferred, line by line, to thermally sensitive paper. This is achieved by using a linear array of very small heating elements. The range of grey tones visible in such prints is about 12, and it is therefore comparable to other types of print. The spatial resolution of this type of imager is adequate for ultrasonic images. These instruments are very compatible with ultrasonic scanning.

Video thermal imagers (colour)

Colour images can be printed by superimposing three images, each in a particular primary colour. To produce each primary-colour image, the heating elements in an array cause dye of the appropriate colour to be transferred to the paper from a sheet of material which is placed between the elements and the recording paper. This type of thermal recorder is very convenient for ultrasonic imaging.

Colour printers

Colour printers are also available which create the colours with primary-colour ink-jets or ribbons. They are found as output devices for computer graphics and Doppler spectra. Since they do not use video signals, they are not compatible with many ultrasonic instruments. One attraction is that the output is a large sheet of paper on which a substantial amount of information can be printed.

ELECTRONIC RECORDING

Video-tape recorder (VTR)

Electronic signals associated with television images have a standardized format. They are commonly generated by a camera pointing at the scene to be televised. The output signals from digital scan converters are also of this standard format. Great flexibility and compatibility exist in equipment consisting of cameras, video-tape recorders, scan converters, character generators, and display units. The standard television format of a line of picture information is shown in Figure 26.5a.

In a video-tape recorder, the picture information is recorded by magnetizing a metal-oxide tape. The electronic image signals are passed to a writing head that produces related variations in a localized magnetic field. As the head crosses the tape, which also moves between reels, each frame of the image is written as a magnetized line across the tape (Fig. 26.5b). On the playback, the head sweeps across the moving tape to detect the variations in magnetization, and so reproduce the picture information. Most video-tape recorders can deal with both black-and-white and colour pictures.

A frame-pause facility stops the tape and causes the reading head to sweep repeatedly over the same line of information. In most inexpensive recorders, the frame-pause image is of low quality, since, with the tape stopped, the recording head does not move exactly along the magnetized line on the tape. More expensive recorders have a superior frame-pause performance. Consider buying those priced just outside the normal domestic range, at the start of the industrial range.

Cassettes employed in video-tape recorders are not compatible with all types of machine. A large domestic market exists for video-tape recorders, so there will, no doubt, be improvements in price and performance.

Video disc

Television images can be recorded on magnetized discs. Usually about 100 frames can be recorded on one disc. An advantage of this approach is that any frame can be selected and displayed as a high-quality image.

Magnetic digital disc

We have seen the advantages of digital techniques in diagnostic ultrasound, the digital scan converter being a particularly important example. An image stored in digital form can be readily transferred to a digital storage disc. Inexpensive discs, known as 'floppy' discs since some are flexible, are well suited to this purpose. Floppy discs typically store a dozen images and could be used for archiving, but film is still most commonly used for this purpose. 'Hard' discs have a larger capacity, typically storing a few hundred images. They are usually fixed in the machine and are used for storing recent scans. A guide to the number of ultrasonic images which may be stored on a disc is obtained

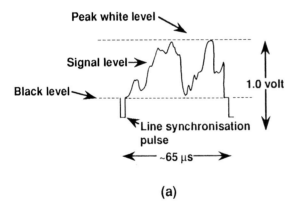

(a)

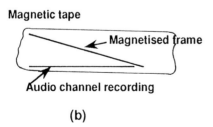

(b)

Fig. 26.5 (a) Standard format of a video line signal; (b) recording of TV image and audio signal on magnetic tape.

by multiplying its capacity (quoted in megabytes) by four; for example, a 20 megabyte disc holds 80 images. Digital discs are not yet widely employed in ultrasonic imaging, but are common in X-ray computed tomography and magnetic resonance imaging.

Digital tape

Magnetic tape, usually in a cassette, can be employed to store large numbers of images at low cost. For example, a 40 megabyte tape stores 160 images.

Optical laser disc

Image information can be stored in digital form on light-sensitive material, the reflectivity or transparency of the material being altered by the recording process. Optical discs have a very large capacity; typically, 5000 ultrasonic images may be accommodated. Unlike magnetic devices, they cannot be erased and reused, at present; but, if we consider the capacity of each disc, their price is reasonable, and they can be used for archiving.

With any of these means of recording and replay, if a system is functioning properly, the directly viewed and replayed images should look similar.

RECORDING REAL-TIME IMAGES

Real-time operation is of central importance to both pulse-echo and colour-flow imaging. Some aspects of recording with specific reference to moving images are therefore worth further study.

Photography

The simplest technique is to photograph several frames of the display with a 35 mm or Polaroid camera. Ideally, the camera shutter should be synchronized electronically with the scanner so that the exposure time matches the duration of a whole number of image frames. If synchronization is not available, it is still possible to record an image with a simple camera, but two problems arise in this situation. With a short exposure time — for example, 0.125 s — an exact whole number

of frames may not be recorded, giving a different brightness level in part of the photograph. On the other hand, if the exposure time is long — for example, 1 s — the influence of any additional fraction of a frame is reduced, but the tissue structures will probably move during the exposure.

Another degree of synchronization found in cardiac systems involves the camera shutter, the ECG, and the image-frame sweep. An image at a selected phase of the cardiac cycle can then be obtained.

Cine-photography

Cine-photography is a practical proposition if an automatic film-developing unit is available. The developed film is studied in detail, either frame by frame or as a projected moving image.

A professional cine-camera often requires 16 mm film and makes exposures at a frame rate of about 24/s. The film is moved in discrete steps, and the shutter is opened between steps to make an exposure. Much of the time (about 50%) is spent moving the film. The exposure time should be equal to that required to present one real-time frame on the display screen. To allow time for film movement, one may be able to photograph only every second real-time frame, which is inadequate to record the detailed movements of heart valves. Detailed study of fast tissue movement or blood flow is best performed by examining successive frames of a digital store cine-loop (Fig. 26.6).

Television video recording

The best approach to real-time recording is to pass the ultrasonic image to a scan converter, and then to read it out to a VTR, line by line, in television format. Because digital scan converters have other valuable features, such as frame-freeze, this is the most logical way to incorporate video recording into equipment.

The attractions of video-tape recording of real-time images are summarized as follows:

1. Ease of recording and replay
2. A sound commentary or, possibly, a physiologic signal may be recorded
3. Tapes and cassettes may be reused or stored

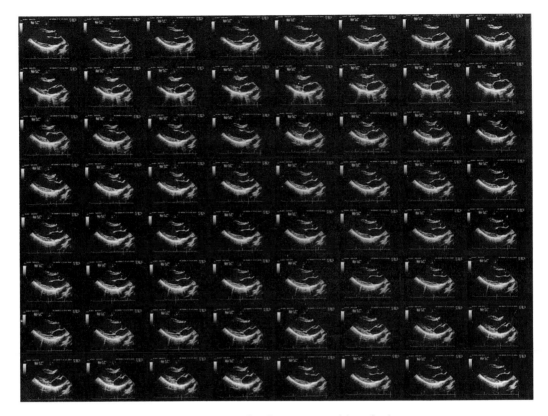

Fig. 26.6   Large series of 64 images as stored in a cine-loop

4. Slow-action replay or frame hold
5. Processing of signals on replay
6. Reasonable cost

Fibre-optic chart recording

If a real-time frame is stored in a scan converter, it is possible to print it out, line by line, via a fibre-optic chart recorder. Real-time frames and related M-mode traces can then be written on the same length of paper.

It is also possible to record a rapid succession of real-time frames on paper using a fibre-optic chart recorder. This is rarely done, as other methods seem more appropriate.

SETTING UP DISPLAY AND RECORDING UNITS

Techniques for setting up displays were discussed in Chapter 7. To optimize the recording of images,

we find it best to vary systematically the factors such as brilliance, contrast, and camera aperture, and then to select the best image from the large number recorded. When the best image is selected, a check should be made to see that the display screen and camera are still sharply focused.

ASSESSMENT OF RECORDING INSTRUMENTS AND MEDIA

The choice of recording technique depends on factors determined by the policies in each clinical department. However, some general statements can be made which act as a guide to selection.

Table 26.1 can be employed to work out approximately the relative costs of some common recording methods. The costs are calculated by taking into account the number of images to be recorded in a year and the depreciation of the recording device. If the number of recordings per annum exceeds 10 000, the device can be ignored,

Table 26.1 Relative costs per shot of recording techniques and of devices. Unit cost taken as that of 1 black and white thermal print.

Medium		Device
Polaroid (black -and-white)	5	6000
Polaroid (colour)	7	6000
Thermal paper (black-and-white)	1	10 000
Thermal paper (colour)	4	20 000
Multiformat film sheet	5	40 000

and the cost of materials predominates. It should be remembered that a sheet of multiformat film records several images, but it has associated development costs. The shelf life of the recorded image should be checked to see if it complies with legal requirements for the retention of diagnostic images.

Table 26.2 gives an indication of the performance of recording media from the points of view of quality of recording, and convenience.

RECORDING DOPPLER DATA

There are a number of reasons for recording a basic Doppler signal, a sonogram, or a colour-flow image.

1. Re-examination of results
2. Later analysis of the signals
3. Collection of a library of typical results
4. Acquisition of teaching material

A large amount of information is contained in a Doppler record of even a few seconds' length, and it is quite common to make records at various sites in the body. Fortunately, methods exist for recording Doppler sounds accurately and quite inexpensively.

Audio-tape recording

A good-quality, domestic, stereophonic cassette recorder is suitable for Doppler signals since they are in the audio frequency range. Such a domestic recorder will operate up to frequencies around 20 kHz. Although this frequency response is adequate, the level of the recording of a signal of constant power varies slightly at different frequencies, a fact which may need to be taken into account if the recorded signal is later used in the quantitative calculation of blood flow (Fig. 26.7). From the point of view of sonogram quality, it is usually difficult to distinguish sonograms which have been produced directly from those which have come via a tape recorder (Fig. 26.8).

Table 26.2 Recording media

Medium	Quality	Convenience
Film (black-and-white, colour)		
35-mm	★★★★★	★★
X-ray	★★★★★	★★★★
Polaroid	★★★	★★★★★
Cine	★★★★	★
Paper		
Photographic	★★★★	★★★
Thermal	★★★★	★★★★★
Magnetic and optical		
Magnetic digital disc	★★★★★	★★★
Magnetic digital tape	★★★★★	★★
Optical digital disc	★★★★★	★★★
Video-tape	★★★	★★★★
Audio-analogue tape	★★★	★★★★
Audio-digital tape	★★★★★	★★★★

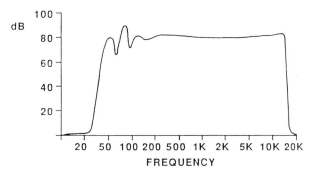

Fig. 26.7 Typical frequency response of an audio-tape recorder. Note that the unit does not store low-frequency signals at equal levels.

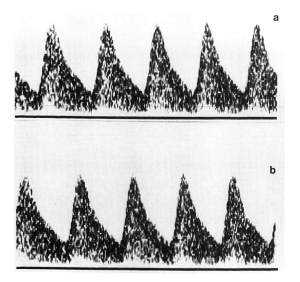

Fig. 26.8 (a) Directly analysed sonogram, (b) sonogram analysed after storage on an audio tape.

A stereophonic system records simultaneously on two channels, so forward flow can be recorded on one channel while reverse flow is recorded on the other. Separate forward and reverse signals must be supplied by the Doppler instrument, as is usually the case. This type of domestic tape recorder will not record quadrature Doppler signals with sufficient accuracy in amplitude and phase for accurate reproduction. It is, however, unlikely that most users of Doppler equipment would want to make such recordings.

A cassette normally stores two stereophonic recordings, each of 30 or 45 minutes' duration, which will typically represent the signals gathered in 20 clinical examinations. Cassettes can be freely transferred between recorders since they all operate on the same international standard. Longer recordings can be made on reel-to-reel units, but they are inconvenient to use, and the searching for previous recordings is time-consuming.

Since a Doppler signal strongly resembles a noise signal, rather than a harmonic musical sound, noise-reduction techniques are best avoided when recording Doppler sounds. The noise-reduction switch, usually labelled with a trade name such as Dolby or ANRS, should be in the 'OFF' position. Noise-reduction techniques are designed to reduce tape hiss, so, if a reasonably strong Doppler sound is being recorded, the result will not be affected by having no noise reduction.

Prior to each Doppler recording, it is desirable to record, with a microphone, information such as patient's name, date, examination site, etc. Otherwise, identification of the recording at a later date depends on careful noting of tape position, using the numeric display on the recorder. Unfortunately, it is becoming increasingly difficult to find recorders with microphone inputs.

Good-quality tapes should be purchased. It is a false economy to use cheap tapes, which can be very poor indeed.

Finally, audio-tape recorders are often susceptible to picking up stray signals from neighbouring equipment. If this is a problem, try moving the recorder to another place. Switching off the other equipment, in turn, should allow the source of the pick-up to be identified.

Desirable features of tape recorders

1. Audio quality
The recorder should handle equally all frequencies of interest. Its frequency response should be flat to within 1 or 2 dB over a frequency range from 50 Hz to 15 kHz. A recorder from any well-known manufacturer costs a small fraction of the cost of the rest of the Doppler system.

2. Recording and playback sound-level indicators

The magnitude of the Doppler signal must be large enough to be well above the background noise, but not so large as to be distorted. The gain of an amplifier in either the Doppler unit or the recorder is adjusted to achieve this. Indicators on the recorder show the level of the signal during record or playback. Because Doppler signals are often very pulsatile, these indicators must have a fast response. LED (light-emitting diodes) arrays are ideal and are generally better than moving-needle meters.

3. Ganged-level controls

The forward- and reverse-flow signals recorded on the separate stereophonic channels must be amplified by the same amount. The two gain-control knobs should therefore be set at the same level. This is often done by linking (ganging) the controls together. In some systems, one control influences both channels.

4. Tape-position counter

This counter shows numerically the position of a recording on the tape. Since many recordings are made on each tape, this is a much-used feature for fast retrieval of recordings. For convenience, it is best to have a counter which does not lose its present value when the instrument is switched off. This avoids having to rewind the tape each time the unit is switched on to re-establish the counter value. Different machines often have different types of counter, making it difficult to locate recordings made on a different cassette deck.

5. Front loading

Front-loading recorders are much more convenient than top-loaders if the unit is to be used in a stack of equipment.

6. Remote control

Remote control is very useful, but not essential.

Digital recording

The audio-tape technique described in the previous section records the Doppler signal as variations in the magnetization of metal-oxide tape (an analogue technique). It is feasible, however, to digitize a Doppler signal, as described for echo signals in Chapter 10, and to store it as a long sequence of binary numbers.

Digital recording is attractive from several points of view; it offers lack of susceptibility to noise, accuracy of reproduction, and compatibility with computers. Digital audio-tape recorders have a performance much superior to that of analogue ones, although, at the moment, they are still relatively expensive.

Video recording

Video recording was discussed earlier in this chapter. At this point, it is worth summarizing the combination of possible simultaneous recordings.

1. Real-time pulse-echo image plus forward- and reverse-flow Doppler signals on the audio channels
2. M-scan plus forward- and reverse-flow Doppler signals on the audio channels
3. Frozen colour-flow image plus forward- and reverse-flow Doppler signals on the audio channels
4. Sonogram plus forward- and reverse-flow Doppler signals on the audio channels

Often a decision has to be made as to the type of recording device and medium to employ. Table 26.2 presents an attempt to compare the types of media in terms of quality and convenience. Costs can be calculated if the number of recordings to be made per annum is known. The cost of the device could be written off over 5 years, and the price of the servicing should be included.

SUMMARY

Display and recording devices play a crucial role in the production of high-quality images. TV tubes are still the method of choice for the presentation of black-and-white or colour images. Film viewed by transmitted light gives the best-quality images, but many new thermal printing devices provide acceptable results and are exceedingly convenient. The cost of each recording method has to be carefully calculated for each workload. Digital recording has much to commend it and may well be the method of choice in the future. Video-tape recorders are well suited to capturing the information content of real-time echo and Doppler images. Audio-tape recorders are also commonly used in Doppler work. The technology of recording is very extensive and changes rapidly.

27. Further details of ultrasonic transducers

Until now, we have mainly thought of the ultrasonic beam as being highly directional, with its intensity strongest along the central axis. This description is adequate for most diagnostic techniques. Nevertheless, the insignificant appearance of the transducer belies its importance, and a more detailed account is worthwhile. In this chapter, we will study various types of transducer used in diagnostic ultrasound and the factors that determine their suitability for particular applications.

The term 'transducer' is used widely in this and other ultrasonics texts. Strictly, 'ultrasonic transducer' would be more correct, because 'transducer' is a general term for a device that can change one form of energy into another.

From the standpoint of diagnostic ultrasound, a transducer is required to produce a narrow directional beam of fairly uniform intensity. It should also be able to generate powers of several watts and detect echoes of microwatt and milliwatt levels. It should be lightweight, small, and electrically safe. These requirements are very demanding, but they can be met through the remarkable properties of materials exhibiting the piezoelectric effect.

THE PIEZOELECTRIC EFFECT

When crystals or plastics with piezoelectric properties are subjected to pressure, an electric charge appears on their surfaces, positive on one side and negative on the other. These materials exhibit this effect because the internal electric neutrality, resulting from negative ions exactly cancelling positive ions, is disturbed when pressure is applied (Fig. 27.1). This imbalance of charge results in a voltage difference appearing between the faces of the material.

Ultrasonic echoes are detected when their pressure fluctuations affect a piezoelectric element and

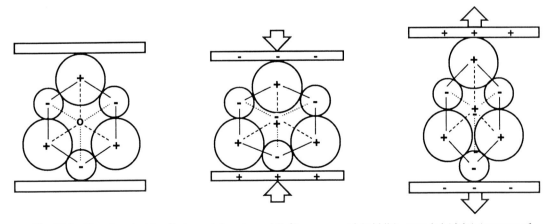

Fig. 27.1 The piezoelectric effect: crystal unstressed (left), compressed (middle), extended (right) (courtesy of Wells PNT).

cause small voltages to be produced. Ultrasound is generated by using the converse of the piezoelectric effect; a fluctuating voltage is applied to an element, causing its thickness to vary. Typically, in a crystal of a 2.5 MHz transducer of 0.75 mm thickness, the application of a pressure of 1.75×10^5 N/m^2 results in 3.3 volts appearing across it (1.75×10^5 N/m^2 = 1.75 atmosphere = the pressure amplitude, p_0, of 1 W/cm^2 ultrasound in soft tissue). When 100 volts are applied to the same crystal, its thickness changes by 3.74×10^{-5} mm. These are typical of some of the higher values of pressure and crystal voltages occurring in diagnostic ultrasonic techniques.

Piezoelectric materials

The piezoelectric effect is exhibited both by naturally occurring crystals and by synthetic ceramic and plastic materials. Examples of natural materials are quartz, lithium sulphate, and Rochelle salt. They rarely find application in diagnostic ultrasound. Most ultrasonic transducers are made from a ceramic solid solution of lead zirconate and lead titanate, known by trade names such as PZT-5. These ceramic materials have some attractive properties; they are cheap, easily shaped, efficient, and can be driven by relatively low voltages. They represented a big advance in the technology of diagnostic ultrasonic instruments when they were introduced. The plastic, polyvinyldifluoride (PVDF), is finding increasing application, particularly at higher frequencies, since it is easy to make and manipulate thin sheets of this material. PVDF has a lower acoustic impedance than ceramic PZT and is therefore better matched to soft tissue. PVDF has reception characteristics similar to those of PZT, but is not as good a transmitter. Composites consisting of a mixture of ceramic and plastic materials are also being evaluated.

STRUCTURE OF DIAGNOSTIC TRANSDUCERS

The active element of a typical, basic ceramic transducer is a disc-shaped piezoelectric element. Dimensions of ceramic elements generally vary from a diameter of 2 cm and a thickness of 1.8 mm for a 1 MHz transducer, to a diameter of 2 mm and a thickness of 0.18 mm for a 10 MHz device. The crystal thickness determines the operating frequency range of the transducer. For a fixed frequency, the beam shape depends primarily on the diameter of the crystal. Plastic elements have similar diameters, but are thinner (e.g. 0.05 mm) and operate over a wider frequency range.

In the production of a ceramic transducer, the required frequency, f, is first ascertained, and from this the corresponding wavelength of ultrasound, λ, in the piezoelectric material is calculated from the relationship, $c = f\lambda$. The thickness of the material is then made to be equal to $\lambda/2$. We noted earlier that a fundamental resonance occurs when ultrasound of the appropriate frequency is propagated in a block of material of thickness $\lambda/2$. This results in efficient generation and detection of ultrasound. It is difficult to make thick elements of PVDF, so they are usually thin and have a correspondingly high resonance frequency (e.g. 40 MHz). The sensitivity of this type of transducer at frequencies below the resonance is uniform, so the same transducer can be operated over a range of frequencies, e.g. from 5 to 15 MHz.

Once a piezoelectric element has been made, a metallic film is put on to both of its surfaces. Wire connections are soldered to each film. It is now possible to apply a voltage to the element or to detect small voltages resulting from incident sonic vibrations. The element is mounted across the end of an electrically and acoustically insulating hollow cylinder; for example, one made from cork (Fig. 27.2). To create short ultrasonic pulses, we must damp the vibrations very quickly after the instant of excitation. This damping is achieved by filling the hollow cylinder with backing material that bonds to the element. A common backing material for ceramic elements is an epoxy resin (Araldite) loaded with tungsten powder; plastic is suitable when PVDF is the active element. Additional electrical damping of the signals is achieved by connecting an induction coil to the wire attached to the back metallic film. The assembly is finally mounted inside a metal or plastic case. When a plastic case is used, its inside wall is lined with a

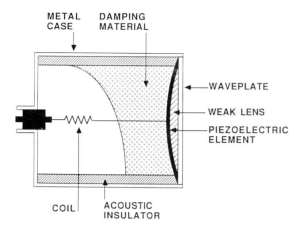

METAL CASE   DAMPING MATERIAL

WAVEPLATE

WEAK LENS

PIEZOELECTRIC ELEMENT

COIL   ACOUSTIC INSULATOR

Fig. 27.2 Structure of a basic single-element transducer. Curvature of the element and the weak lens provide focusing

thin sheet of metal to provide shielding from RF electromagnetic radiation, which is often transmitted from neighbouring equipment or broadcasting aerials. The wire from the front film on the element is then connected to earth, and the back connection taken out through a socket. On most PZT transducers, a layer of plastic is attached to the front face of the crystal. Later, we will see that this both protects the crystal and helps in transmission of ultrasound across the tissue–transducer interface.

This design of transducer is aimed at the generation and detection of short pulses, for example, those with 2 or 3 cycles of vibration. Transducers for continuous-wave operation have little or no backing material behind the element. CW Doppler transducers are included in this category.

Our studies of real-time scanners have shown that many transducers are in the form of arrays. The elements of these arrays are piezoelectric ceramics or plastics. A significant problem in the design of arrays is to maintain acoustic insulation of an element from its neighbours. The two approaches to this ideal are to make the array from completely separate elements, and to make it from one piece of material with grooves cut between the elements. The former is difficult when the elements are small; the latter gives inferior acoustic insulation. The performance of an array is also dependent on the design of the front waveplate and the backing layer. The designer also has to make

decisions on the number, area, and separation of the elements. It can be seen that there is considerable scope for variation in array performance.

GENERATION OF ULTRASOUND

Excitation of the piezoelectric element

The manner in which a fluctuating voltage is applied to an element in order to generate ultrasound depends on the nature of the wave to be produced; that is, whether it is short pulsed, long pulsed, or continuous wave. To generate a continuous wave of particular intensity and frequency, one uses a continuously alternating electric voltage of the same frequency and suitable amplitude. This type of wave is generated by CW Doppler instruments.

A few techniques, for example, pulsed-Doppler systems and colour-flow imagers, require the generation of long-pulsed waves. Such long pulses result from the application of long-pulsed electrical signals.

The very short pulses required for A, B, and M modes of scanning are created by exciting the element with a very short, sharp electric voltage that shocks it into a brief burst of vibration (Fig. 27.3). The applied voltage normally has a maximum value of a few hundred volts and the generated pulses are 1 or 2 cycles long. This shock excitation is analogous to striking a bell to make it ring.

Ultrasonic transmission across the transducer–tissue interface

There is a large difference between the acoustic impedance of the material of a crystal transducer and that of soft tissue. The problem is less severe with plastic transducers. This acoustic mismatch creates problems for both the efficient transmission and the reception of ultrasound. When an echo strikes a soft-tissue/crystal boundary, 80% of the incident energy is reflected back into the tissue. One consequence is that larger pulses have to be generated initially by the transducer. Another is that the large reflected portion of an echo may produce reverberation artefacts.

It is possible to reduce the large acoustic mismatch at the skin of the patient by inserting a layer of material between the crystal and the tissue. In

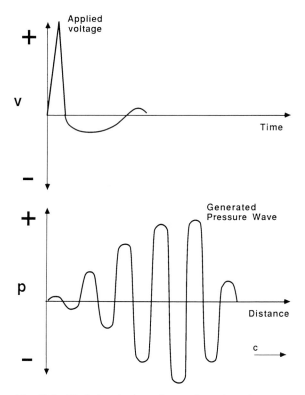

Fig. 27.3   Typical excitation voltage spike and resultant pulse wave from a transducer.

fact, it can be shown that if this matching layer has a suitably chosen acoustic impedance and is of thickness equal to a quarter of the wavelength of ultrasound ($\lambda/4$) in the layer, the transmission of ultrasound from the transducer to the soft tissue can be 100%. Plastic or tungsten-loaded Araldite has been used to make matching quarter-wavelength layers. This matching technique is most successful in Doppler instruments that operate at a well-defined wavelength. Since pulsed ultrasound contains a range of wavelengths corresponding to its bandwidth, a layer of material cannot be of thickness equal to $\lambda/4$ for all the frequency components. A matching layer is less effective, therefore, for pulsed ultrasound, but it is still well worthwhile.

Consideration of the transmission between the transducer and tissue casts some light on the question of the best coupling medium. It can be shown theoretically that the effect of a very thin layer of material between the transducer and skin is negligible, provided that the acoustic impedance of the material is not very low, such as that of air. The choice of coupling medium is therefore determined by factors of cost, acceptability, and corrosive properties.

DIAGNOSTIC ULTRASONIC BEAMS

In Chapters 1 and 5, we noted that highly directional ultrasonic beams can be generated by simple hand-held transducers. Later, in Chapter 12, we noted that it was the effective beam shape that was important in diagnostic ultrasound rather than the actual ultrasonic field. The effective beam shape was seen to influence resolution and to vary with the settings of the sensitivity controls. The intensity distribution, that is, the ultrasonic field, in front of the crystal is obviously one of the main factors determining the effective beam shape. In Chapter 1, it was indicated that the the term 'field' would be reserved for transmitted ultrasound, and that the term 'beam' would be used when the result of transmission and reception was being considered, as is usually the case in scanning.

Few studies have been undertaken to ascertain the deformation undergone by an ultrasonic beam in tissue. The intensity distribution in tissue is assumed to approximate that measured in oil or water.

Field from a perfect piston source

Initially, we will examine the idealized case of the field produced by a piston source in a non-absorbing medium, and then discuss field distributions occurring in practice. We can consider a moving crystal as a perfect piston that transmits a continuous wave of ultrasound into water. The dominant features of the theoretical shape can be considered to be like those shown in Figure 27.4. This shape consists of a gradually narrowing conical region followed by one in which there is divergence. The region of conical shape is known as the near field, or 'Fresnel zone', and that of the diverging shape as the far field, or 'Fraunhofer zone'. Outside the field shape indicated, intensity falls off rapidly.

The length of the Fresnel zone is $D^2/4\lambda$ where D is the diameter of the element, and λ the wavelength of the ultrasound in the propagating

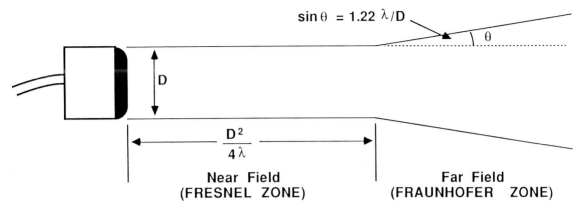

Fig. 27.4 Simplified field shape from a sinusoidally excited flat-disc transducer element generating a continuous wave.

medium. Column 2 of Table 27.1 shows a selection of values of Fresnel zone lengths. In the Fraunhofer zone, the angular divergence is given by $\sin \theta = 1.22\lambda/D$. Column 3 shows some typical values for the angle θ.

These two formulae can be used to answer two questions that frequently are asked. First, can narrower fields of ultrasound be made by reducing the diameter of the crystal? From the above formulae for Fresnel zone length and $\sin \theta$, it is evident that a decrease in D reduces the length of the Fresnel zone and increases the angle θ. Thus, by reducing the crystal diameter, the overall field actually increases in width. An optimum value for the diameter D has therefore to be calculated to give an acceptable field shape at each frequency.

The second question is: why can better lateral resolution be obtained at higher frequencies? The reader should recall that high frequencies correspond to short wavelengths. Again from the two

formulae, we see that the smaller the wavelength λ, the longer is the Fresnel zone, and the smaller the angle of divergence. Thus, it is easier to produce narrower fields with short wavelengths, that is, with high frequencies.

Intensity distribution within the field

Let us now consider the intensity distribution within the continuous-wave field shape just described. A plot of intensity along the central axis shows large fluctuations, as illustrated in Figure 27.5a. Violent fluctuations occur in the Fresnel zone, but in the Fraunhofer zone the intensity falls off smoothly with distance from the transducer. Remember that this plot is for an idealized piston action and is along the central axis of the beam. If one moves a small probe perpendicularly to the central axis at any point in the Fresnel zone, the intensity distribution would be found to consist of

Table 27.1 Fresnel zone lengths and Fraunhofer zone angles of divergence as occurring with tranducers of dimensions and frequencies used in diagnosis

Frequency/crystal diameter	Fresnel zone length, $D^2/4\lambda$ (mm)	Fraunhofer zone divergence, θ
1 MHz/20 mm	65	5°23'
2 MHz/15 mm	73	3°35'
5 MHz/8 mm	52	2° 43'
10 MHz/5mm	42	2°6'
15 MHz/3 mm	22	2°20'
25 MHz/2 mm	16	2°10'

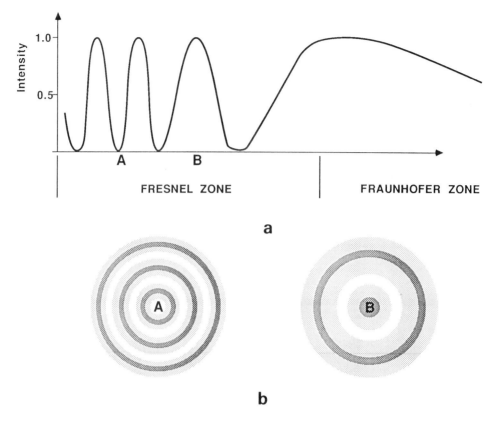

Fig. 27.5   Intensity pattern of a continuous wave from a flat disc. (**a**) Distribution of intensity along the central axis, (**b**) intensity patterns in planes perpendicular to the central axis at A and B. The dark areas represent high intensity.

a series of rings of high and low intensity. Figure 27.5b shows this for areas around the points A and B, which are located perpendicularly to the central axis. In the Fraunhofer zone, there is a more gradual variation in intensity in planes at right angles to the central axis.

At first glance, these fluctuations are alarming, and, indeed, they have occasionally been used (probably incorrectly) to explain the difficulties associated with imaging structures within a few centimetres of the transducer face. Apart from the fact that transducer crystals do not perform a perfect piston movement, there are two factors that reduce the importance of these fluctuations.

1. The distance between the off-axis rings of high and low intensity is of the order of a wavelength, that is, less than 1 mm. Most reflecting surfaces therefore intersect several rings.

2. Pulses of ultrasound contain a range of frequencies, each of which has its own pattern of maximum and minimum intensity. Because these patterns do not coincide, there is an overall smoothing of the intensity distribution of the beam.

Theoretical calculation and experimental measurement confirm that for short pulses the intensity distribution exhibits reduced fluctuations (Fig. 27.6).

The same favourable circumstances do not hold for the fields produced by CW or PW Doppler instruments. For example, a CW blood-flow detector operates at a well-defined frequency and is concerned with detecting signals from cells. The field from a Doppler instrument generating long pulses, e.g. 10 cycles in length, is very similar to a CW field of the same frequency. Doppler instru-

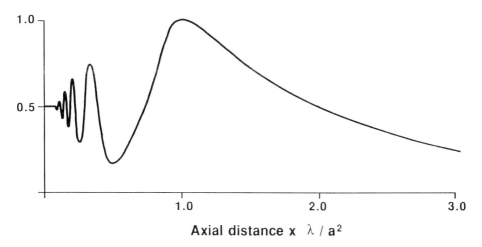

Axial distance x λ / a^2

Fig. 27.6 The intensity along the axis of a flat-disc transducer emitting a three-cycle pulse (courtesy of Pye D).

ments may have fluctuations in their intensity patterns, a fact which adds to the problems of measuring blood flow quantitatively.

Side-lobes of an ultrasonic beam (grating-lobes)

As well as the main central field of the transducer, less intense divergent side-lobes of the field are also present. The reception zone also has side-lobes. Theoretical calculations of the intensity of ultrasound in one of the more significant side-lobes indicate that it can be one-hundredth of that in the main field (20 dB lower), that is, an amplitude of one-tenth. This intensity is sufficiently high to produce detectable echoes from strong reflectors situated well off the central axis of the main beam. The intensity of the side-lobes is dependent on the details of the motion of the vibrating element. Side-lobes could obviously be a source of artefact echoes. Side-lobes are essentially part of the overall beam pattern of a transducer. When the transducer consists of an array structure of elements, i.e. a grating, the lobes are commonly called 'grating-lobes'. Grating-lobes can be a particular problem in the design of array transducers since they are often larger than the typical side-lobes of single-element devices.

A technique known as 'apodization' is often employed to reduce side-lobes or grating-lobes. The contributions to transmission and reception are made greatest from the central area of the element or array, and decrease to the sides. Apodization is most easily implemented with array transducers.

Measurement of fields and beams from echo-imaging and Doppler transducers is described in Appendix 4. It is possible to have field shapes measured at non-destructive testing laboratories that offer this service.

ULTRASOUND BEAM FOCUSING AND DEFOCUSING

Ultrasound, like light, can be focused and defocused by devices such as lenses and mirrors. Earlier we noted that the degree of focusing may be classified as weak, medium, or strong (Ch. 1) and also studied electronic focusing (Ch. 5). The analogy between light and ultrasound cannot be taken too far since optical wavelengths are about 1000 times smaller than those used in diagnostic ultrasound. Diffraction of the ultrasonic waves is therefore more obvious and results in less sharp focusing.

Lenses

An acoustic lens can be inserted into a transducer beam to provide focusing. The position of the focus may be altered by changing the lens rather than the whole transducer (Fig. 27.7). A variety

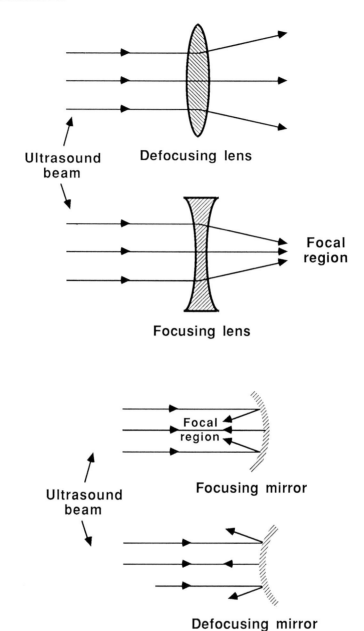

Fig. 27.7 Focusing and defocusing of ultrasound by lenses and mirrors.

of materials have been used to make lenses, for example, plastic, rubber, and aluminium. Focusing by means of a lens is used widely in diagnostic instruments.

Focusing and defocusing lenses are usually of the curvature opposite to that of their optical equivalents. This is because ultrasound travels faster in the solid lens material than in the surrounding liquid or tissue; light, on the other hand, travels slower in glass than in air. In Chapter 4, we noted that refraction at interfaces is dependent on the wave velocity in each medium. Rubber acoustic lenses have the same curvature as optical lenses. They are often seen on arrays where they focus the beam in the out-of-plane direction.

Shaped elements

Figure 1.5 illustrates beam focusing by shaping the element of the transducer. This method is commonly employed with ceramic and PVDF elements. The curvature of medium- and strong-focusing transducers is such that they are most conveniently used in a water-bath. Even with weak-focusing concave crystals, contact with the skin is problematic. The solution adopted has been to level off the curved surface with a plastic material. Although this plastic effectively forms a defocusing lens in front of the crystal, the curvature of the crystal is arranged so that the overall effect is still weak-focusing. Transducers constructed in this way are sometimes said to have 'internal focusing'.

Mirrors

Concave and convex mirrors focus and defocus ultrasound effectively (Fig. 27.7). Efficient reflection can be achieved at air and steel boundaries if the ultrasound is travelling in water.

Zone plates

It is possible to design a complex circular aperture that blocks selected parts of an ultrasonic field (Fig. 27.8). The remaining portions of the field spread out as a result of diffraction on passing through the aperture, and interference produces a high-intensity focus at a point. The reception zone of such a device is also focused. It will be useful to recall the focusing action of a complex circular aperture when holography is discussed in Chapter 28.

Zone lenses

A zone lens consists of a series of concentric rings of material of different thickness. The velocity of sound in the material of the lens is different from that of the surrounding liquid. On passing through the zone lens, the sound waves from each ring are no longer in step, that is, they are out of phase. Again, the resulting diffraction and interference produces a high-intensity focus. So far as I know, however, neither zone plates nor lenses have been used in diagnosis.

SPECIAL TRANSDUCERS

A number of special transducers have been made for particular applications. Those described below illustrate the simple variations possible in transducer design.

Stand-off transducers

Owing to the large-amplitude transmission pulse, a transducer cannot detect echoes from reflecting interfaces very close to it. There is therefore a dead space of a few millimetres immediately in front of the transducer. Typically, for a 3 MHz device this dead space is 2–5 mm in depth. One technique for detecting surfaces in the dead space is to insert a layer of material between the transducer face and the outside surface of the body. A water-bath or a layer of silicon gel material can perform this function. The inserted layer of a basic stand-off probe is usually water or oil contained in a hollow tube. One end of the tube is sealed by the transducer; the other, by a thin membrane.

Stand-off probes are used mostly in ophthalmology when measurements of dimensions are being made, and it is desired to distinguish all structures from the cornea to the retina. They also find ap-

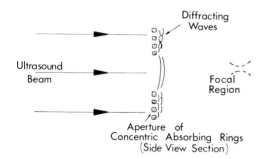

Fig. 27.8   Focusing of an ultrasonic beam, using an aperture consisting of concentric rings (zone plate).

plication in scanning neonates and in measuring tissue strata just under the skin.

Ophthalmic transducers

Transducers employed in ophthalmic applications are usually of the single-element or array-focusing types. They may, however, be regarded as somewhat special in that they are of small dimensions and operate at high frequencies (e.g. 5–20 MHz). At such high frequencies, crystals are cut thinly — for example, 0.12 mm thickness at 15 MHz — resulting in a fragility that can create constructional problems. It is easier to make high-frequency transducers with plastic piezoelectric elements. Transducers used in ophthalmologic applications of ultrasound can also be designed to allow access to the orbit or ocular system by a variety of routes.

Variable angle and soft-head transducers

If it is necessary to hold the transducer at large angles to the perpendicular from the surface of the skin, or if contact is difficult because of bone immediately below the surface, it may be possible to attach a small bag of fluid to the front of the transducer. Reverberation echoes within the bag can be reduced by keeping the thickness of the fluid layer to a minimum and by using a fluid that absorbs ultrasound, such as castor oil.

Transducers plus mechanical manipulators

Occasionally, transducers are linked with implements such as forceps to remove foreign bodies from the eye. Echoes from the tip of the forceps and the foreign body are both observed on the display screen.

SELECTION OF A TRANSDUCER FOR A PARTICULAR APPLICATION

The choice of transducer for a particular application usually boils down to selection of the highest frequency that will give the necessary penetration. Frequency apart, other considerations may make one transducer more suitable than another. The shape of the emitted beam is of particular relevance. To achieve the best overall resolution,

use an electronically focused array. However to examine structures in a particular depth range, we find that a strong-focusing, single-element transducer produces the best results.

Often, more mundane considerations determine the suitability of a transducer. For example, a device with a large-diameter crystal may be inconvenient for directing an ultrasonic beam between rib spaces. The physical size of a transducer is important when infants are examined. Similarly, contact between a concave transducer and the skin may be especially difficult in some situations.

To summarize, the three main factors influencing the selection of a transducer are penetration, beam shape, and transducer structure. Table 27.2 indicates the fields of application of transducers with frequencies in the diagnostic range.

DAMAGE TO TRANSDUCERS

Because transducers are subject to a great deal of handling, it is essential to remember that they are expensive and readily damaged. This damage is obvious if the unit ceases to function, but partial failure may result in spurious pulses being generated. The latter may possibly be observed by holding the transducer in the air and examining the display.

Ceramic crystals are brittle, and the points of connection of the wires to the metal film on the crystal are also weak. Transducers should not be subjected to violent shocks, for example, by being dropped. The window material of a mechanical device may be brittle or soft and easily punctured. The cable from the rear of a transducer can be damaged by bending it through large angles. If this cable is sealed into the body of the transducer, it may be difficult and expensive to replace. Bubble formation in the liquid of a transducer is common. At the time of purchase, it is worth checking that they can be removed easily or inexpensively. Faults in a transducer, particularly in electrical connections, may be revealed by an X-ray image.

Immersion for long periods in water or oil should be avoided, if possible, because these fluids can corrode or weaken the material of the transducer, in particular, the lens, the bonding cement, and the acoustic insulator.

Table 27.2 Transducer frequencies and their fields of application

Application	Frequency (MHz)	Comments
Head	1–3	Suitable for coupling on to skin with bone close to surface
Heart	1–5	Crystal size suitable for transmitting between ribs
Eye	5–25	Suitable for immersion scanning?
Kidney	2–5	
Obstetrics	1–5	
Abdomen	1–5	
Infants	3–7	
Liver	1–5	
Breast	2–10	Suitable for immersion scanning?
Blood vessels	3–10	
Thyroid	5–7	Suitable for immersion scanning?
Invasive	5–20	

Sooner or later, the question of sterilizing the probe may arise. Although temperatures near 100°C will not affect the piezoelectric properties of the crystals, such temperatures can have a drastic effect on the bonding cements. Gamma radiation will also damage plastics and bonding materials. Only low-temperature techniques for sterilizing should be employed, for example, that using ethylene oxide.

Transducers should be cleaned only with liquids which will not affect their surfaces. Water is probably the safest.

NON-PIEZOELECTRIC ULTRASONIC TRANSDUCERS

It is interesting to note other methods for generating and detecting ultrasound.

Magnetostrictive transducers

Magnetostrictive transducers make use of the fact that some magnetic materials, such as iron and nickel, change their dimensions when subjected to a magnetic field. The material is surrounded by a wire coil through which a varying current is passed to produce a fluctuating magnetic field. This field generates vibrations in the material. Conversely, sonic waves striking the magnetic material cause it to vibrate. Changes in the magnetic field of the material result from these vibrations and cause a current to flow in a surrounding wire. By this means, ultrasonic waves can be detected.

Magnetostrictive transducers are used in cleaning baths, where they generate high-power ultrasound, for example, 100 W at frequencies around 30 kHz. They are also found in surgical devices sometimes referred to as 'sonic scalpels'.

Electromagnetic and electrostatic transducers

Transducers can be designed to make use of the electromagnetic forces that act between wires carrying electric current. Varying the currents causes the wires to vibrate. Another interesting type depends on the forces between electrostatically charged metal plates. Electrostatic transducers are highly sensitive over a wide frequency range and could find application in diagnostic ultrasonics.

Mechanical transducers

Whistles and sirens, which generate ultrasound by passing high-pressure gas through orifices, can be made to generate high-powered ultrasound of frequencies up to 100 kHz.

One of the first ultrasonic transducers was a whistle used by Galton in 1883 to study the limits of hearing.

SUMMARY

New piezoelectric materials are being produced, contributing to the improved performance of transducers. The structure of transducers was discussed. Since the performance of transducers is dependent on many design and production factors, the clinical performance of each must be individually checked. To provide further insight into the generation of ultrasound and beam shapes, we considered these topics from a theoretical point of view. Further information on focusing of beams was outlined. The possibility of making transducers for special purposes was demonstrated. Finally, the high cost and ease of damage of some modern transducers were emphasized.

REFERENCES

Silk M G 1984 Ultrasonic transducers for nondestructive testing. Adam Hilger, Bristol
Tarnoczy T 1965 Sound focussing lenses and waveguides. Ultrasonics 3: 115–127
Wealthall S R, Todd J H 1972 A soft ended probe for echo-encephalography. Br J Radiol 45: 867

28. Trends in technical developments

Past developments in ultrasonics have often come as a surprise to workers in the field. Nevertheless, some clinically useful developments can be anticipated by studying current research in technology. This chapter presents a brief résumé of work in the scientific literature or presented at conferences.

Transducers

Recent years have seen the production of transducers with plastic piezoelectric elements (e.g. PVDF) which offer a better acoustic match to tissue than the harder ceramic elements. At present, piezoelectric plastic elements are more suited to reception than to transmission, but new materials are still being developed. Some transducers have been produced with a combination of plastic and ceramic elements for reception and transmission, respectively. The use of composite materials consisting of rods of ceramic elements embedded in piezoelectric plastic is also being explored.

Polymers such as PVDF can be readily shaped and made into arrays. Their function in the latter capacity is helped by the fact that the transmission of ultrasound between the elements is more attenuated in plastic than in ceramic.

These developments in transducers should lead to greater sensitivity and dynamic range plus improved beam shapes. Greater variation in overall transducer-assembly design is also possible. Given the central role of transducers, improved performance will be of direct relevance in both pulse-echo imaging and Doppler techniques.

Improvements can be expected in annular, linear, and phased arrays. Two-dimensional linear

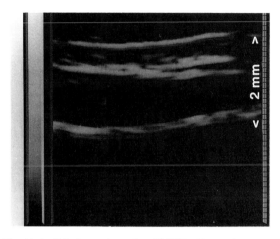

Fig. 28.1 Skin layers imaged at 25 MHz. Top surface, outside skin; middle surface, dermis/fat interface; Bottom surface, fat/muscle interface. Total thickness approximately 2 mm (courtesy of Cutech).

and phased arrays have been produced which focus in the out-of-plane direction to reduce the slice thickness. Arrays operating at higher frequencies than at present will, no doubt, appear in due course. Figure 28.1 presents an image of skin layers created by a 25 MHz scanner using a single element transducer.

Real-time B-scanners

The types of scanner can be expected to increase in number at both the expensive and inexpensive ends of the range. Arrays with large numbers of elements and computers which can handle many signals simultaneously are very compatible. Examples of this type of instrument are already on the market. In the future, we will see many variations in the way in which the computer controls the transducer array and processes the echo signals. For example, each individual element may be excited independently and the echoes stored before being combined to produce an image. A large amount of research and development is underway to find out which of the many options will improve image quality.

As electronics, display units, and transducers become cheaper, we can expect to see the impact on small portable scanners.

Invasive scanners

Although invasive transducers have been around since the earliest days of diagnostic ultrasound, it is only within the last few years that there has been an explosion in their popularity. We can expect to see improvements in design to adapt them better for specific tasks and to increase the flexibility of scanning action. Prototypes have been made of very small devices for imaging inside arteries. Very high-frequency devices (up to 40 MHz) have been reported.

Circumferential scanners

If ultrasonic beams can be directed into the body from many points on its circumference, a very complete image may be obtained. Such scanners have been produced on several occasions in the past, but they have never found widespread application. Increasing interest in imaging muscle in the limbs has revived interest in these specialized units. One recent experimental unit consisted of six linear arrays placed round the circumference of the water-tank in which the limb was immersed.

Image processing

There is considerable activity in the field of image processing. This is primarily aimed at improving spatial and contrast resolution. Attempts are being made to improve spatial resolution by compensating for the finite length of the ultrasonic pulse and the beam width. Contrast resolution can be improved by reducing speckle noise in images. By using adaptive filters which smooth only regions where speckle has been identified, one can reduce noise without blurring genuine tissue interfaces (Fig. 28.2). Processing may also provide a step

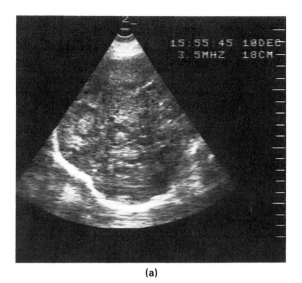

(a)

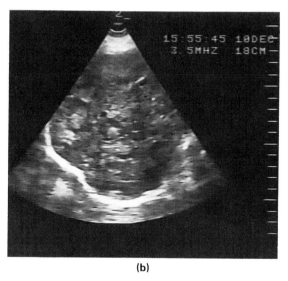

(b)

Fig. 28.2 (a) Image of metastasis in liver. (b) the top image smoothed to reduce noise and preserve boundaries using adaptive filtering (courtesy of Loupas T).

forward in the identification of tissue types from images; for example, by analysing the small motions in the speckle patterns of different tissues.

Computer control

We have already noted the manner in which more and more computer power has been applied to control array transducers. Computers can be installed to look after almost any function of the instrument, for example, the recording unit or the sensitivity. Early systems aimed at automatically controlling the TGC of a scanner showed that such control was feasible, but these systems were prone to instability and the filling in of cystic images with small signals. More sophisticated computer-controlled units have overcome these problems and now manipulate the sensitivity rapidly as the beam direction and the scan plane change. Even an expert operator could not hope to optimize the sensitivity throughout the image at this rate.

Guidance techniques

Two features make ultrasonic imaging ideally suited to guiding needles and catheters within the body, namely the ability to depict motion and the lack of hazard to patient or operator. Research and development continue into better means of obtaining biopsy specimens, for instance, with endoscopic scanners. There is also interest in guiding other devices, such as angioplasty balloons or optical fibres, to convey laser light to internal tissues.

The problem of making the tip of a fine needle more visible has been tackled in several ways. One approach has been to increase the reflectivity of the tip. Difficulties are still experienced with such needles when the tip is in strongly reflecting tissue. Other techniques have involved making the needles sonically sensitive so that a signal is detected when the ultrasound beam strikes the tip. To achieve this, one can attach a crystal either to the tip or to the part which remains outside the body (Fig. 28.3). The latter method makes use of the fact that needles or their stylets act as waveguides and conduct ultrasound readily along their length. Knowing the direction of the beam and the time at which the signal is detected permits a marker spot to be superimposed on the image at the location of the needle tip. This technique also works with flexible catheters.

Doppler waveform analysis

Analysis of Doppler velocity waveforms has already been shown to be of value in classifying vascular disease. Many methods of analysing waveforms are available from the field of signal

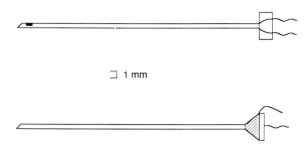

Fig. 28.3 Sonically sensitive needles with piezoelectric elements at tip or at outside end. Ultrasound is conducted along the shaft to the element in the latter case.

processing in engineering. Some of these methods are under investigation at present for analysis of Doppler signals.

In addition to velocity waveforms, more attention may be paid to acceleration and quantitative flow waveforms in the future.

Spectrum analysers

Spectrum analysers which generate sonograms perform reasonably well. Developments are underway to improve their power, temporal and frequency resolution. It is possible to generate spectra at 1 ms intervals, rather than at the 5–10 ms used at present. Improved frequency resolution may be valuable only in situations where there is no spectral broadening caused by cells moving quickly through a narrow beam.

The noise in sonograms may also be smoothed in ways which do not blur their detailed structure. This processing makes it easier for the computer to identify such features as the maximum velocity envelope.

Doppler quantitative flow measurement

The fundamental importance of the quantity of blood supplied to tissue results in continuing interest in devising techniques which can measure flow with increased accuracy. The more complex instruments now available for measuring velocity profiles or mean velocity at many points in a vessel may lead to better quantitative flow measurement.

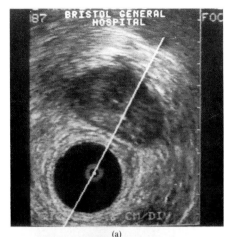

(a)

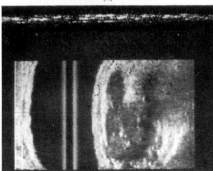

Fig. 28.4   Top: transverse image of the prostate obtained with a rotating transducer rectal scanner; bottom: longitudinal image of prostate reconstructed from a series of transverse images (courtesy of Halliwell M, Jenkins D, Jackson P C and Wells P N T (1989) Brit J Radiol 62: 824–829).

Duplex systems

In the fullness of time, the duplex technique may be merely a mode of operation of a colour-flow imager. Meanwhile, duplex systems are being developed to suit particular clinical applications. The best results are obtained when a system has been specifically designed for a field of study. For example, cardiac systems are not best for obstetric studies.

Doppler colour-flow imaging

Colour-flow imaging is in its infancy. Further improvements may be possible in areas such as the method of estimation and presentation of the velocity information, the noise level in the images,

image-artefact reduction, and increasing sensitivity to slow flow. It should be possible to reduce the cost of this equipment, since after the development has been paid for, the manufacture of a few boards is relatively inexpensive.

Tissue characterization

Tissue characterization has been a goal of diagnostic ultrasound since the earliest days, yet no technique is in routine clinical use. Activity in the field is still quite high, but the problem of the variable effects among patients of the overlying tissues has not been solved. Fat and muscle can have strong effects on any ultrasonic beam which is used to interrogate tissue.

Observation of a pulse-echo image can provide some information about the attenuating or scattering properties of tissue. It may therefore be possible to extend this approach to create images of other properties of tissues; for example, by portraying the fine motions of tissue when it is compressed by the cardiac pulse or by an external agent. Rapid signal processing in modern computers makes such approaches feasible. Depicting properties in images is also helpful in the identification of artefact results.

Three-dimensional imaging

Several scanners have been made in the past in which the ultrasound beam moves in three dimensions to collect echoes, rather than being restricted to one scan plane. Technically, it is fairly easy to move the beam throughout 3-D space to record echoes and their location in the volume scanned. The problem has always been to devise a good way of displaying the data. The basic difficulty is that echoes from the outer regions of the structure obscure those from the inside. With the advent of cheap computer memory, it is now possible to store all of the echoes from the structure and display those in any plane which is selected by the operator. This enables sections to be displayed which are not accessible in normal 2-D scanning (Fig. 28.4). Since we can store echo information from 3-D tissue anatomy in our minds as real-time B-scanning is performed, the value of computer storage systems has still to be ascertained.

Contrast agents

The injection of indocyanine green containing microbubbles into the heart played a major part in identifying the chambers and moving structures depicted in M-scanning. To obtain more reproducible results, researchers have steadily pursued a more scientific approach to encapsulating microbubbles in protein material. Clinical trials of these agents are now underway in cardiology and other fields (Fig. 28.5). Other approaches are also under investigation, in particular, the reaction to uptake of perfluorocarbons in tumours.

The development of colour-flow imaging may reduce the value of contrast agents in vascular studies; however, microbubbles have been shown to enhance weak Doppler signals.

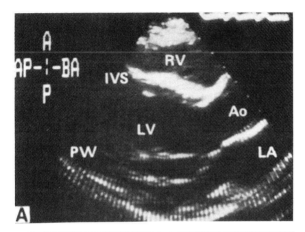

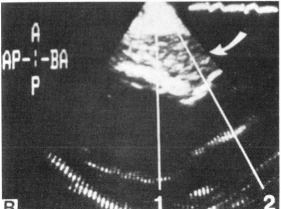

Fig. 28.5 Microbubble contrast agent appearing in the right ventricle (courtesy of Roelandt J). M-scans can be taken along selected beam paths to time events

Transmission imaging

Ultrasound can be employed in a manner analogous to that of conventional X-ray imaging. It is passed through the body and produces an image representing the attenuation experienced in different paths. There is no efficient ultrasonic equivalent of the film used to detect X-rays, but detectors can be made to record the distribution of transmitted ultrasound. More fundamental difficulties are that ultrasound is completely blocked by gas in the body and very strongly attenuated by bone. This limits the areas of possible application. Further problems are added by the fact that ultrasound is deviated by phenomena such as refraction and diffraction. Nevertheless, very intriguing images have been published of limbs and neonates. Commercially manufactured machines for transmission imaging have been very rare.

Holography

Optical holograms, which are quite common, store information about a light wave front reflected from an object or scene. This information (the amplitude and phase of the wave front at each point on it) is stored in a very fine interference pattern on photographic film. When light is shone on or through a hologram, the wave front is reconstructed, and, if it enters the eye, a 3-D image of the original object or scene is observed.

Ultrasonic holograms can also be made if the amplitude and phase information at each point in a reflected ultrasonic wave front is stored. Since no good ultrasonic film exists, the wave front is recorded by a variety of other techniques, such as point-by-point detection with a piezoelectric crystal, or through distortions of a thin film of oil. The ultrasonic wave front is reconstructed as an optical one by illuminating the hologram with light. Hence, the structure originally insonated can be viewed as an optical image.

There are problems in ultrasonic holography related to the large difference in the wavelengths of ultrasound and light, and to the fact that the ultrasound comes from within the structure and not just from the surface, as in optical holography. However, in theory, ultrasonic holography can produce high-resolution real-time images. There is still interest in this field, and progress may occur as transducer arrays are made larger and better able to record ultrasound over an area.

Ultrasonic CT

A beam of ultrasound can be passed through the body in many directions, and the attenuation may be measured for each path in a manner similar to that for X-rays in CT scanning (Fig. 28.6). An image may then be produced of a section through the body in which each pixel shade represents the attenuation of the tissue at that point. Indeed, ultrasonic CT scanning is potentially more versatile than that of X-rays, since images can be produced depicting the speed of ultrasound or the

Doppler flow phantoms are being refined to make artificial blood more realistic in terms of its scattering power of each element of tissue. Unfortunately, ultrasonic beams are deviated more than X-ray beams by refraction and reflection; and, in addition, many paths through the body are blocked by bone and gas. Development work continues to try to overcome these difficulties.

Dosimetry

Equipment, in the form of hydrophones and force balances to determine intensity, power, and pressure, has improved dramatically in the last 10 years. Attention is now being paid to means of measuring effects in tissue, in particular, temperature rise and the level of cavitation. This is related to the view that proper safety standards can be es-

tablished only after the relevant mechanisms in tissue are fully understood.

Quality assurance

Although test-objects exist which can demonstrate the constancy of performance of equipment and allow measurement of some performance factors, such as depth of penetration or dynamic range of the whole imaging system, work continues to develop phantoms which more closely mimic tissue. These would allow more accurate assessment and comparison of machines. For example, the contrast resolution of an instrument or its ability to detect small cystic structures in tissue are of direct interest in an assessment.

particle size and scattering power. The elastic and acoustic properties of the tube walls are also being improved. Greater convenience of use is also being achieved. Finally, phantoms which can generate physiologic flow waveforms have been built. Computer control of the pump allows a wide range of waveforms to be readily produced.

Propagation in tissue

As knowledge of the distortion of pulse and beam shapes in tissue is accumulated, this information is being allowed for in the design of machines. Recently, units have been marketed which allow for the fact that the high-frequency components of pulses are preferentially attenuated as they pass through tissue. Allowance has still to be made for the effect of non-linear propagation. Greater understanding of the distortion of pulses and beams should lead to improved imaging and Doppler performances.

SUMMARY

Real-time B-scan technology was seen to be a mature technology which is still improving through transducer design and computer processing of echo data. Doppler technology is less mature, and significant improvements can be expected. Research and development continue in a number of additional fields such as contrast agents, tissue characterization, dosimetry, propagation effects, and novel imaging modes.

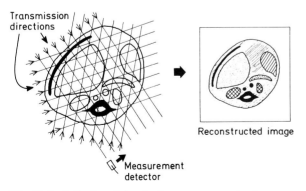

Fig. 28.6 Collection of data for image reconstruction by computerized tomography.

REFERENCES

Aldridge E E, Clare A B, Lloyd G A S et al 1971 A preliminary investigation of the use of ultrasonic holography in ophthalomology. Brit J Radiol 44: 126–130

Fritzsch Th, Hilmann J, Mützel W, Lange L 1986 Right-heart echocontrast in anesthetized dog after i.v. administration of a new standarized sonographic contrast agent. Arzenheim. Forsch./Drug Res. 36 (ii): 1030–1033

Glover G H 1977 Computerised time-of-flight ultrasonic tomography for breast examination. Ultrasound Med Biol 3: 117–127

Halliwell M, Key H, Jenkins D, Jackson P C, Wells P N T 1989 New scans from old: digital reformatting of ultrasound images. Brit J Radiol. 62: 824–829

Hill C R 1973 Medical ultrasonics: An historical review. Brit J Radiol 46: 899–905

Ishiyama K, Yanagawa T, Sato T, Yano M, Yoshikawa N 1985 Development of small radius convex scanning system with view angle of 98 degrees. Proc. 4th Meeting World Federation Ultrasound Medicine Biology, Eds. Gill R W, Dadd M J, Sydney

Keller M W, Feinstein S B, Briller R A, Powsner S M 1986 Automated production and analysis of echo contrast agents. J Ultrasound Med. 5: 493–498

Kessler L W 1974 Review of progress and applications in acoustic microscopy. J Acoust Soc Am 55: 909–918

Linzer M (ed) 1976 Ultrasonic tissue characterization. Special Publication 453. National Bureau of Standards, Washington, DC

Loupas T, McDicken W N, Allan P L 1987 Noise reduction in ultrasonic images by digital filtering. Brit J Radiol. 60: 389–392

McDicken W N, Anderson T, Allan P 1985 The development of sonically-sensitive needles for biopsy by ultrasonic guidance. Proc. 4th Meeting World Federation Ultrasound Medicine and Biology, eds. Gill R W, Dadd M J, Sydney

Marich K W, Zatz L M, Green P S et al 1975 Real-time imaging with a new ultrasonic camera: Part 1. In vitro experimental studies on transmission imaging of biological structures. JCU 3: 5–16

Newerla K 1987 Ultrasound reflection tomography using six modern linear transducer arrays. Proc. 6th Cong European Federation Societies Ultrasound Medicine Biology, Eds Bondestam S, Alanen A, Jouppila P, Helsinki

Pye S D, Wild S R, McDicken W N 1988 Clinical trial of a new adaptive TGC system for ultrasound imaging. Brit J Radiol. 61: 523–526

Wells P N T, Halliwell M, Skidmore R et al 1977 Tumour detection by ultrasonic Doppler blood-flow signals. Ultrasonics 15: 231–232

Appendix 1 Quality assurance for echo imaging

Echo-imaging systems

The medical user's approach to quality assurance should be different from that of the physicist or service engineer who investigates a system to ascertain its technical performance or to institute repairs. The latter require test-objects (phantoms) or devices which indicate the performance of specific parts of the scanner. The medical user is more concerned to answer the questions, 'Is the overall system performance as good as it should be?' and 'Has the system performance changed over recent months?' These two questions can be answered with relatively simple test-objects and procedures which can be carried out quickly, say, in 10 minutes.

A suitable test-object consists of structures embedded in a block of tissue-mimicking material. An example of such material is agar gel containing carbon particles the amount of which is arranged to give attenuation and scattering similar to that in soft tissue. The velocity of ultrasound in the material is made equal to 1540 m/s by adding alcohol. Several such test-objects are commercially available.

The following structures are embedded in the

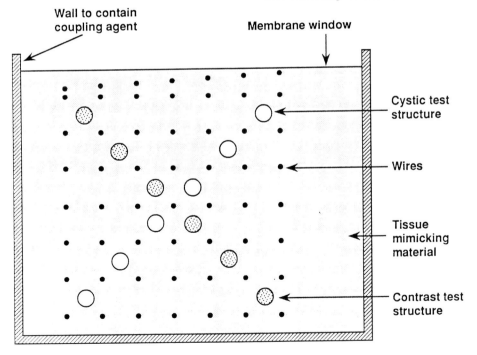

Fig. A1.1 A tissue-mimicking test-object. Considerable variation is found in commercially available objects in terms of structure, content, and suitability for testing machines.

material to enable basic tests to be performed (Fig. A1.1).

1. A regularly spaced array of fine wires or threads

2. Clear cystic-type structures at different depths

3. Small spherical, cylindrical, or conical regions of reflectivity slightly different from the rest of the tissue-mimicking material

To carry out a quality-assurance procedure, one sets the machine controls at well-defined and reproducible positions, which should be as near as possible to those employed in clinical practice. The scan plane is then made to cut perpendicularly across the wires in the test-object, and an image is recorded. The images of the wires give a value for the axial and lateral resolution at different depths (Fig. A1.2). Note that these values are not absolute; they refer to the particular wires being scanned in the particular tissue-mimicking material. However, they do allow machines to be compared and changes to be detected. Techniques which attempt to measure axial and lateral resolution with pairs of closely spaced wires have fallen out of favour, since it is difficult to make test-ob-

jects with many pairs of wires at slightly different separation. Examination of a series of wire images at different depths shows the change in beam shape; in particular, the focal point and focal depth may be identified.

The image of a regular array of wires can also be used to check for distortion, which could arise in several parts of a scanner, but which is most likely to be in the TV display tube. Finally, the calliper can be checked in both horizontal and vertical directions by placing the marker spots at the centres of the images of wires of known separation. The circumference- and area-measuring facilities may be checked by tracing round a known area which is delineated by the wires in the image.

Scanning the cystic structures provides a good test of the level of background noise in the image. A high noise level may be caused by a wide beam, side-lobes, or electronic noise produced in the scanner or picked up from other electrical equipment. Although such background noise may not be visible in non-cystic regions of the image, it still degrades the image in these regions.

The regions of different reflectivity provide checks on the grey-tone presentation and on the contrast resolution of the machine. Test-objects of

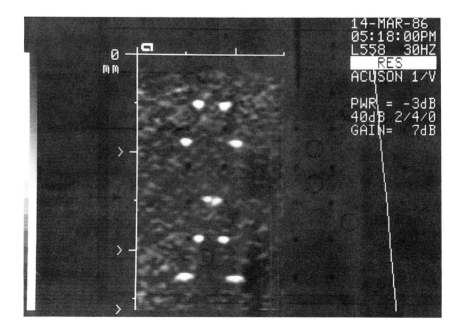

Fig. A1.2 Images of wires in a test-object which allow axial and lateral resolution to be measured.

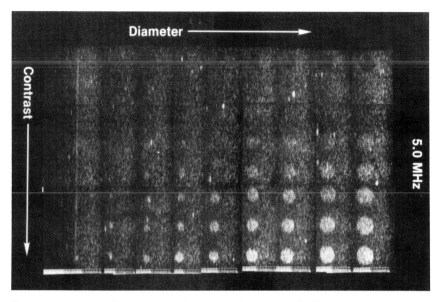

Fig. A1.3 Image from a contrast test-object which contains a range of structures of different sizes and scattering strengths (courtesy of Nuclear Associates).

this type are still being developed. Few exist for which the reflecting powers of the internal structures are accurately known. Figure A1.3 shows the image from a contrast-resolution test-object in which the size and reflectivity of the enclosed structures are systematically varied.

The maximum depth in the test-object at which echoes can just be detected is also of interest as a measure of scanner sensitivity. With transmitted-power, gain, and TGC controls at their highest settings, the depth of penetration is measured. The ultrasound beam should also be focused as deeply as possible when this test is performed.

The sensitivity and grey-tone presentation of a scanner can also be tested by injecting ultrasonic signals of known magnitude into the transducer. This type of device is usually used by a physicist or engineer.

Video systems

The above test utilizing a tissue-mimicking phantom allows the grey-tone display, the recording device, and the film processor to be checked. However, it is also easy to use an electronic pattern generator for this purpose (Fig. A1.4). Pattern generators may be built into the scanner

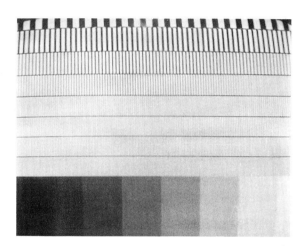

Fig. A1.4 Pattern from an electronic generator used for checking spatial and contrast resolution of display and recording systems.

or be independent units which provide a TV signal for feeding into the display unit or recorder. Typical uses of patterns are listed below:

1. A two-dimensional array of dots enables the focusing of the display and recording units to be assessed.

2. A pattern of lines of decreasing separation al-

lows checks of the resolution of the display and recording units.

3. A grey bar pattern, say of 16 or more levels, allows the grey-shade presentation to be checked.

4. Distortion may be observed with a pattern of horizontal and vertical lines.

5. Dirt on a screen will produce blotches in what should be a single grey tone.

6. Uniformity of exposure or light leakage may be checked in a recorded image of the test pattern.

REFERENCES

Clark P 1988 Performance checks. In: Practical ultrasound (Ch. 5), Ed. Lerski R A IRL Press, Oxford
Hoskins P R, Anderson T, McDicken W N 1989 A computer controlled flow phantom for generation of physiological Doppler waveforms. Phys Med Biol 34, 1709–1717

Appendix 2   Quality assurance for Doppler techniques

A number of prototype Doppler test-objects have been reported, and two or three are commercially available. They normally consist of a block of tissue-mimicking material containing one or more thin-walled tubes through which artificial blood is pumped (Fig. A2.1). The artificial blood is typically dextrose particles in a mixture of 4 parts water and 5 parts glycerol. The particles simulate blood cells, and the glycerol is included to attain the correct viscosity. The concentration of dextrose particles is not critical; 50 g/litre results in realistic blood-flow signals.

When a computer is employed to control the pump, a wide range of continuous and pulsatile flow patterns can be produced. Few flow test-objects attempt to mimic the clinical situation exactly. For example, the elasticity of blood ves-

sels or their complex structure is rarely included.

With all of the sensitivity controls in noted positions, close to those of clinical practice, a sonogram or flow image is recorded. The constancy of performance of the Doppler system is checked. Such a procedure is of value for CW, PW, and colour-flow imaging instruments. The sensitivity of the system is measured by noting the maximum depth at which flow in a vessel is detected. Further development is required to make phantoms for resolution measurements in Doppler devices. If the flow rate through the test-object is known, a check of quantitative flow calculations by the machine can be made.

Doppler test phantoms have also been produced based on the detection of a moving string or thread in a water-bath. Scattering from the string or

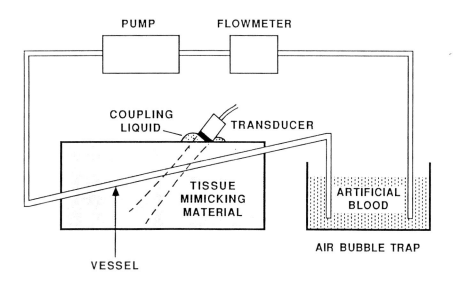

Fig. A2.1   A schematic diagram of a Doppler test-object. Doppler test-objects are at an early stage of development.

thread simulates that from blood approximately. Continuous or pulsed wave blood flow can be mimicked. Such a device can be used to check velocity measurement, range gate registration, angle correction and wall filter level. A string phantom can also be employed to plot sample volume dimensions.

The frequency with which quality-assurance tests should be undertaken depends on the stability of the machine in question. Modern electronics in pulse-echo imaging instruments are usually very stable, so one test per month is probably adequate. Doppler systems are also stable, but there are often several ill-defined controls which could be in the wrong position. Until one obtains extensive experience, it is probably advisable to perform a quick test at the start of each session to ensure that the sensitivity and recording levels are correct.

REFERENCE

Evans D H, McDicken W N, Skidmore R, Woodcock J P 1989 Doppler test phantoms and quality control. In: Doppler ultrasound: Physics, instrumentation and clinical applications (Ch. 12). Wiley, Chichester, England

Appendix 3   The decibel (dB) notation

A measure of the size of one quantity (Q_1) relative to another (Q_2) is the ratio Q_1/Q_2. Ratios of two quantities can be very large numbers, if for instance, the denominator, Q_2, is small. Since large numbers can be difficult to handle, the logarithms of the numbers are sometimes worked with, since it reduces their range; for example, the logarithms of 100 and 100 000 are 2 and 5, respectively. Another advantage when working with logarithms is that multiplication and division are replaced by the simpler processes of addition and subtraction, respectively. Hence,

$$\log (xy) = \log x + \log y$$
$$\log (xx) = \log (x^2) = \log x + \log x = 2 \log x$$
$$\log (x/y) = \log x - \log y$$

At the end of a calculation, the final numeric result is obtained by reconverting from the logarithm format. This ease of calculation was more important in the precomputer era, but the use of logarithms is still retained in engineering. This is not as unfortunate as it may seem, because once quantities are converted into the logarithms, we can then work with a small range of values; for instance, we can label an amplifier gain control, without ever needing to convert back to the normal quantities.

The bel notation uses logarithms. Consider a transmitter which can put out a series of intensity levels I_1, I_2, I_3 watt/cm^2, etc. A measure of I_2 relative to I_1 is the ratio I_2/I_1, as is the $\log (I_2/I_1)$. We can label the output at the control position corresponding to I_2 as

$$\begin{aligned} \text{Output at } I_2 \text{ position} &= \log (I_2/I_1) \text{ bel units} \\ &= 10 \log (I_2/I_1) \text{ decibel} \\ &\quad \text{units} \end{aligned}$$

The decibel is just a tenth of a bel. For example, if I_2/I_1 is 10 000, the I_2 control position would be labelled 40 dB.

If I_1 is the minimum output, then I_2 is greater than I_1 and the decibels are positive: with I_1 the maximum, the decibels are negative. Table A3.1 shows ratio values of intensity and corresponding decibel values. The other control positions I_3, I_4, I_5, etc can be similarly labelled in decibels. It is quite common for the intensity, or power, output of a scanner to be labelled 0, 10, 20, 30, 40, 50 dB, or 0, 2, 4, 6, 8, 10 dB. The operator develops an understanding for the type of image produced at the different settings. It is not necessary to convert logarithmic to absolute intensity values unless safety calibrations are being undertaken.

The decibel notation is encountered in a number of situations. For example, consider an amplifier in which the input voltage signal is V_1 and the output is V_2. The gain of the amplifier is V_2/V_1. The gain can be expressed in decibels:

$$\text{Gain in dB} = 20 \log (V_2/V_1)$$

The number 20 appears rather than 10 when this formula is derived from that for intensity. It is V^2 which is proportional to intensity I or power P. Hence, $10 \log I$ is related to $10 \log V^2$, that is, to $20 \log V$. Table A3.2 presents voltage ratios and corresponding decibel values.

Recall that the TGC controls often make the gain increase with depth. The rate of increase of the gain, the TGC slope, is then labelled in dB/cm. For example, with 3 MHz of ultrasound, a slope of 6 dB/cm is typical. For both gain and TGC labelling in decibels, it is not necessary to convert back to the original gain ratios, but merely to understand how the machine functions at different settings.

Table A3.1   The decibel notation applied to intensity (or power)

Decibel (dB)	Intensity ratio (I_1/I_0) and $I_1 > I_0$	Decibel (dB)	Intensity ratio (I_1/I_0) $I_1 < I_0$
+1	1.259	−1	0.794
+2	1.585	−2	0.631
+3	1.995	−3	0.501
+5	3.162	−5	0.316
+6	3.981	−6	0.251
+10	10.0	−10	0.1
+15	31.62	−15	0.031 6
+20	100.0	−20	0.01
+25	316.2	−25	0.003 2
+30	1 000	−30	0.001
+35	3 162	−35	0.000 32
+40	10 000	−40	0.000 1
+45	31 620	−45	0.000 032
+50	100 000	−50	0.000 01
+55	316 200	−55	0.000 003 2
+60	1 000 000	−60	0.000 001

I_0 = Reference level I_0 = Reference level
Positive decibels $(I_1 > I_0)$ Negative decibels $(I_1 < I_0)$

Table A3.2   The decibel notation applied to voltage (or echo amplitude)

Decibel (dB)	Amplitude ratio (V_1/V_0) $V_1 > V_0$	Decibel (dB)	Amplitude ratio (V_1/V_0) $V_1 < V_0$
+1	1.122	−1	0.891
+2	1.259	−2	0.794
+3	1.413	−3	0.708
+5	1.778	−5	0.562
+6	1.995	−6	0.501
+10	3.162	−10	0.32
+20	10.0	−20	0.100
+30	31.62	−30	0.032
+40	100	−40	0.01
+50	316.2	−50	0.003 2
+60	1 000	−60	0.001
+70	3 162	−70	0.000 32
+80	10 000	−80	0.000 1
+90	31 620	−90	0.000 032
+100	100 000	−100	0.000 01

V_0 = Reference level V_0 = Reference level
Positive decibels $(V_1 > V_0)$ Negative decibels $(V_1 < V_0)$

A ratio of pressure amplitudes may also be expressed in decibels. If a wave has a pressure amplitude p_1 on one side of a tissue layer, and a pressure p_2 when it emerges at the other side, the change in pressure amplitude, expressed in decibels, is:

$$\text{Amplitude change} = 20 \log (p_2/p_1) \text{ dB}$$

If the layer has a thickness x, the rate of change of pressure is:

$$\frac{20}{x} \log \left(\frac{p_2}{p_1} \right)$$

$$20 \log (p_2/p_1)/x = \text{Attenuation coefficient in dB/cm}$$

$$= \frac{10}{x} \log \left(\frac{I_x}{I_0} \right)$$

From this discussion it can be seen that any ratio can be expressed in decibels simply by taking logarithms. The denominator of the ratio is usually a special reference level or an input level of the quantity being considered. Because decibel labels merely refer one level to an arbitrary reference or input level, values quoted for one machine cannot be used on another of different design and be expected to give a similar result.

Decibels are most commonly met with in everyday life when noise is being discussed. For noise measurements, the reference level is taken to be the threshold of hearing, that is, 0 dB. A conversation sound level is then typically +70 dB; a factory floor, +80 dB; and a jet aircraft, +120 dB. Pain is experienced at levels of +140 dB and above.

Appendix 4   Measurement of ultrasonic pressure, intensity, power, fields, zones, and beams

The methods described below are valid or can be adapted to suit both pulse-echo imaging and Doppler transducers.

Pressure

The ultrasonic pressure waveform at a point in a transmitted field is best measured with a probe called a 'hydrophone'. A hydrophone is basically a very small transducer whose piezoelectric element detects the pressure fluctuations at the point of interest (Fig. A4.1). The sensitive element in a hydrophone is typically 1 mm or less in diameter. It may be mounted on the tip of a needle, which supports it without disturbing the field. Alternatively, a hydrophone can be constructed with a thin membrane of piezoelectric plastic, which is arranged to be sensitive only at a small central spot (Fig. A4.2).

Intensity

The intensity at points near the focus and in the far field of a transducer can be calculated from the pressure amplitude by using the formula:

$$I = p_0^2/2\rho c$$

The assumptions made in the derivation of this

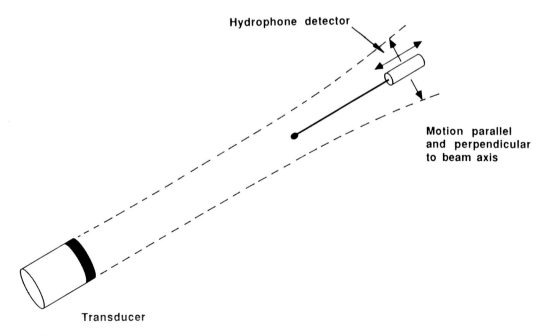

Hydrophone detector

Motion parallel and perpendicular to beam axis

Transducer

Fig. A4.1   A hydrophone transducer; typically, the piezoelectric element is less than 1 mm in diameter.

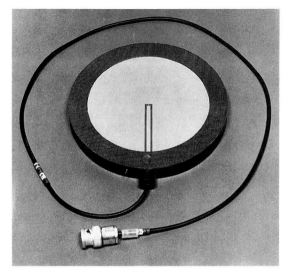

Fig. A4.2 A membrane hydrophone. The thin plastic membrane is sensitive at a small spot of a diameter less than 1 mm at the centre (courtesy of Preston R C).

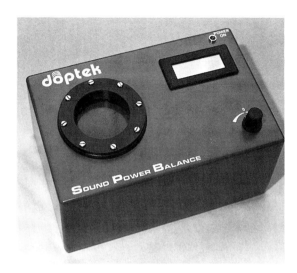

Fig. A4.3 A portable power balance (courtesy of Dôptek).

formula mean that it is not strictly valid in the near field, where only an estimate of the intensity can be obtained.

The exact definition of the intensity being calculated must be made clear (Table 8.1). For example, if the maximum pressure amplitude of p_0 is measured in a pulse, then the corresponding maximum instantaneous intensity is given by:

$$I \text{ (temporal peak)} = [p^2 \text{ (temporal peak)}]/2 \, \rho c$$

An average intensity along the pulse may be calculated by working out intensities at other times throughout the pulse. This calculation gives I (pulse average), Ipa, at the point in the field selected. If this point is at the spatial peak of the pressure in the field (probably the focus), we obtain the I (spatial peak, pulse average), Isppa. The other intensities quoted in Chapter 8 can be obtained by similar means. A common example is the I (spatial peak, temporal average), Ispta, which is derived by averaging instantaneous intensities at the spatial peak over the whole duration of the PRF cycle (Fig. 3.8). Averages are also taken over the cross section of the field to obtain spatial averages, for instance, I (spatial average, temporal average), Isata.

Power

The power of an ultrasonic field may be obtained by adding the intensities at small areas throughout the cross section of the field. However, more often, power is measured directly with a radiation-force balance (Fig. A4.3). The field is directed into the balance to intersect a target which normally either totally absorbs or reflects it. Associated with the flow of energy in the field, there is a flow of momentum. Since the target absorbs or reflects the field, it causes a change of momentum, and, hence, it experiences a force, the radiation force. The power (W) is related to the force (F) on a reflecting target by the formula:

$$\text{Power (W)} = Fc/2$$

where c is the velocity of sound in the propagating medium, usually water. For example, if a force of 0.135 mg (1.3×10^{-6} N) is recorded the power is given by

$$W = 1.3 \times 10^{-6} \times 1540/2 = 1\text{mW}$$

For an absorbing target, the force is halved since the momentum change is half of the reflection case.

Hydrophones and power balances are commercially available. Their calibration should be carefully checked before they are used to make ab-

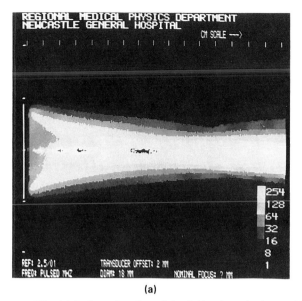 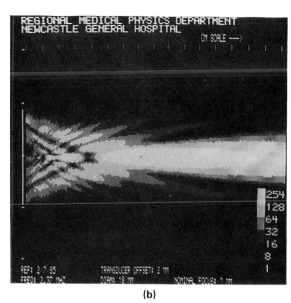

(a)   (b)

Fig. A4.4 Intensity plots of the fields of a pulsed wave (**a**) and continuous wave (**b**) (courtesy of Whittingham T A).

solute measurements of intensity and power. The accurate measurement of intensity is difficult since errors can easily occur; for instance, in placing the hydrophone at the spatial peak of the field.

Field shape

To determine the shape of an ultrasonic field, we measure the pressure amplitude systematically at a large number of points in front of the transducer. The results are normally presented from measurements in a plane which lies along and passes through the axis of the field. Plots perpendicular to the axis are also of value since they show the symmetry or lack of it in the field. An intensity pattern is calculated from a pressure-amplitude plot (Fig. A4.4).

Instruments which consist of a linear array of small hydrophones are available. Such instruments provide simultaneous values of pressure across the field; in other words, they provide a profile across the field (Fig. 5.14). Accurate measurement of the spatial peak pressure amplitude, and, hence, the corresponding intensity, is more readily achieved with this approach.

An elegant optical technique for observing ultrasonic fields is the 'schlieren' method. When ultrasound passes through water, the pressure fluctuations alter its optical refractive index at points in the field. The regions of altered refractive index are observed by shining light into the tank and using a system of lenses and apertures. The schlieren method can be adapted to suit both CW and PW fields. The attraction of this method is that it shows the field shapes in real-time, and the effects of manipulating features, such as the focus or number of active elements, in the transducer (Fig. A4.5).

Reception zones

Reception zones are rarely measured, but they could be measured with a small point transmitter which is systematically moved in front of the transducer. In the case of transducers which comprise a single element, the reception zone is usually assumed to have the same shape as the transmitted field. When electronic focusing with an array transducer is employed, this assumption is no longer valid.

Beam shape

We noted in Chapter 1 that the shape of a scan-

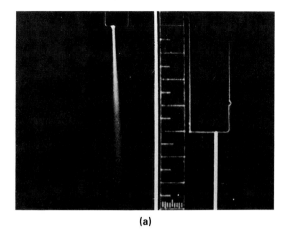

(a)

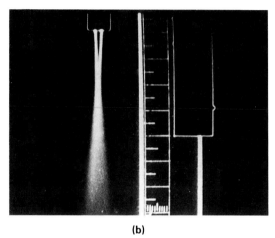

(b)

Fig. A4.5 Schlieren photographs of ultrasound transmitted from a 10 MHz Doppler transducer. (**a**), single crystal transmitting; (**b**), both crystals transmitting. This gives an appreaciation of the region of overlap of the transmission field and the reception zone, since both have the same shape (courtesy Follett D H).

ning beam is determined by both the transmitted field and the reception zone. Determination of the beam shape of a pulse-echo imaging transducer is performed by systematically moving a reflecting target, for example, a 1 cm ball bearing, throughout the space in front of the transducer. The echo amplitude from the target is recorded at each point (Fig. A4.6). To reduce the time of data

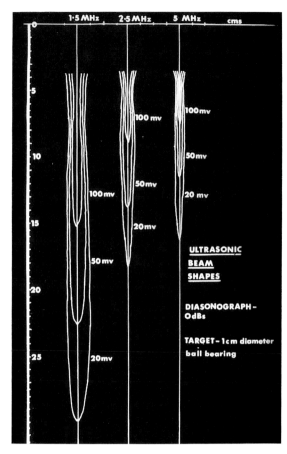

Fig. A4.6 Iso-echo contours of beams from single-element transducers that are weakly focused (courtesy of England M).

collection, one makes measurements usually only in a plane along the transducer axis and at one or two planes perpendicular to the axis.

Determination of the shape of a continuous- or pulsed-Doppler beam is normally performed with a small moving target, which is systematically placed at points in front of the transducer. Typical targets are oscillating ball bearings, moving threads, or small jets of liquid containing particle scatterers. The beam shapes of continuous and pulsed transducers are normally plotted along and across the central axis (Fig. A4.7, Fig. A4.8).

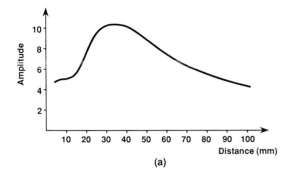

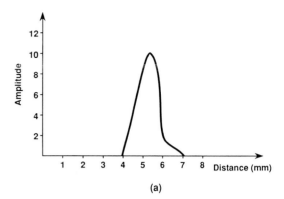

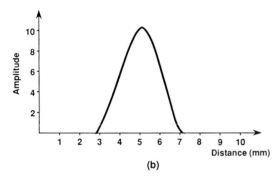

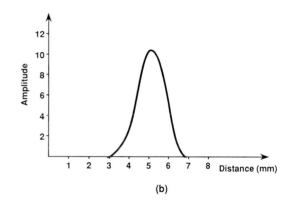

Fig. A4.7 Signal level received from a small moving target by a PW Doppler device: (**a**) along the central axis, (**b**) perpendicular to the axis.

Fig. A4.8 Signal level received from a small moving target by a PcW Doppler device: (**a**) along the central axis, (**b**)

REFERENCES

Croot C F J, Robbins R 1967 Schlieren photography of an ultrasound beam. Med Biol Illust 17: 202–207

Duck F A 1981 The pulsed ultrasonic field. In: Moores B M, Parker R P, Pullan B R (eds) Physical aspects of medical imaging (Ch. 3), Wiley, Chichester, England

Follett D H 1986 Light diffraction by ultrasound as evidence of finite amplitude distortion. Proc Inst Acoustics 8: 55–62

Hoeks A P G, Ruissen C J, Hick P, Reneman R S 1984 Methods to evaluate the sample volume of pulsed Doppler systems. Ultrasound Med Biol 10: 427–434

Lewin P A 1981 Miniature piezoelectric polymer ultrasonic hydrophone probes. Ultrasonics 19: 213–216

Preston R C, Bacon D R, Livett A J, Rajendran K 1983 PVDF membrane hydrophone performance properties and their relevance to the measurement of the acoustic output of medical ultrasound equipment. J Phys E: Sci Instrum 16: 786–796

Walker A R, Phillips D J, Powers J E 1982 Evaluating Doppler devices using a moving string test target. Journal of Clinical Ultrasound 10: 25–30

Appendix 5 Labelling planes of scan

A simple method for labelling longitudinal and transverse planes of scan is described at the end of Chapter 12. A method like that one is usually adopted for convenience.

With many B-scan machines, at the start of the examination, the mechanical gantry is placed in a central position, as for a vertical longitudinal scan through the centre of the abdomen, for example. Circuitry that records the position of the gantry is then zeroed. Thereafter, displacements of the mechanics from the zero reference are tracked and output numerically on the display screen; for example, 2 cm to the right of midline (R + 2), 30° tilt to vertical (V + 30g), 45° rotation (R − 45°). It is worth studying this tracking facility to see if it uniquely defines the plane of scan or only allows simple displacements to be recorded.

The AIUM interim standard listed in the references gives a simple method of labelling transverse, longitudinal (sagittal), and coronal image planes. The references also provide two similar proposals for labelling all planes of scan. As this is fairly time-consuming, it is only done in special circumstances.

REFERENCES

American Institute of Ultrasound in Medicine standard presentation and labelling of ultrasound images. 1976 JCU 4: 393–398

McDicken W N, Evans D H 1975 Labelling planes of scan and calculating location coordinates in diagnostic ultrasonics. Br J Radiol 48: 392–395

Appendix 6   Miscellaneous wave phenomena

Not all possible ultrasonic wave phenomena or wave types are exploited in diagnostic ultrasound. Brief descriptions of some common phenomena and types of wave are given here to provide familiarity with them.

HIGH-FREQUENCY MECHANICAL WAVES

Until now, this text has dealt primarily with longitudinal waves. Other types of mechanical wave motions have not been used in diagnostic techniques because they are difficult to propagate in tissue. It could be that they will one day find some specialized applications, however.

Shear waves

Shear waves are transverse waves in which the particles vibrate at right angles to the direction of wave travel. They are similar to waves on the surface of water, but particles throughout the medium perform oscillations, rather than just those close to the surface. Shear waves are extremely difficult to propagate in liquids because of high absorption and are unlikely to be of value for examining soft tissue. Attempts have been made to use them to detect fractures in bone. The velocity of a shear wave is about half that of a longitudinal wave in the same medium.

Torsion waves

If the driving source performs an oscillatory twisting action about an axis, torsional waves can be propagated. The propagating medium is usually in the form of a rod or wire.

Rayleigh waves

Rayleigh waves are transverse waves similar to shear waves, but they travel across the surface of solid material like waves on water. They can be used to detect flaws on surfaces.

Love waves

These travel across a surface and cause the particles to vibrate parallel to the plane of the surface, that is, at right angles to the plane of vibration of the particles in Rayleigh waves.

Lamb waves

In thin sheets of materials, it is possible to generate Lamb waves that result in flexural vibrations of the sheet.

MODE CONVERSION

Mode conversion occurs when one type of wave gives rise to another; for example, when a longitudinal wave strikes a solid surface at an angle. A complex mechanical interaction occurs at the interface, resulting in both longitudinal and transverse waves being propagated in the solid medium. Mode conversion could occur in diagnostic ultrasonics at a bone/soft-tissue interface. Inside the bone, a shear wave, that is, a transverse type of wave, is generated and could produce spurious echoes because it travels at a different speed and in a different direction from the longitudinal wave. Mode conversion has not been reported in practice as a source of spurious echoes, probably because of the presence of many other difficulties where bone is concerned.

POLARIZATION

In transverse waves, the direction of oscillation of each particle — for example, vertically for waves on water — and the direction of propagation of the wave define a plane. If these two defining directions do not alter, the plane is fixed and is called the 'plane of polarization'. In sound waves, on the other hand, because the particles oscillate in the same direction as that of propagation, no plane is defined. Ultrasound waves, therefore, cannot be polarized.

Appendix 7 Absorption and attenuation coefficients

In Chapter 4, it was noted that attenuation processes remove energy from an ultrasound beam. A fixed fraction of the field energy at a point is removed over the following centimetre of path length. The size of the fraction is dependent on the strengths of the attenuating processes. The continual removal of a fraction of the energy of a plane wave results in the intensity decreasing along the path in an exponential manner (Fig. A7.1a).

$$I_x = I_0 e^{-\mu x}$$

The coefficient of attenuation, μ, is the fraction of energy removed from a plane wave by attenuation in unit path length (usually in 1 cm path length). We can rearrange the above equation to give

$$\mu = \frac{10}{x} \log \left(\frac{I_x}{I_0}\right)$$

This expression provides the attenuation in dB/cm, which is the normal unit of attenuation in diagnostic ultrasound. Table A7.1 presents some values

Table A7.1 Attenuation coefficients for common tissues in dBcm^{-1} at 1 MHz. The value at a higher frequency may be obtained approximately, by multiplying by the frequency in MHz.

Tissue	Attenuation (or absorption) coefficient (dBcm^{-1})
Blood	0.2
Muscle	1.5
Liver	0.7
Brain (adult)	0.8
Brain (infant)	0.3
Bone	10.0
Fat	0.6
Water	0.002 (absorption)
Soft tissue (average)	0.7
Castor oil	1.0 (absorption)

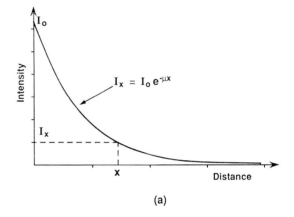

(a)

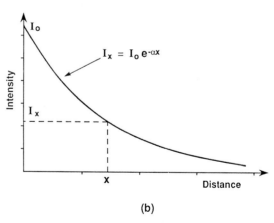

(b)

Fig. A7.1 Exponential reduction of intensity as a result of (a) attenuation and (b) absorption.

for attenuation coefficients in a range of tissues.

We noted earlier that liquids involve absorption on its own. The exponential decrease of the energy of a plane wave is therefore due to absorption (Fig. A7.1b). The absorption coefficient, α, is the fraction of wave energy absorbed in unit path length.

343

$$\alpha = \frac{10}{x} \log \left(\frac{I_x}{I_0} \right)$$

Table A7.1 shows absorption coefficients of some common liquids.

REFERENCES

Bamber J C 1986 Attenuation and absorption. In: Hill C R (ed) Physical principles of medical ultrasonics (Ch. 4), Ellis Horwood, Chichester, England

Appendix 8   Definitions

The *absorption* of ultrasound by a medium is the conversion of the energy of the wave into heat within the medium.

The *acoustic impedance* is the ratio of the wave pressure, p, over the particle velocity, u, i.e. $Z = p/u$. For a plane wave front $Z = \rho c$ where ρ is the density of the medium and c is the velocity of sound.

Aliasing is the erroneous reconstruction of a signal from a series of samples, due to the sampling rate of the signal having been too low. The reconstruction of a Doppler shift signal from too few pulsed wave samples results in a Doppler signal of the wrong frequency being produced.

An *algorithm* is a computer program which carries out a specific computational procedure.

The *amplitude* of an ultrasonic wave or electronic signal is the maximum change from the baseline value of the parameter describing it, e.g. the maximum change in the pressure or voltage.

An *analogue signal* is one in which the value of one physical variable (e.g. pressure or light intensity) is represented in an analogous way by another physical variable (e.g. voltage or film density).

The *aperture* of a transducer is the sine of half the angle subtended by the active portion of its front face at the focal point.

Apodization is the weighting of the contributions, from different parts of a transducer face before they are combined in the formation of an ultrasound transmission field or reception zone.

An *artefact* is a spurious signal which does not truly represent the physical conditions existing in the tissues being examined.

An *A-scan* is a pulsed-echo scan performed with the ultrasound beam pointing in one direction and in which echoes are displayed as vertical deflections of the trace on a CRT screen at locations corresponding to the interfaces which produced the echoes.

The *attenuation* of ultrasound is the reduction of the energy of the wave due to all of the phenomena which reduce its intensity, e.g. absorption, scattering, reflection and field divergence.

Autocorrelation is a technique for rapidly detecting cyclic changes in a signal.

Axial resolution is the minimum separation of two targets, in the direction along the beam axis, for which separate signals can be detected.

Backscatter is scattering of ultrasound at an angle of 180° to the beam direction, i.e. back towards the transducer.

A *bit* (binary digit) is a number in the binary number system; it can take the value 1 or 0.

A *B-scan* is a pulsed-echo scan in which the beam sweeps across a plane through tissue and the echoes are presented as grey tone spots on a CRT screen at locations corresponding to those of interfaces in the scan plane which produced the echoes.

Cavitation of the stable sort is the enhanced oscillation in the volume of bubbles due to the pressure fluctuations of a sound wave.

345

Cavitation of the transient sort is the growth and collapse of bubbles under the influence of the pressure fluctuations of a sound wave.

Colour flow imaging (mapping) is an ultrasonic technique which uses the Doppler effect to measure the velocities of moving targets and then presents the magnitude and direction of the velocities as colour-coded pixels at locations on a display screen corresponding to the positions of the targets.

Compound scanning is a technique is which the tissues are interrogated from several beam directions as the image is built up.

Compressibility is a measure of the ease with which a material alters in volume when pressure is applied. High compressibility describes materials which alter their volume readily.

Contrast resolution is the minimum change in the physical quantity depicted in an image which can be identified.

The *decibel* is a measure of the intensity of an ultrasonic field obtained by taking ten times the logarithm of the ratio of the intensity over a reference value. The decibel notation can be applied to many quantities, e.g. pressure or voltage.

Diffraction is the spreading of an ultrasonic wave after it interacts with an obstacle or is emitted from a source.

A *digital scan converter* is a digital storage device which accepts echo signals in scan lines and feeds them out in TV raster lines.

A *digital signal* is one in which the quantity of interest is represented as a binary word by a sequence of voltages pulses which normally take the values 5 or 0 volts.

Digitization is the conversion of an analogue voltage signal into a series of binary numbers which represent its changing value.

The *Doppler effect* is a change in the observed frequency of a wave due to motion of the source, observer or reflector.

A *duplex scan* is an ultrasonic technique in which a pulse-echo B-scan is used to identify the site of blood flow and then a Doppler beam is used to detect the velocities at that site.

Dynamic range is the range of signal magnitudes which is generated by or can be handled by a system without distortion.

The *exposure* of a patient to ultrasound is the product of the power of the transmitted field and the duration for which the field is applied.

Fast Fourier transform (FFT) — *see* Frequency analysis.

The *focus* of an ultrasonic field is that point on the transducer axis at which the field width is a minimum.

Fourier analysis — *see* Frequency analysis.

Fourier spectrum — *see* Frequency spectrum.

Fourier transform — *see* Frequency spectrum.

Frame-rate is the number of complete sweeps per second of the ultrasonic beam through the field of view.

Frequency analysis is the analysis of a signal into its frequency components.

The *frequency bandwidth* is the range of frequency components in a signal or the range of frequencies which an electronic instrument can accommodate.

A *frequency spectrum* is the presentation of the frequency components of a signal. A spectrum should be distinguished from a sonogram.

The *frequency of ultrasound* is the number of cycles of oscillation performed per second by the particles of the medium in which the ultrasound is travelling.

A *grating-lobe* is part of the ultrasonic beam pattern at the side of the main beam from an array transducer.

A *grey shade* image is one in which the magnitude of a physical quantity, e.g. the amplitude of an echo, is related to the shade of grey at the related point in the image.

A *harmonic* frequency is one which is related to the

fundamental frequency of a signal by a simple arithmetic relationship.

Heterodyne detection is an electronic process which extracts a Doppler shift signal and preserves the direction of flow information by mixing the received ultrasonic signal with a reference signal of frequency different from that of the transmitted ultrasonic wave.

The *hue* of a colour is the characteristic which allows it to be separated into groups such as red, green, purple, blue etc. The words hue and colour are often used synonymously.

A *hydrophone* is an instrument for measuring the parameters of an ultrasonic field.

The *intensity* at a point in an ultrasonic field is the rate of flow of energy through unit area placed at right angles to the field at that point.

Interference is the process by which one wave adds to a second wave in the propagating medium to produce a new waveform.

Lateral resolution is the minimum separation of two targets in the direction across the beam for which two separate identifiable signals can be obtained.

Line density is the number of lines per unit distance or per degree in an ultrasonic image.

A *longitudinal wave* is one in which the particle motion is parallel to the direction of wave propagation.

An *M-scan* is a pulsed-echo scan which is performed with the beam pointing in one direction and in which the echoes from interfaces are plotted against time to show the variations of the positions of the interfaces.

Noise is random fluctuation in a signal or image.

Non-linear propagation occurs in high amplitude waves when the particle velocity is no longer proportional to the particle pressure.

The *Nyquist* limit is the highest frequency which can be reconstructed without error from the samples of a signal. It is equal to half of the pulse repetition frequency.

A *parameter* is a quantity which can take on a range of values and hence helps to define the state of a system.

The *particle displacement* due to an ultrasonic wave is the instantaneous displacement of a particle of the medium from its rest position.

The *particle pressure* due to an ultrasonic wave is the instantaneous pressure experienced by a particle of the medium.

The *particle velocity* due to an ultrasonic wave is the instantaneous velocity of a particle of the medium.

Phase is the stage reached in the cycle of wave motion at a point in the propagating medium.

The *piezoelectric effect* is the appearance of electric charge on the surfaces of a material when pressure is applied.

A *pixel* is a picture element.

A *plane wave* is one in which the wavefront is flat.

Postprocessing is the manipulation of echo signals on transfer from a scan-converter to a display.

The *power* of an ultrasonic field is the rate of flow of energy through the whole cross-section of the field.

Preprocessing is the manipulation of echo signals prior to the storage of echo data in a scan-converter.

The *principle of superposition* states that the resultant wave formed by the overlap of two or more waves is obtained by adding the contributions from each wave at each point.

Propagation is the process of transmission of wave oscillations through a medium.

Pulse repetition frequency (PRF) is the number of ultrasonic pulses per second transmitted by the transducer.

Pulse wave velocity (PWV) is the velocity of the pressure wave generated by the heart along an artery.

Quadrature signal processing is an electronic technique for the extraction of the direction of flow information in a Doppler signal by generating and processing two signals which are 90° out of phase with one another

Radiation force (pressure) is the force experienced by an object when placed in an ultrasonic field due to the object interrupting the flow of momentum in the field.

A *radio frequency signal* is one whose frequency is in the MHz range.

Real-time B-scanning is an imaging technique in which several frames per second are produced, typically the frame rate is greater than 5 per second.

A *real-time procedure* is one in which the results are presented during the procedure.

A *reception zone* is the region in front of a transducer from which ultrasound can be detected.

A *rectified echo signal* is one which has been smoothed so as to follow the magnitude of the pressure amplitude.

Reflection is the interaction of a wave at the interface between two media where there is a change of impedance, with the result that some wave energy is directed back into the first medium.

The *reflectivity* of a tissue is a measure of its ability to produce echoes and is related to the acoustic impedance changes that exist within the tissue.

Refraction is the deviation of an ultrasonic beam at an interface between two media in which the velocities of sound are different.

Resonance is the enhanced oscillation in a structure due to its dimensions being such that there is a build up of the resultant wave amplitude in it as a result of constructive interference of internally reflected waves.

The *sample volume* is the region in the ultrasonic beam from which Doppler signals are detected.

Saturation of a colour is the amount of white light that is mixed with it to change its appearance, e.g. paleness or darkness. Complete saturation corresponds to pure colour with no white light.

Saturation of a signal is a state in which the large values of the signal cannot be accommodated by an instrument and they have become compressed.

Scattering is the interaction of a wave with small structures in the propagating medium causing wave energy to be dispersed in many directions.

A *shock wave* is one in which sharp discontinuities exist in its pressure waveform.

A *side-lobe* is part of the ultrasonic beam pattern at the side of the main beam from a transducer.

A *sonogram* is the presentation on a display of successive spectra derived from the analysis of Doppler signal.

Speckle is the noise in an image or sonogram due to fluctuations in the echo signals produced by small closely spaced targets.

Spectral analysis (Fourier or frequency analysis) is the analysis of a signal into its frequency components.

A *spectrum* is the presentation of the frequency components in a signal.

A *swept focus* (dynamic focus) is one which is rapidly moved along the beam axis to coincide with the range from which echoes are being received at that instant.

Temporal resolution is the minimum separation in time for which two separate events can be identified.

Time gain compensation (TGC) is electronic compensation for the attenuation which affects different echo signals due to being generated at different depths in tissue.

Tissue characterisation is the use of ultrasonic information to identify the type or properties of tissue.

A *transducer* (probe) is a device for the conversion of one form of energy to another, e.g. ultrasonic energy to electrical energy.

A *transverse wave* is one in which the particle motion is perpendicular to the direction of wave propagation.

An *ultrasonic beam* is the region in front of a transducer from which echoes are detected when it is operating in a pulse-echo mode.

An *ultrasonic field* is the region in front of a transducer into which sonic energy is transmitted.

Ultrasound is sound of frequency greater than that of the upper limit of the human audible range.

An *unrectified echo signal* is one in which the positive and negative fluctuations of the pressure wave have been preserved.

The *variance* is a statistical measure of the spread of values in a number of measurements. It is equal to the square of the standard deviation.

Velocity resolution is the minimum difference in velocity which can be measured.

A *video signal* is an electrical signal which is in a suitable form for the generation of an image.

A *wavefront* is an imaginary surface in a ultrasonic field over which a wave parameter such as pressure has the same value.

Index

351